Praise for *The Smarter Sci*

D1495834

THE SMARTER SCIENCE OF SLIM is a proven and practical guide to fighting the big problem of obesity. Simplifying a bunch of biology while making decades of academic obesity research accessible to everyone, Bailor gives a complete and captivating explanation of the science of losing weight permanently.

Dr. Theodoros Kelesidis, Division of Endocrinology, Diabetes, & Metabolism, Harvard Medical School & Department of Medicine, UCLA School of Medicine

THE SMARTER SCIENCE OF SLIM challenges the diet dogma and offers a sensible path to good health. Bailor's insightful book is smart, health promoting, and deserves to be hot, hot, hot!

Dr. JoAnn E. Manson, Chief, Division of Preventive Medicine, Brigham and Women's Hospital, Professor of Medicine, Harvard Medical School

In THE SMARTER SCIENCE OF SLIM, Bailor demolishes the dietary and nutritional nonsense that has contributed to the epidemics of obesity and diabetes in our country. In its place he erects a simple program anyone can follow that is based on solid science and common sense. THE SMARTER SCIENCE OF SLIM is likely to be the last diet book you will ever need to buy. Unless you enjoy failed diets, do the right thing—the healthy thing—and read this book.

Dr. Larry Dossey, *Oprah* medical expert, *New York Times* best-selling author, and Former Chief of Staff of Medical City Dallas Hospital

THE SMARTER SCIENCE OF SLIM reveals some of the latest and best scientific research on the real story of diet, exercise, and their effects on us. Bailor's concept of high-quality exercise is rapidly gaining support in the medical community and has repeatedly delivered clinical results which seem almost too good to be true. I heartily recommend this book to people who want to take responsibility for their own health.

Dr. John J. Ratey, Clinical Professor of Psychiatry at Harvard Medical School and author of *Spark: The Revolutionary New Science of Exercise and the Brain*

THE SMARTER SCIENCE OF SLIM sheds light on the surprising discrepancy between the way healthy nutrition has been presented to the public and the science that underlies it. The idea that fat in the diet translates into fat on the body has dominated nutritional discussions for decades. This work challenges this central idea, and offers clues about why diabetes has been on the rise, and why so many people who are intent on losing weight have found it so difficult to do so. It is an important piece of work.

Dr. Anthony Accurso, Johns Hopkins Bayview Medical Center

As someone who takes fitness and health seriously and has written extensively on this topic over some 30 years, I am generally underwhelmed whenever I see a new "how to" book enter the marketplace. Most are celebrity driven, and most celebrities simply do what their personal trainers tell them to do with little regard for physiologic fact. I am pleased to say that THE SMARTER SCIENCE OF SLIM represents something different. Strikingly different in fact.

Author Jonathan Bailor has that rare gift of being able to take highly technical scientific data and interpret it in a way that the average person can understand instantly. In addition, he is able to do so in a manner that makes entertaining and compelling reading while clearly indicating how (and why) the last 40 years of fitness and nutrition advice have made us fatter and more at risk for disease than at any other point in our species' history. But most importantly, he is able to take that mountain of scientific data and divine the practical and simple direction it is pointing to in terms of advancing human health and fitness. The book you are holding in your hands can be said to represent the thinking person's guide to exercise and diet in the 21st Century. No fads. No gimmicks. No celebrity-driven pitching of nonsense. Finally, a book that is worth reading; not only for the sheer pleasure of it, but also for its ability to dramatically and positively change your health, strength and life.

John Little, Author of *Max Contraction Training*, Co-Author of *Body By Science*

Revolutionary. Thoroughly researched, rigorously simplified, and downright fun, Bailor's work stands head-and-shoulders above the mass of fat loss myths lining bookstore shelves. In his surprising and scientifically sound exposé of the modern fat loss mythology, Bailor reveals the sources of our fat loss struggles and provides straight-forward, practical solutions. Everyone, and I mean everyone, will learn and laugh a lot while reading THE SMARTER SCIENCE OF SLIM.

Dr. Jan Fridén, Distinguished professor and head of a muscle research program at the University of Gothenburg, Sweden

When it comes to the most important part of your life, your health, Bailor has written a book that is a must-read for knowing the truth about evaporating body fat. I am a firm believer in achieving the body you have always dreamed of, and Bailor opens the black box of fat loss and makes it simple for you to explore the facts. Read this book today in order to live your best life.

Joel Harper, *Dr. Oz Show* fitness expert, NYC celebrity personal trainer, joelharperfitness.com

WOW! This book will blow your mind and is a must-read for anyone who wants to learn how to be healthy the 21st century way. In THE SMARTER SCIENCE OF SLIM, Bailor exposes the dietary myths of why we as a nation are still overweight despite years of best-selling diet books. Calories, fat, exercise and hormones—it is all in this book and finally someone got it right. The diabesity epidemic stops here.

Dr. Fred Pescatore, Author of the *Hamptons Diet*

THE SMARTER SCIENCE OF SLIM redefines and updates the science of weight loss and bravely takes on long held beliefs about body change. This book provides a groundbreaking paradigm shift for all of those who have struggled with weight loss. I have used this science in my clinic for years. It gets results and changes lives.

Jade Teta, ND, CSCS, author of *The New ME Diet*

Poignant, applicable and easy to read, Bailor's relevant work couldn't have come at a better time. If you've struggled with weight loss, this could be the magic bullet you're looking for.

David Barr, Exercise Science Writer for *Muscle & Fitness*, Editor in Chief of Strength and Science, CSCS, CISSN

In THE SMARTER SCIENCE OF SLIM, Bailor entertains as much as he educates. Simplifying and integrating an amazing amount of important scientific and clinical research, Bailor presents a well-conceived, well-researched and well-written book, in addition to a very sensible, practical, and successful approach to losing fat. This book will undoubtedly change the way you think and look, while keeping you smiling all along the way.

Dr. Wayne Westcott, Quincy College Fitness Research Director and author of *Get Stronger, Feel Younger*

THE SMARTER SCIENCE OF SLIM is the go-to source for all that is practical, realistic, and effective when it comes to weight loss. Bailor brilliantly brings together all the outdated myths (i.e. eat less, exercise more) and dispels them one at a time in a fun, easy to understand way. This book changes the future of permanent weight loss forever!

Cynthia Pasquella, Board Certified Clinical Nutritionist, CHLC, CWC, cynthiapasquella.com

Fat loss theories are everywhere; except here. THE SMARTER SCIENCE OF SLIM is the source for the fat loss facts. Bailor has taken a lot of amazingly complex medical research and turned it into a simple, clinically proven fat loss program that will change the way we think about fat loss.

Dr. William Dunn, specializing in the obesity/cancer link

Stimulating and provocative.

Dr. Søren Toubro, Professor at the Centre for Advanced Food Research at the University of Copenhagen

Strikingly beautiful and accessible.

Reinhard Engels, Author of the *No S Diet*, nosdiet.com

Brilliant. THE SMARTER SCIENCE OF SLIM is a masterful compilation of nutritional and exercise science disproving the archaic fat loss theory of "eat less, exercise more." Bailor persuasively packages a wealth of research along with his personal and professional experience into an easily understood and applied framework that will change the way you live, look, and feel. For all those who feel left behind in the nutritional battles and exercise gimmicks of the last ten years, look no further, Bailor will end your confusion once and for all.

Dr. William Davis, Fellowship of the American College of Cardiology

This is not just another diet book. Bailor has assembled a wealth of scientific evidence showing how our "healthy" diet and exercise obsession are making us fat and sick. THE SMARTER SCIENCE OF SLIM is a scientifically backed, paradigm shifting, and entertaining exposé that disproves our basic ideas of eating and exercise. If you buy one health book this decade, make it THE SMARTER SCIENCE OF SLIM.

Marion G. Volk, MHSc, Obesity researcher

As a World Cup and Olympic athlete I have read hundreds of health and fitness books; Bailor's work stands alone. I have never seen such a simple and entertaining presentation of so much fat loss science. Debunking the myths sabotaging the weight loss efforts of millions, Bailor will change the way you think of fat loss and the way you look in less time than you ever thought possible.

Maik Wiedenbach, World Cup and Olympic Athlete, CEO of Adlertraining, National Academy of Sports Medicine certified trainer

Through a combination of detailed research, shocking facts, and time spent in the fat-loss trenches, Bailor has passionately produced an essential guide to transforming the human body. We urgently need an unbiased solution to making our bodies look and feel better. THE SMARTER SCIENCE OF SLIM is that solution.

Ben Greenfield, National Personal Trainer of the Year, National Strength and Conditioning Association- BenGreenfieldFitness.com, nutritionalmagnesium.org

From preface-to-conclusion, Bailor cleverly articulates the misinformation that has inundated Americans' views on fat loss for the last 30 years. His book is not just an enjoyable read, but his ability to incorporate scientific-backed research with his no-nonsense, often humorous at times-approach makes this a book every intelligent American should read, especially those who are frustrated with yo-yo dieting and unsuccessful attempts at fat loss. THE SMARTER SCIENCE OF SLIM is at the top of my recommended reading list for each of my clients and employees.

Lindsay Vastola, CEO Body Project Fitness and Health, Certified Fitness Trainer

THE SMARTER SCIENCE OF SLIM says it all! As a former athlete and NFL referee it was—and still is—my goal to be in the best physical condition possible. It takes discipline and effort, but with the plan that author Bailor presents, obtaining and maintaining your best physical being is achievable.

Dr. Jim Tunney, former NFL Referee, Author of *It's the Will, Not the Skill*

THE SMARTER SCIENCE OF SLIM is both fun and informative. It challenges the central dogma of diet and weight control and provides a sensible alternative to the current less food, more exercise strategy. Bailor provides a compelling, simple, and practical solution to the challenge of obesity. Try it!

Dr. Steve Yeaman, Deputy Director, Institute of Cellular Medicine, Newcastle University

Skeptics will be disappointed. The ideas presented in THE SMARTER SCIENCE OF SLIM seem both like common sense and mind-blowing revelations. Almost as if these are things all of us knew but have forgotten in the haze of disinformation. More than a dozen times while reading Bailor's book, the phrase "Too good to be true" popped into my head. But even cynics must cave in the light of factual data. The real impact, though, comes when the reader reconciles the decades of half-truths with the scientific research, and realizes that there is still hope. All we needed was someone to help us remember.

Robby Reining, Amazon.com Top Reviewer

Jonathan Bailor spent ten years summarizing the last forty years of nutrition and exercise research—and we will all be better off because of it. Bailor uses these thousands of pages of academic research to show us why what we are currently doing is not working, along with an exciting and proven way to fix it. He rightly calls this fix THE SMARTER SCIENCE OF SLIM.

While showing a genuine concern for his reader, Bailor reveals how small—but scientifically proven—lifestyle changes dramatically change the way our bodies look and work. Bailor's book is bar-none the best health related publication I've ever read, and the easiest to implement. You can't help but change the way you think about eating and exercise after reading this book. Give Bailor a few hours and he'll change your mind and your life, forever, for the better.

Julie Spiegel, Amazon.com Top Reviewer

If you are going to read one book on how to eat and exercise, read this one. THE SMARTER SCIENCE OF SLIM had an immediate and dramatic impact on how I eat and how I feel. This book will significantly and permanently improve your life.

The Reverend Craig Stephans, Anglican Priest and Amazon.com Top Reviewer

In an absorbing book that you will not want to put down, Bailor will change the way you think about diet and exercise. Using an astonishing collection of academic research, THE SMARTER SCIENCE OF SLIM shows why so many diets fail and the scientifically proven way to change that. Extensively researched and easy to understand, THE SMARTER SCIENCE OF SLIM is a must-read for anyone ready to live a healthier life.

Angela Streiff, Amazon.com Vine Voice Reviewer

It is obvious that Bailor has done his homework while creating this important publication that turns current thinking on weight loss on its ear. When I first saw his premise that the common theory of weight loss—eat less and exercise more to lose weight—is all wrong, I couldn't believe it. What he is telling us is that there is a smarter way to fat loss—eat more, exercise less—smarter. Now that sounded like my kind of program to lose fat and improve my health. I am just an average guy trying to keep his weight in check in my golden years. I have tried many diets out there and most left me hungry all the time and feeling deprived, and I would eventually give up. When I saw this book, it gave me hope again.

Bailor has a writing style that makes it seem he is talking directly to you—like he was your neighbor and friend. His humor gets his points across easily and his extensive research and references in the book make it easy to see how he cannot be wrong. I loved the book and highly recommend it to anyone who has tried to diet the conventional way and ended up hungry and miserable during the process, and eventually just gaining the weight back. The book provides you a path to lower your body's weight set point and unclog your metabolism so it actually burns stored fat. It will change your view of weight loss completely.

Alan Hukle, Amazon.com Top Reviewer

THE SMARTER SCIENCE OF SLIM takes the pain out of gain. The science will amaze you and Bailor's solution will forever change you. Truly, you do not need to waste your time or money on another health or fitness book...THE SMARTER SCIENCE OF SLIM is your answer to living with optimum health.

Cherie Hill, Bestselling Kindle Author in Christian Non-fiction and Amazon. com Top Reviewer

Reading THE SMARTER SCIENCE OF SLIM, Bailor's passion for his topic and his amazing level of research are immediately apparent. What I appreciated most is that the book gave me information to which the average person does not have access--information that the government and big business would rather be kept locked away.

Sheri Ackerman, Amazon.com Top Reviewer

Jonathan Bailor has put a lot of time into his work in this arena. He provides compelling data regarding exercise and nutrition and our collective view on these subjects. After everything you've already tried to get in shape, isn't it worth giving it another shot? I think it is.

Gunnar Peterson CSCS

Bailor explodes common diet beliefs with THE SMARTER SCIENCE OF SLIM. This is solid information, backed by scientific studies that can help you reach your goal weight without dieting or depriving yourself.

Bill Cashell, Author of *The Emotional Diet*

If you want the "real skinny" on getting and staying skinny you must read THE SMARTER SCIENCE OF SLIM. This book cuts through the fat and gives you the science of being fit from the world's top authorities. Bailor has masterfully woven together all the scientific facts from the top thought leaders in this space to provide us with a clear, lose the fat and keep it off blueprint for life.

Michael Altshuler, Motivational Speaker and CEO of Texting Pays

If you want to learn how to eat right, exercise more effectively and shed fat, I can't think of a better book.

J.W.K., Amazon.com Top Reviewer

In his book THE SMARTER SCIENCE OF SLIM Jonathan Bailor presents much more than advice on lifestyle and diet. This is a complete argument relating themes of nutrition, exercise, digestion and food to their associated consequence, weight. Unlike many works in the area of diet, THE SMARTER SCIENCE OF SLIM presents informed consideration of the subject, offers no quick fix, no formulaic or unsubstantiated, quasi-religious claims. What the book does do is argue a coherent, rationally-constructed and evidence-justified position which identifies an approach to diet and lifestyle rather than a prescription. It is to the author's credit that the book achieves its aims in a fluent, readable style that engages and entertains as well as informs.

Philip Spires, Author of *Mission* and *A Fool's Knot*

THE SMARTER SCIENCE OF SLIM is extremely informative, well-researched, and easy to read. If you want to know anything about being slim—this is the book for you.

Dr. Wolfgang Riebe

With remarkable scientific evidence Jonathan Bailor leads you from the pain and slavery of obesity to the happiness and freedom of permanent fitness. His words gain universal value and will motivate you to change your life forever.

Dr. Bruno Cortis, Author of *Heal Your Cancer–Emotional and Spiritual Pathways*

Also by Jonathan Bailor

The Smarter Science of Slim Workbook:
The Five-Week Harvard Medical School, Johns Hopkins, and UCLA
Endorsed Program to Burn Fat Permanently

The Smarter Science of Slim Journal:
A Smarter Way to Track Your Weight Loss

THE SMARTER SCIENCE OF SLIM

What the Actual Experts Have Proven About
Weight Loss, Health, and Fitness

Jonathan Bailor

Aavia Publishing
Fewer, better books™

New York • Seattle

© 2012 by Jonathan Bailor. All rights reserved.

Published in the United States, Canada, and the U.K. by Aavia Publishing. New York. Seattle. www.AaviaPublishing.com.

No part of this work may be reproduced, stored, or distributed in any form or by any means except as permitted under Section 107 or 108 of the 1976 United States Copyright Act, without first obtaining written permission of the Publisher, or authorization through payment of the appropriate per-copy fee to the Copyright Clearance Center, 222 Rosewood Drive, Danvers, MA, 01923, (978) 750-8400, or on the web at www.copyright.com. Requests to the Publisher for permission should be sent to http://www.AaviaPublishing.com/contact.

Aavia Publishing books can be purchased at quantity discounts to use as premiums, promotions, or for corporate training programs. For more information on bulk pricing please email Aavia Publishing at http://www.AaviaPublishing.com/contact.

Editors: John Paine, Hillel Black, Mary Rose Bailor
Interior Design: Adina Cucicov, Flamingo Designs
Exterior Design: Michael David McGuire
Cover Photo: Douglas Gorenstein
Illustrations: Alex McVey
Consultants: Sheri Ackerman, John Coss, Caitlin Ashley-Rollman, LeAnne Marshall, Angela Streiff, Robby Reining, Robert Bailor, Angela Bailor, Melinda Knight, Alan Hukle, Craig Stephans, Cherie Hill, Julie Spiegel, Bill Cashell, Lydia Allen, Angie Boyter, John Roberto, Tara Hopwood

A special thanks to Dr. JoAnn E. Manson and Dr. Theodoros Kelesidis for their life-changing research and boundless support. Also, I cannot thank my wonderful editors John Paine, Hillel Black, and Mary Rose Bailor enough. Your ability to help make dense academic research simple and compelling is unparalleled.

And special appreciation to Michael David McGuire and his media team in New York. McGuire's unique insights and guidance helped greatly strengthen this project.

Publisher's Cataloging-in-Publication

Bailor, Jonathan.
The Smarter Science of Slim: What the Actual Experts Have Proven About Weight Loss, Health, and Fitness/ Jonathan Bailor.—1st ed.
p. cm.
Includes bibliographical references.
Library of Congress Control Number: 2011905665
ISBN 978-0-9835208-0-1, 978-0-9835208-1-8 (electronic), 978-0-9835208-2-5 (audio)
1. Health 2. Weight Loss 3. Physical Fitness 4. Exercise 5. Diet 6. Nutrition 7. Self-Help
I. Bailor, Jonathan II. Title.

Manufactured in the United States of America. First Edition.

The information expressed here is intended for educational purposes only. This information is provided with the understanding that neither Jonathan Bailor nor Aavia Publishing are rendering medical advice of any kind. This information is not intended to supersede or replace medical advice, nor to diagnose, prescribe or treat any disease, condition, illness or injury. It is critical before beginning any eating or exercise program, including those described in this and related works, that readers receive full medical clearance from a licensed physician.

Jonathan Bailor and Aavia Publishing are not liable to anyone or anything impacted negatively, or purported to have been impacted negatively, directly or indirectly, by leveraging this or related information. By continuing to read this and related works the reader accepts all liability and disclaims Jonathan Bailor and Aavia Publishing from any and all legal matters. If these terms are not acceptable, visit http://www.AaviaPublishing.com/contact to return this book for a full refund.

Acknowledgments

This book is the result of more than ten years of collaboration with hundreds of brilliant and inspiring researchers and reviewers. To everyone who helped bring this science to the surface, I cannot thank you enough for your time, insight, and support. Together we will make the world a healthier and happier place. Truly and deeply, thank you.

Dedication

To my best friend and wife Angela and my heroes and parents Mary Rose and Robert. All that I am and ever will be is thanks to your love, example, and support.

Table of Contents

Foreword

By JoAnn E. Manson, M.D, M.PH., Dr.P.H
**Professor of Medicine and the
Michael and Lee Bell Professor of Women's Health
Harvard Medical School
Chief, Division of Preventive Medicine
Brigham and Women's Hospital**

The dual epidemics of obesity and type 2 diabetes are the looming public health crises of the 21st century. All around us today, in all walks of life, are people who struggle with weight control. The growing prevalence of obesity in the United States and around the world, especially among children and adolescents, portends an enormous global burden of chronic disease in the future. The crystal ball shows not only more people with diabetes, but also enormous numbers of people with hypertension, heart disease, stroke, and even cancer. Although medical research has made strides in treating and controlling some of the health consequences of obesity, the prevention and management of obesity truly hold the key to improved health. Of particular importance, we now know that people suffering from overweight or obesity can take charge of their health—if they are willing to make even modest changes in their lifestyle.

Throughout my career in preventive medicine and epidemiology, I have valued the importance of empowering the public through information and shared decision making. Together with my colleagues, our research has focused on prevention of cardiovascular disease and diabetes, including assessing the role of lifestyle factors in reducing risks. We have examined the "power of prevention" in several large-scale clinical studies, including the Harvard Nurses' Health Study, the Women's Health Initiative, the Women's Health Study, the VITamin D and OmegA-3 TriaL (VITAL), and other research projects. One of the major findings from our large population-based studies is that type 2 diabetes and heart disease are largely preventable through lifestyle modifications, which are powerful determinants of our risk of chronic disease. For example, we've published papers from the Nurses' Health Study indicating that at least 90% of cases of type 2 diabetes and at least 80% of heart attacks can be prevented by lifestyle changes, including being physically active, maintaining a healthy weight, and following a diet high in fruits, vegetables, and whole grains, and low in saturated and trans fats and refined carbohydrates.

We've made efforts to inform the public of these findings, as well as of the work of other researchers around the world, often writing columns in magazines and working closely with print and electronic media over the years. Yet the scientific findings of so many researchers and other dedicated individuals in academia remain largely unknown by the general public. Part of the problem is the pervasive and overpowering impact of mass marketing by the food industry. Another problem is the often confusing and contradictory messages about nutrition and health on the internet and various mass media outlets. Even the dietary guidelines from the federal government may seem confusing and at odds with some of the research studies that have attracted attention. How is the general public supposed to know which scientific studies to believe?

That's why Jonathan Bailor has performed an invaluable service with his book, *The Smarter Science of Slim*. Jonathan has studied thousands and thousands of pages of academic research on health and weight-loss, and he has put the results into terms that the everyday person can understand. We have made great strides over the years in understanding how the body responds to different types of food. Yet all too often a popular author selectively cites the scientific evidence, emphasizing only those aspects of the wide-ranging research that support the diet plan he or she is promoting. Jonathan's work is far from "just another diet book."

The Smarter Science of Slim dismantles the myths that have contributed enormously to the health and weight problems that many people have, and replaces them with easy-to-understand facts that will change the way you think about eating and exercise. On the eating side, he shows why changes in a person's metabolism affect weight gain, and how to get your metabolism burning rather than storing body fat. He provides a sensible formula for eating the right kinds of food that produce satiety—that fill you up so much that you won't have room for the types of foods that are fueling the obesity and diabetes epidemics. He shows how balance is the key to long term health and weight loss. He also clarifies what the scientific literature suggests are the best ways to exercise. Short bursts of vigorous and forceful activity can provide all of the stimulation needed to get your metabolism back on track. But moderate exercise also has a role.

The scientific community now knows a great deal about how the human body works. In culling the literature and gathering the results of so many clinical studies, Jonathan Bailor presents a weight-loss program that is based on rigorous science. We can make the right choices that will help us to avoid becoming overweight or obese. As a treasure trove of reliable information and sound facts, *The Smarter Science of Slim* can help you take charge of your destiny and turn the tide on weight gain.

Preface

By Theodoros Kelesidis, M.D,
Division of Endocrinology, Diabetes, & Metabolism, Harvard Medical School
Department of Medicine, UCLA School of Medicine

While researching and practicing at the Division of Endocrinology, Diabetes, & Metabolism at the Harvard Medical School and the UCLA School of Medicine, I would often be asked when there will be a proven prescription for weight loss. *The Smarter Science of Slim* is that prescription.

Jonathan Bailor's easy-to-understand and engaging style disguises an astonishing amount of otherwise incredibly complex scientific information. You will not realize you are learning so much because you will be so involved in what you are reading. The pages you are holding will change the way you feel and look faster than any pill ever could. It is incredibly rare to find anything as thoroughly researched and carefully analyzed, yet so clearly and engagingly presented in the context of everyday living—and eating. For anyone who has struggled with managing weight or maintaining energy, you do not need pills. You need this book.

Having conducted research across four continents, I appreciate Bailor's meticulous methodology, but it's what he does with the information that made the book one I will "prescribe" to colleagues, patients, students, family, friends—and you. He points out that in so many cases what scientists have proven in the lab IS NOT how you have been told to eat or exercise. No, this isn't a conspiracy diatribe; it's just a smart writer pointing out the disconnect between the science and our lifestyle and then showing how you can eat more food and do less exercise, while improving how you look and feel, once you know and apply the science.

Here is a sample of some of what you will discover in *The Smarter Science of Slim*: Most people can manage to temporarily lose weight via traditional techniques, but Bailor reveals the biology of why these techniques lead to long term weight *gain* 95% of the time. Bailor then provides a proven way to burn fat *long term*. With this information, you can avoid "yo-yo'ing" forever. Another one of my personal favorites: Ever notice how more people are members of gyms and how there are more "health" supplements than ever before in human history, yet the "civilized" world has never been so heavy or suffered from so many lifestyle diseases? Bailor leverages reams of research to suggest a simple approach that will get your biology working for you rather than against you. He rightly prescribes solving problems—fixing the deep metabolic issues underlying weight gain—instead of treating symptoms by starving yourself. And he does so without going to ridiculous extremes, like so many of the fad diets you see every day. This collection of research reveals a wholly different cause and wholly proven solution to the weight and health issues plaguing us today.

For a fresh perspective on why and how to make simple and practical life-enhancing adjustments to your eating and exercise habits, read Bailor's book. You will learn how some mis-information is probably responsible for the "weighty" matters of epidemic rates of obesity and heart disease. You will also be given simple, scientifically sound guidelines on how to eat more food and exercise less—but smarter, while burning fat and boosting your health.

The Smarter Science of Slim is a proven and practical guide to fighting the big problem of obesity. Simplifying a bunch of biology while making decades of academic obesity research accessible to everyone, Bailor gives a complete and captivating explanation of the science of losing weight permanently.

Enjoy reading this book, but more importantly, apply what you will learn.

Simple Surprising Science

"Hippocrates [the father of Western medicine] wrote that the obese should 'eat only once a day and...walk naked as long as possible.' Progress in this area [fat loss] will require that we move beyond this 2,000-year-old prescription and instead develop strategies that are based on twenty-first-century science."

J.M. FRIEDMAN, ROCKEFELLER UNIVERSITY[1]

As our knowledge of the human body becomes ever more exact, scientists have made remarkable leaps forward in many fields. We have completed the study of the human genome. We can combat horrible diseases such as childhood leukemia with terrific success rates. Yet for one question that many of us would like answered—what causes the body to burn fat?—we find all sorts of confusing claims. One guru advises an all-fat diet. Another wants you to eat only vegetables. Since we know so much about how our body works, can't science tell us the answer?

As it turns out, science already has.

I have spent over ten years reading thousands of fat-loss studies. Not theories promoted by diet gurus. Not what magazines say. Not what TV tells us, often while selling a pharmaceutical product. Only the proven data. Just the facts.

My investigation uncovered all kinds of scientific findings:

- Studies stating how certain foods cripple our ability to burn fat
- Scientists showing how to burn fat while eating more food
- Researchers revealing how to get all the benefits of traditional exercise in a tenth of the time
- Physiologists finding out how eating less sets us up to *gain* fat in the long run
- Doctors discussing how a few minutes of a new form of exercise immunizes us against fat gain
- Endocrinologists explaining how we fix the underlying condition causing us to gain fat

We deserve to know the proven facts about fat loss, but who has time to read tens of thousands of pages of scientific studies? The investigation took me more than a decade. It should not take you that long—because the facts have been summarized in this book. They have also been simplified, so anyone who wants to lose weight can understand them. Make no mistake. Tons of clinical studies have shown the best way to trim off those unwanted pounds.

It is time to stop listening to marketing myths about how to lose weight. We tried it. It failed. It is time to move on to a smarter science of slim.

For example, since the 1970s we have been told to eat less and exercise more. Today, nearly half of all women and a third of all men are following some diet plan, and studies from the University of Southern Denmark show we have significantly increased the amount of exercise we get. In other words, we have taken the "eat less, exercise more" theory to heart. Here is what that has done to our hearts (and waistlines):[2]

Millions of Non-Fatal Heart Disease Incidents in the U.S.

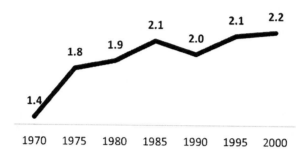

Millions of Hospital Discharges for Cardiovascular Diseases in the U.S.

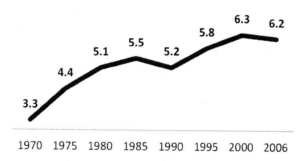

Percent of Americans at Least Overweight

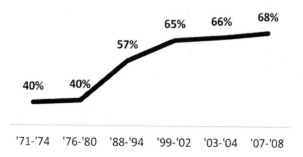

Millions of Americans with Diabetes

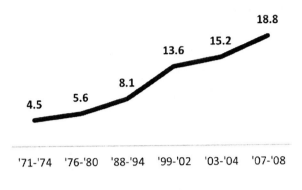

'71-'74	'76-'80	'88-'94	'99-'02	'03-'04	'07-'08
4.5	5.6	8.1	13.6	15.2	18.8

3

Judging by these results, attempting to eat less and exercise more is not effective. Researcher S.C. Wooley from the University of Cincinnati wrote: "The failure of [heavy] people to achieve a goal they seem to want—and to want almost above all else—must now be admitted for what it is: a failure not of those people but of the methods of treatment that are used."[4]

Hundreds of the most brilliant academic health and fat loss researchers from around the world agree with Dr. Wooley. Albert Stunkard at the University of Pennsylvania said: "How may the medical profession regain its proper role in the treatment of obesity? We can begin by looking at the situation as it exists and not as we would like it to be...If we do not feel obliged to excuse our failures, we may be able to investigate them."[5]

Why should you and I care? Those same scientists have released thousands of pages of revolutionary fat-loss research over the past few decades. The only catch has been that the research was accessible only to academics. Fortunately, this book simplifies the last forty years of fat-loss facts so you can use them for your own benefit.

Let's take an example: The *Calories In—Calories Out* theory of weight loss. This *theory* has been proven wrong in study after study, but you do not need to wade through all those facts. All you need is some plain common sense. A pound of body fat contains 3,500 calories. Cutting a measly 100 calories—less than one cup of reduced-fat milk—per day would cut 365,000 calories over ten years. If *Calories In—Calories Out* is correct, a 150-pound woman who drinks one less cup of reduced-fat milk per day will lose 104 pounds and weigh 46 pounds ten years later. That is absurd.

Or take the classic myth: *a calorie is a calorie*. Researchers have discovered that calorie quality varies wildly. High-quality calories from non-starchy vegetables, lean protein, and natural fats trigger hormones that cause our body to burn fat. Low-quality calories from starches and sweets trigger hormones that cause our body to store fat. According to clinical studies, by eating *more* high-quality calories we burn more body fat.

Here is another old weight loss myth: *calories are all that matter*. Scientists know that is false. Take the simple example of diabetics—people who cannot effectively get energy into their cells because they are missing the hormone insulin. Why are they injecting themselves with the hormone insulin if calories are all that matter? Hormones—not how much we eat or exercise—determine whether we are burning or storing body fat.

Finally, let's look at the government's *Dietary Guidelines*—both their pyramid and the more modern plate graphics. The Chair of the Department of Nutrition at the Harvard School of Public Health has stated: "...the USDA Pyramid is wrong...at best, the USDA Pyramid offers wishy-washy, scientifically unfounded advice...it ignores the evidence that has been carefully assembled over the past forty years." The *Journal of the American College of Cardiology* goes even further: "The low-fat-high-carbohydrate diet, promulgated [encouraged] vigorously by the...food pyramid may well have played an unintended role in the current epidemics of obesity...diabetes, and metabolic syndromes." Our primary source of nutrition information—the U.S. Department of Agriculture (USDA)—is hurting rather than helping us. Is it any wonder we are struggling with our health and weight?[6]

On the bright side, researchers at top universities around the world have discovered a dramatically different set of dietary guidelines that make us thin and fit instead of heavy and sick. These guidelines have dramatically improved my life, and they will improve your life too. All you need is access to the right information.

Make no mistake: the food, fitness, and pharmaceutical industries have known these facts for decades. Why haven't they come forward and made the information available to the general public? Because there is a lot more money to be made off of sick, stocky, and sad people than off of healthy, happy people. The bigger we are, the bigger the profits of the $3.1 trillion food, $150 billion fitness, and $500 billion pharmaceutical industries. Big food, fitness, and pharma want us to stay slim like big tobacco wants us to stop smoking. And just as big tobacco tried to hide the scientific facts of smoking, big food, fitness, and pharma are trying to keep the science of slim from surfacing. As Yale University researcher Kelly Brownell puts it: "By 1964, there was sufficient scientific evidence...[but] many years passed and many millions died before decisive action was taken to [turn the tide against smoking]...Repeating this history with food and obesity would be tragic."[7]

Once you have empowered yourself with proven fat-loss facts, your body will burn fat automatically. Does that sound too good to be true? Have you ever met anyone who eats as much as they want, does not exercise, and still stays skinny? Put differently, have you ever met anyone who's body burns fat for them automatically? We all have. So the question is not: "Is automatic lifelong fat loss possible?" Millions of naturally thin people have already demonstrated that it is. The question is: "How can you and I burn fat automatically, like naturally thin people?"

Researchers have revealed a simple and surprising answer: Eat more. Exercise less. Smarter.

Smarter is the key. By eating more—but higher-quality food—and exercising less—but with higher-quality—we provide our body a unique combination of nutrition and hormones which reprograms it to behave more like the body of a naturally thin person. Our body starts burning—instead of storing—fat. It's not magic. It's the smarter science of slim.

The Smarter Science of Slim

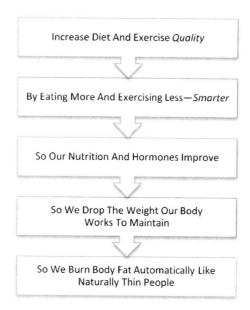

Let's look at a point-by-point comparison of common weight loss theory and what researchers have proven. On the left you'll find the advice you've read dozens of times. Now look at the right-hand column. There is quite a difference.

Common Theory vs. Smarter Science

Common Theory Eat Less, Exercise More—Harder	Smarter Science Eat More, Exercise Less—Smarter
• Focuses on calorie quantity and ignores calorie quality	• Leverages calorie quality to take care of calorie quantity
• Fights against our "set-point weight"	• Lowers our "set-point weight"
• Provides the temporary need to burn something	• Provides the permanent need to burn body fat
• Slows down our metabolism	• Speeds up our metabolism
• Ignores hormonal issues	• Focuses on hormonal issues
• Destroys our ability to burn body fat	• Restores our ability to burn body fat
• Profitable for the "food," fitness, and pharmaceutical industries	• Not profitable for the "food," fitness, and pharmaceutical industries

To be clear, the last forty years of fat-loss research reveals that the traditional approach *can* work—just not very often. Eating less and exercising more does not keep body fat off long-term 95% of the time. To put this 95% failure rate into perspective, quitting smoking cold turkey has a 94.5% failure rate. In other words, more people are able to quit smoking cold turkey than are able to keep body fat off using the traditional approach.[8]

% of People Who Lose Weight Long-Term Using the Traditional Approach[9]

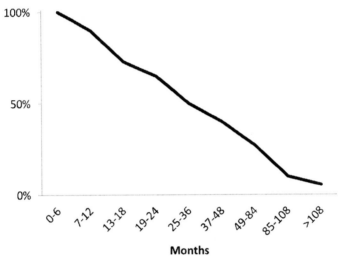

The smarter scientific approach to fat loss is much more effective.[10]

For example, researchers at Skidmore College compared a traditional "eat less, exercise more—harder" program against an "eat more, exercise less—smarter" program. Let's call the groups in the study the Harder Group and the Smarter Group.

The Harder Group ate the traditional diet of 60% carbohydrates, 15% protein, and 25% fat while doing low-quality cardiovascular exercise for forty minutes per day, six days per week. Low-quality cardiovascular exercise refers to exercises like walking, biking, and jogging, which must be done for hours to impact our health and weight. The Smarter Group ate a higher-quality diet of 40% carbohydrate, 40% protein, and 20% fat while exercising only 60% as much, but with higher-quality. The study lasted for 12 weeks and included 34 women and 29 men between the ages of 20 and 60.[11]

At the end of the study, the Harder Group "successfully" ate less and exercised eighteen hours more than the Smarter Group. After examining the results though, the researchers concluded:

> *The primary finding of the current study is that a lifestyle modification program consisting of high-intensity cardiovascular and resistance training combined with a balanced carbohydrate and protein diet results in greater improvement in body composition, cardiovascular risk factors, and muscular strength than a program comprised of a traditional diet and moderate-intensity exercise regimen commonly recommended for weight loss.*

Less academically speaking, eating more and exercising less—smarter—was more effective than the traditional approach. Here is the data.

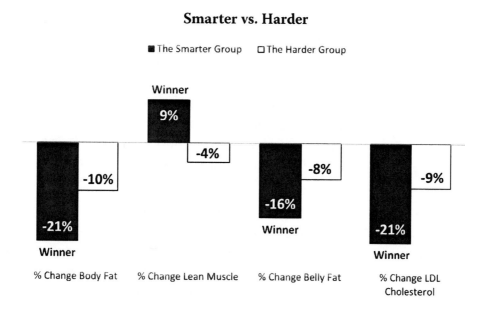

Smarter vs. Harder

■ The Smarter Group   □ The Harder Group

Intrigued? It gets better. The program in this book takes the strategies used by the Smarter Group to the next level. We'll cover this program in seven parts.

Part 1—Myth: Calories In—Calories Out

We'll start by reviewing research revealing how our weight is controlled. We'll discover that our weight revolves around a "set-point"—a range of about ten pounds that our body works to keep us within. Low-quality food creates a hormonal "clog" that raises our set-point. That's how we gain weight.

Next we will explore how this hormonal clog causes our body to want to weigh more regardless of how little we eat or how much we exercise. Then we will get to the good news: Once we unclog our metabolism, our set-point falls, and our lowered set-point keeps us slim regardless of how much we eat or exercise. Millions of naturally thin people already do this. We can too.

Finally, you and I will see that the first step to enabling our bodies to burn fat for us is to free our minds from the myths of calorie and exercise *quantity*. Instead of focusing on counting the calories we take in and exercise off, we will focus on increasing the *quality* of our calories and exercise. We will eat *more* and exercise *less*, but smarter. This will unclog our metabolism, and our body will take care of fat loss for us.

Part 2—Myth: A Calorie Is a Calorie

We'll see that in order to eat *more*—smarter, we need to eat more high-quality foods. They help heal the hormones that control our body's ability to burn fat. That is the key to clearing the clog that prevents us from losing weight long term.

We will find that the quality of calories is determined by four factors: Satiety, Aggression, Nutrition, and Efficiency. Satiety is how quickly calories fill us up. Aggression is how likely calories are to be stored as body fat. Nutrition is how many vitamins, minerals, amino acids, essential fatty acids, etc., calories provide. Efficiency is how easily calories are converted into body fat. Whether a calorie is high-quality or low-quality depends on where it fits on the SANEity spectrum.

High-quality calories are on the healthy end of the SANEity spectrum. They are Satisfying, unAggressive, Nutritious, and inEfficient. They fill us up quickly and keep us full for a long time. They provide a lot of nutrients, and few of them can be converted into body fat. Even better, they trigger the release of body-fat-burning hormones, clear clogs, and lower our set-point. In short, they are SANE.

Low-quality calories are just the opposite. They are on the unhealthy end of the SANEity spectrum. They are unSatisfying, Aggressive, non-Nutritious, and Efficient. They trigger the release of body-fat-storing hormones, cause clogs, and raise our set-point. In short, they are inSANE.

Lastly, we will see that SANE eating is simple. When you eat high-quality food—such as non-starchy vegetables, seafood, lean meat, fat-free or low-fat cottage cheese, fat-free or low-fat *plain Greek* yogurt, fruit, eggs, nuts, and seeds—you will be too full for low-quality food such as starches and sweets. Eating *more* SANE calories causes the quality of our diet to rise. That lowers our set-point. And a lower set-point keeps us slim automatically.

Part 3—Myth: Calories Are All That Matter

You and I will walk through the science showing why understanding and improving the quality of our calories is so important. We will discover that calorie *quality* controls the hormones that control our set-point, while summarizing shocking studies where calorie *quantity* had little if anything to do with long-term body weight.

We'll explore how our metabolism relies heavily on hormones, and how eating SANE high-quality calories keeps things running smoothly, while eating inSANE low-quality calories causes us to produce too many body-fat-storing hormones and too few body-fat-burning hormones.

Finally, we'll review how we can heal our hormones by eating *more* and exercising *less*—smarter—instead of eating less and exercising more—harder. We will see that since in-SANE low-quality calories caused our clog, eating less of them will not clear it, while eating more SANE high-quality calories will.

Parts 4 & 5—Government Guidelines and Graphics, Big Profits and People

We will discover that the clogged-up and myth-filled world of today has a long history. One of the lowest-quality sources of calories in the world is starch, but our government somehow does not know this fact. In their pyramid, the starch group appears at the very base, as though it should be the foundation of a healthy diet:

Government's Food Guide Pyramid

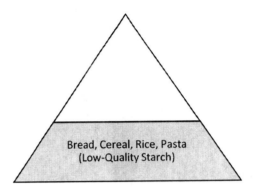

Bread, Cereal, Rice, Pasta
(Low-Quality Starch)

Government's MyPlate

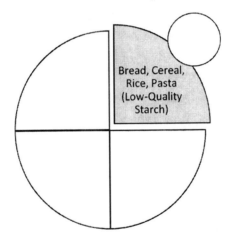

Bread, Cereal,
Rice, Pasta
(Low-Quality
Starch)

Then, you and I will uncover how USDA bureaucrats recommend starch as the backbone of our diet, while biologists have proven that the body needs absolutely no starch and that a surplus of starch removes our body's ability to burn body fat. We ate no starch for 99.8% of our evolutionary history, but today's typical diet is saturated with it. This dramatic change in our diet has led to the dramatic change in our appearance.

Lastly, we'll see how big food, fitness, and pharmaceutical corporations have made things worse. They exploit the government's guidelines and graphics to keep people and profits fat. Their most powerful weapon is the single most inSANE clog-causing substance in the world: added sweeteners. You and I will see how added sweeteners further prevent our body from burning fat, and how returning to the diet that kept us healthy and slim for hundreds-of-thousands of years is the key to staying healthy and slim today.

Part 6—Solution: Eat More—Smarter™

We will find that long-term fat loss has nothing to do with dieting and everything to do with eating so many more non-starchy vegetables, fish, meat, select dairy products, fruits, nuts, and seeds that we are too full for starches and sweets. Low-fat, low-carbohydrate, and high-protein diets are unnecessary. If we simply return to our natural balanced way of eating, we will return to our normal weight—along with good health.

I will suggest five steps to eating more—smarter:

1. Eat so many non-starchy vegetables and so much protein that you are too full for starches and sweets.
2. Remember your ancestors.
3. Buy groceries in bulk to save money.
4. Drink lots of water and green tea.
5. Do what works for you.

Part 7—Solution: Exercise Less—Smarter™

We'll explore how exercising to enable our body to burn fat for us long term is completely different than exercising to burn a few calories right now. While calorie-focused exercise is done frequently, for a long time, and uses a little resistance, exercise which focuses on long-term fat loss is done infrequently, for a short period of time, and uses a lot of resistance.

Together we will find that just as high Satiety, low Aggression, high Nutrition, and low Efficiency calories dramatically increase the quality of eating, deep, hormonal, infrequent, eccentric, and brief movements dramatically increase the quality of exercise. We will see how moving our body a little, but forcefully, makes our metabolism work more like the metabolism of a naturally thin person.

We'll also discover that this smarter scientific exercise program takes at most twenty minutes per week, is safer than traditional exercise programs, and can be done at home with no expensive equipment.

And finally, you and I will put all of this science together to see how:

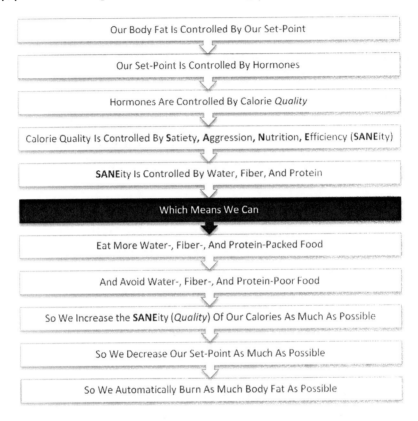

The problem is complex. The solution is simple. The science is surprising. And the results are amazing.

Let's get started.

PART 1

Myth: Calories In—Calories Out

"In other fields, when bridges do not stand, when aircraft do not fly, when machines do not work, when treatments do not cure, despite all conscientious efforts on the part of many persons to make them do so, one begins to question the basic assumptions, principles, theories, and hypotheses that guide one's efforts."

ARTHUR JENSEN, UNIVERSITY OF CALIFORNIA[1]

CHAPTER 1

The Fat Metabolism System

"The best data available suggest that the obese...eat no more than the lean."
S.C. WOOLEY, UNIVERSITY OF CINCINNATI[2]

Think back to high school biology class. We all learned how we pump blood with our circulatory system, how we breathe with our respiratory system, and how men think with their reproductive system. (Actually, maybe they didn't teach that last part.) But there is another major system which did not make it into our high school biology textbooks. This system lies at the heart of the obesity, diabetes, cardiovascular disease, and heart disease epidemics. It is also the system completely ignored by the typical approach to fat loss. It is our *fat metabolism system*.

> **The Fat Metabolism System:** A series of signals from our hormones and brain which control how much we eat, how many calories we burn, and how much body fat we store. Researcher P.J. Havel from the University of California defines it more academically: "...a variety of nutrient, endocrine [hormonal], and neural [brain] signals...[regulating] food intake, energy expenditure, and body fat stores."[3] [1]

---

1   You will see words in brackets [like this] in quotes from researchers. I do this to make academic writing easy to understand while maintaining the original intent of the researcher.

We've been told that the key to fat loss is manually controlling "calories in" and "calories out." Yet our fat metabolism system is an automatic internal calorie controller. How all its parts work together within the body is complicated, but knowledge of biology is not needed to understand its effects. We use metabolism all the time to explain why that guy who eats whatever he wants looks like a beanpole, while other people pack on the pounds after smelling a cheesecake. We say, "Sam's so lucky to have a fast metabolism." Or, "Poor Jane. She must have a slow metabolism."[4]

Instead of going through life hungry or spending countless hours in a gym, we can fix the issue that underlies fat gain: a hormonal clog in our fat metabolism system. By unclogging, we can change the way our fat metabolism system works. We can make it burn—instead of store—body fat.

> **The Clog:** The inability of our fat metabolism system to respond to signals from our hormones and our brain which otherwise enable us to burn body fat. Academics also refer to "the clog" as metabolic dysregulation, and it is the underlying cause of long term weight gain. UCLA and Harvard Medical School researcher T. Kelesidis puts it more academically: "The circulating [hormone] level...directs the central nervous system in regulating energy [balance]...[However] the vast majority of obese humans... are resistant...to its weight-reducing effects."[5]

Think about trying to remove body fat from a clogged fat metabolism system like trying to drain water from a clogged sink. Eating less is like turning down the faucet. Exercising more is like scooping out the overflowing water. Both are temporary ways to deal with the symptoms of the problem. Neither does anything about the root cause. That is why they both fail long term.

The problem is the clog. The solution is clearing the clog. And clearing the clog requires thinking in terms of *quality*, not *quantity*.

Fiddling with the quantity of food we eat and the quantity of exercise we get will never clear our hormonal clog. *Quality*—low-quality food and low-quality exercise—is the cause of the backup. A sink does not get clogged by putting too much water into it. It gets clogged when we put the wrong stuff into it.

As M.F. Rolland-Cachera, a researcher at the French National Institute of Health and Medical Research puts it: "Many studies have failed to show a correlation between individual energy intake and obesity." H. Keen, a researcher at King's College London goes one step further and tells us [my emphasis here and throughout]: "The association of increased adiposity [body fat] with low food energy consumption may indicate an underlying 'low energy throughput' state [clog]." More simply, the theory that weight gain is caused by too many calories has been disproven. Researchers now know the real cause of weight gain is a clog in our fat metabolism system.[6]

The Need and Ability to Burn Body Fat

Let's imagine a world where calorie *quantity* is actually the key to long-term fat loss. Now let's try an experiment. We'll divide a group of people in half. We'll feed one half 120 extra calories per day for eight years. What would happen? If weight was ruled by calorie quantity, the math is pretty easy. Multiply 120 extra calories per day times 365 days in a year, times eight years, and the total equals 350,400 extra calories. Take that sum and divide it by the 3,500 calories in a pound of body fat, and we can predict that these people will gain 100 pounds. The equation is easy, but unfortunately, it's incorrect.

Instead, let's look at a real-life study: the $700 million Women's Health Initiative. This study tracked nearly 49,000 women for eight years. Just like our experiment, the women in one group ate an average of 120 more calories a day than the other group. Remember, that adds up to 350,400 more calories. How many more pounds did the women who ate 350,400 more calories gain?

0.88 pounds.[7]

That is not a typo. Eating 350,400 more calories caused the women to gain an average of less than a pound. Hmmmm. It seems that something is wrong with the *Calories In— Calories Out* equation.

This quantity-focused fat loss myth incorrectly assumes that taking less calories in, or exercising more calories off, forces our fat metabolism system to burn body fat. That has been clinically proven to be false. It does not force us to burn body fat. It forces us to burn less calories. That is why dieters walk around tired and crabby all day. Their bodies and brains have slowed down.[8]

When our fat metabolism system needs calories and none are around, it is forced to make a decision: Go through all the hassle of converting calories from body fat or just slow down on burning calories. Given the choice, slowing down wins. University of Wisconsin researcher R.E. Kessey puts it more academically: "Metabolism [is] sharply reduced when an organism falls into negative energy balance."[9]

More importantly, the *need* to burn body fat does not mean body fat is burned. If you are clogged, the *need* to burn body fat is not enough. Your fat metabolism system does not have the *ability* to burn body fat, and you do not burn body fat efficiently. From researcher J.M. Friedman at the Rockefeller University: "The implication is that something metabolically different about [overweight] individuals results in obesity independent of their caloric intake." Consider a study done at St. Joseph's Hospital and Medical Center in Phoenix, Arizona. Researchers examined both heavy and thin people to see how their fat metabolism systems behaved when they were given no calories. As expected, everyone's system slowed down. Because these people were on zero-calorie diets, everyone burned body fat, but here's the kicker. Thin people burned off nearly 50% more body fat than heavy people.[10]

Think about that for a second. Despite having *more* body fat, the heavy people burned *less* body fat. In the words of the researchers, "...obese patients could not take advantage of their most abundant fat fuel sources but have to depend on the efficient use of...the breakdown products of body protein [muscle]."[11]

Where Patients' Fat Metabolism Systems Got Energy

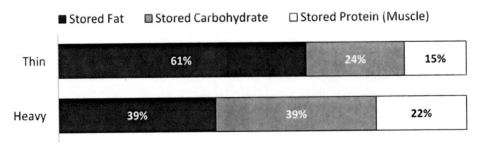

	■ Stored Fat	▦ Stored Carbohydrate	☐ Stored Protein (Muscle)
Thin	61%	24%	15%
Heavy	39%	39%	22%

That finding is depressing. The heavy people burned what relatively little muscle tissue they had rather than burning the excess body fat they were drowning in. They *needed* to burn body fat, but did not burn body fat effectively. This is where the idea of a clog comes into play. The researchers put the problem like this: "Profound metabolic disturbances [clogs] exist in the obese state that constantly interfere with normal hormonal responses [the ability to burn body fat]." As long as you and I are clogged, our ability to burn body fat will be severely compromised.[12]

Fiddling with the quantity of calories in or out does not create the *ability* to burn body fat. We need to shift our focus to eating more—but higher-quality—food and doing less—but higher-quality—exercise.

Eating more high-quality food provides more nutrition while preventing overeating. That helps clear our hormonal clog while creating the need *and* the ability to burn body fat. If we add high-quality exercise, then we activate clog-clearing hormones, and burning body fat goes from being a struggle to being simple. And since we will eat as much high-quality food as we want while doing only ten to twenty minutes of high-quality exercise per week, we can keep this up permanently. That permanent need *and* ability to burn body fat is our bullet train to long-term fat loss.[13]

Get Your Fat Metabolism System to Burn Body Fat for You

Despite being proven wrong, eating less and exercising more is still the most common approach to weight loss. We are led to believe that our fat metabolism system sits back while we consciously regulate our weight. That is not how our body works. After W.C. Miller of Indiana University ran a clinical test of this principle, he concluded: "This study examined the relationships among body fat...energy intake, and exercise...There was *no* relationship between energy intake [calories in] and adiposity [body fat]"[14]

Think about any other system in our body—our respiratory system, our immune system, etc. We do not manually control our bodily systems. We can try to hold our breath. We can try to avoid colds. But the respiratory and immune systems are in control and will do what they want. The fat metabolism system works the same way. Researcher J.M. Friedman from the Rockefeller University explains, "The average human consumes one million...calories a year, yet weight changes very little...These facts lead to the conclusion that energy balance is regulated with a precision of greater than 99.5%, which far exceeds what can be consciously monitored."[15]

When you think about how hard our body systems work to make sure we stay on an even keel health-wise, this point makes perfect sense. Yet here is what the American Heart Association advises: "How can you manage your weight in a healthful way? The answer is simple: balance the calories you take in with the calories you burn." Which seems odd considering they also said: "Few reliable data are available on the relative contributions to this obesity epidemic by energy intake and energy expenditure." I might be missing something, but if "few reliable data are available," then how did they come up with this answer?[16]

We don't have to worry about beating our hearts thanks to our circulatory system, and we also don't have to worry about balancing our calories thanks to our fat metabolism system. The key to weight loss and health in general is keeping all of our body's systems "clog-free" by eating more high-quality food. In the case of our fat metabolism system, this lowers our set-point weight and keeps us slim as reliably as our elevated set-point currently keeps us heavy. Chapter 2 shows how our set-point works and how we will get it to burn body fat for us.

CHAPTER 2

Your Set-Point Weight

"The set-point theory of body weight regulation is based on a large body of empiric evidence."
D.S. WEIGLE, UNIVERSITY OF WASHINGTON[1]

Our fat metabolism system automatically regulates our weight around a "set-point." That set-point is why no matter how little we eat or how much we exercise, we generally end up weighing the same. It is why you can get sick, lose weight, but then gain it all back. It is also why heavy people do not keep getting heavier and heavier until they explode.

> **Set-Point Weight:** The weight that our fat metabolism system automatically works to keep us at regardless of the quantity of calories we take in or exercise off.

I know that last part sounds silly, but let's look at this point seriously. Why don't obese people gain weight forever? If the quantity of calories they ate and exercised off raised them to 450 pounds, why doesn't it raise them to 4,500 pounds? These individuals somehow *automatically* stop gaining weight. How does that work under the *Calories In—Calories Out* theory?

It doesn't.

Here is how weight gain works in the real world: A person's set-point rises and then their fat metabolism system fights to keep them weighing more regardless of how little they eat or how much they exercise. D.S. Weigle at the University of Washington notes: "Obesity is not a disorder of body weight regulation. Most obese patients regulate their weight appropriately about an elevated set-point weight." A heavy person's higher set-point keeps them at that higher weight like a thin person's lower set-point keeps them at a lower weight. We all have a set-point. The issue is how high it is. Long-term fat loss comes from lowering it, not from starving it.[2]

The set-point takes *whatever* quantity of calories we eat plus *whatever* quantity of calories we burn and balances us out automatically. That is why manually balancing calories fails 95% of the time over the long term. It is trying to override our set-point, and we generally do not win battles against our basic biological functions. As researcher Keith Frayn of Oxford University noted: "We should not be surprised that dieting is difficult because it is a fight against mechanisms which have evolved over many millions of years precisely to minimize its effects."[3]

In a series of studies, University of Cincinnati researchers surgically removed and added body fat to various animals. Animals with body fat surgically removed then replaced "exactly the mass of fat which was taken." Animals with body fat surgically added automatically burned more body fat until their body fat returned to its set-point.[4]

In other studies, individuals intentionally overate. All these studies show that people:[5]
  1. Gain less weight than predicted by *Calories In—Calories Out*
  2. Stop weight gain completely at a certain point
  3. Return to their original weight automatically when overeating stops

You can see the pivotal role that a set-point plays in our metabolism. Study after study makes the same point. In studies at the University of Vermont, students ate up to five times more than normal but could not increase their weight by more than 12%. They would overeat and overeat, but their fat metabolism systems would not let them gain weight beyond a certain point. Studies were also conducted where prison inmates voluntarily ate up to 10,000 calories a day—they literally ate until they vomited. None of the prisoners could increase their weight by more than 25%.[6]

Knowing that our initial set-point is determined by our genetics, researchers tested twins to definitively prove the power of the set-point. Twins share the same genes and therefore the same initial set-point. One study tested two sets: let's call them the Smith twins and the Thomas twins. Given 1,000 excess calories per day, would the Smith twins and Thomas twins all gain the same amount of body fat? Or would the set-point for the Smiths produce a different weight gain than the Thomases?[7]

Different. Very different.

The Smiths both gained the same amount of weight because they had the same set-point. So did the Thomases. But weight gain varied by nearly three times between the two sets of twins because they had different set-points. While the Smiths each gained two pounds, the Thomas twins each gained eight pounds.

J.M. Friedman of the Rockefeller University sums up the set-point: "[The simplistic notion] that weight can be controlled by 'deciding' to eat less and exercise more...is at odds with substantial scientific evidence illuminating a precise and powerful biologic system that maintains body weight within a relatively narrow range." This point is also emphasized by P.J. Havel at the University of California: "Body weight...[is] tightly regulated over relatively long periods of time. Even after large alterations of body fat resulting from restriction of energy intake...body weight and fat stores tend to return to pre-intervention levels."[8]

Our body does not want us to starve. To lose weight, we need to lower the "relatively narrow range" where our "powerful biologic system" operates. In order to do that, we need to find out what causes the set-point to rise in the first place.[9]

How Our Set-Point Rises

Our fat metabolism system keeps us at our set-point the same way it does everything else: hormones. The two most commonly talked about are insulin and leptin. Insulin determines whether we are storing or burning body fat. Leptin regulates how much food we eat, how much energy we burn, and the amount of body fat specified by our set-point.

Let's assume we are unclogged. When our weight starts rising above our set-point, hormonal signals cause our metabolism to go up, our appetite to go down, and our body fat to get burned. This prevents excess body fat from sticking around for long. We stay at our set-point without trying.[10]

But when we fill our body with low-quality foods, the fat metabolism system gets clogged. It is unable to effectively respond to these hormones. Without those hormonal "burn body fat" signals getting through, the metabolic processes that otherwise automatically keep us thin do not happen.

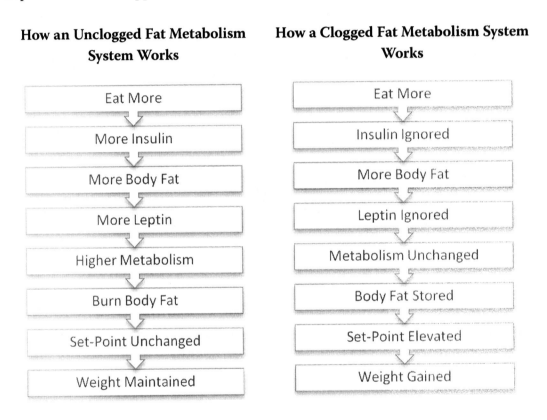

How an Unclogged Fat Metabolism System Works	**How a Clogged Fat Metabolism System Works**
Eat More	Eat More
More Insulin	Insulin Ignored
More Body Fat	More Body Fat
More Leptin	Leptin Ignored
Higher Metabolism	Metabolism Unchanged
Burn Body Fat	Body Fat Stored
Set-Point Unchanged	Set-Point Elevated
Weight Maintained	Weight Gained

Once our fat metabolism system is not effectively responding to hormones like leptin and insulin, we are clogged. When the current level of hormones do not get the job done, our fat metabolism system produces more of them. Chronically high levels of these hormones make our fat metabolism system think that an abnormally high level of body fat is normal. Since our fat metabolism system automatically keeps us at what it thinks is normal, it keeps us at an abnormally high level of body fat. By eating poorly, we can raise our set-point.[11]

> **Raised Set-Point:** Abnormal levels of hormones making the fat metabolism system think abnormal levels of body fat are normal.

The set-point won't go back down to normal until we get our hormone levels back to normal. We do that by unclogging ourselves. That means increasing the quality of our eating and exercise. And increasing the quality of our eating and exercise is easy when we eat more and exercise less—smarter.

University of Wisconsin researcher R.E. Keesey makes this point more academically: "If the goal is substantial and sustainable weight loss...a more promising approach would be one based upon a strategy of directly altering the set-point...The physiologic adjustments that ordinarily act to *resist* weight change...would instead *facilitate* the achievement and subsequent maintenance of a lower weight."[12]

The set-point can be frustrating. It's why eating less of our current diet and doing more traditional exercise doesn't work 95% of the time. But by understanding the science of the set-point, it can become our ultimate source of hope. Instead of fighting against our raised set-point by working harder, we can eat and exercise smarter, unclog, lower our set-point, and enable our fat metabolism system to burn body fat for us automatically. Chapter 3 shows how we do that.[13]

CHAPTER 3

How to Lower Your Set-Point Weight

"Set-points are not fixed."
R.E. KEESEY, UNIVERSITY OF WISCONSIN[1]

A s we have seen, you can stray from your set-point temporarily by lowering the *quantity* of food you eat and raising the *quantity* of exercise you do. Yet you cannot adjust your set-point itself unless you focus on changing the *quality* of the food and exercise. The higher the quality, the lower your set-point.

How Quality Influences Our Set-Point

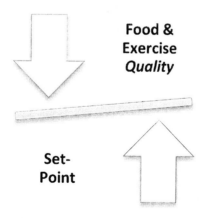

Food &
Exercise
Quality

Set-
Point

Consider B.J. Rolls' research at the University of Oxford. She took rats and divided them into two groups:

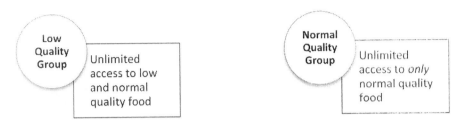

As expected, the Low Quality Group got heavy and the Normal Quality Group did not. But here is where the study gets interesting. After the Low Quality Group got heavy, Rolls took the low-quality food (processed starches such as such as chips, cookies, and crackers) away from them. Now both the overweight Low Quality Group and the regular-weight Normal Quality Group had access to the same food. The Low Quality Group, though, stayed at their heavy weight.

Wait a second. How can the same diet keep one group of rats heavy and keep another group slim? Because they changed their set-points.

The Normal Quality Group started with a normal set-point, remained at a normal set-point thanks to a normal quality diet, and therefore maintained a normal weight. The Low Quality group started with a normal set-point, increased their set-point thanks to a low-quality diet, and thereafter maintained a heavy weight. In Rolls' words: "Because the experimental rats are maintaining excess weight above the control rats, despite eating the same amount...it is possible that the obese rats have undergone *a long-lasting endocrine or metabolic change*." That change is a clog in their fat metabolism system.

The study gets even more interesting. Rolls then took half of the heavy Low Quality Group and kept them eating only normal quality food, but much less of it. In other words, she made the heavy rats eat less. Lowering the *quantity* of food caused the rats to *temporarily* lose weight. However, as soon as Rolls stopped starving the Low Quality Group, they returned to the heavy weight targeted by their recently raised set-point. They did not return to a standard rat weight. The low-quality food they ate at the start of the study created a clog in their fat metabolism system that raised their set-point and put them on a path of long-term weight gain.[2]

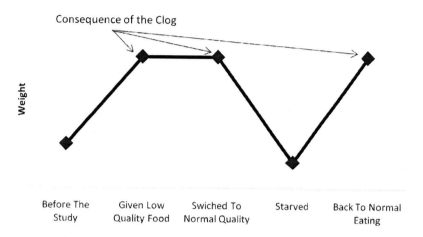

The Impact of Low Quality Food

Consequence of the Clog

Weight

| Before The Study | Given Low Quality Food | Swiched To Normal Quality | Starved | Back To Normal Eating |

These eye-opening results have been repeated over and over. University of Utah researcher J.W. Peck devised a test similar to Rolls' study, dividing normal rats into three groups. Each group could eat an unlimited quantity of calories. The only difference was the quality of the calories.

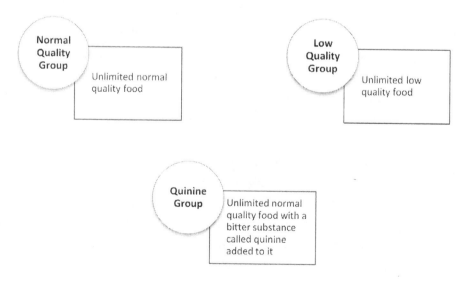

As expected, the Normal Quality Group maintained a standard weight, the Low Quality Group gained weight, and the Quinine Group lost weight. Peck then made each group of rats eat less of their type of food. All of the rats temporarily lost about 10% of their body weight. Now for the unexpected part.

Peck then stopped starving the rats, and they all went back to eating an unlimited amount of their chosen food. The Normal Quality Group automatically returned to their standard rat weight. The Low Quality Group automatically returned to their heavier weight. And the Quinine Group automatically returned to their reduced weight. Like Rolls' study, after eating less, all the rats automatically regained weight, but how much they regained depended on their set-point, which depended on the quality of their diet. In other words, food *quantity* temporarily moved them away from their set-point, but food *quality* determined the set-point itself.

Peck was not done. He wanted to see what impact exercise quantity would have on the various set-points, so he had his furry friends burn off calories by shivering away all day in a very cold room. All of the rats automatically increased how much they ate to offset how much they exercised. Burning more calories simply made the rats eat more calories. Their set-point was unchanged.

Peck then freed the rats from the cold conditions, but continued the experiment. He kept all the groups on their respective diets while feeding them additional calories through a stomach tube. He wanted to see if a higher *quantity* of the same *quality* of calories would impact the rats' set-points. It did not. All of the rats automatically adjusted the amount of normal quality, low-quality, or bitter food they ate in order to maintain the normal, higher, or lower weights targeted by their set-points.

Eating less did not cause long-term weight loss. The set-point won. Exercising more did not cause long-term weight loss. The set-point won. Having additional calories pumped directly into the stomach did not cause long-term weight gain. The set-point won. The only factor that did impact rats' long-term weight was the quality of their calories. That worked because it changed their set-point. Fortunately, recent research reveals a more enjoyable way of changing the quality of our diet. No quinine-laced food for us. Just a lot more natural foods rich in water, fiber, and protein like non-starchy vegetables, seafood, lean meat, eggs, fat-free or low-fat cottage cheese, or fat-free or low-fat *plain Greek* yogurt, fruits, nuts, and seeds.[3]

One more study proves this point. In Dr. Nancy J. Rothwell's study at St. George's Hospital Medical School in London, growing rats were divided into Low-Quality American Diet and High-Quality Natural Rat Diet groups. Rothwell let all of the growing rats eat as much as they wanted for sixteen days. On the seventeenth day the rats continued eating as much as they wanted, but Rothwell switched the Low-Quality American Diet rats to the high-quality natural rat diet. Here is what happened:[4]

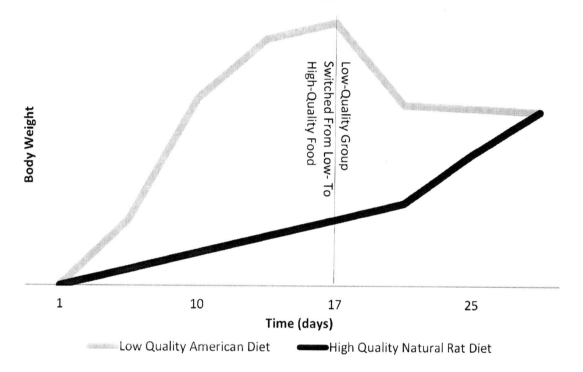

The heavier young rats quickly dropped all their excess weight automatically when the *quality* of their diet improved. And so will you once you stop focusing on quantity and start applying the science of quality. So let's look at the four major problems of the traditional quantity-focused fat-loss approach:[5]

1. Eating less does *not* cause long-term fat loss.
2. Exercising more does *not* cause long-term fat loss.

3. Exercising less does *not* cause long-term fat gain.
4. Eating more does *not* cause long-term fat gain.

In chapter 4, we'll look at what scientists have to say about each of these statements. They already know the answers, and they can prove it. That's good for you, because by knowing the facts, you can finally start to lose weight—for good.

CHAPTER 4

Eating Less Does *Not* Cause Long-Term Fat Loss

"The reduction of energy intake continues to be the basis of...weight reduction programs...[The results] are known to be poor and not long-lasting."
GEORGE BRAY, PENNINGTON BIOMEDICAL RESEARCH CENTER[1]

Eating less does *not* create the need to burn body fat. It creates the need for the body to slow down. Contrary to popular opinion, the body hangs on to body fat. Instead, it burns muscle tissue, and that worsens the clog problem. Only as a last resort, if the body has no other option, it may also burn a bit of body fat.[2]

Why does the body hang on to body fat and burn muscle? To answer that question, let's look at it another way. What does our fat metabolism system want more of when it thinks we are starving? Stored energy. What is a great source of stored energy? Body fat. So when our fat metabolism system thinks we are starving, does it want to get rid of or hold on to body fat? It wants to hold on.

Next, what does our fat metabolism system want less of when we are starving? It wants less tissue which burns a lot of calories. What type of tissue burns a lot of calories? Muscle tissue. So when our fat metabolism system thinks we are starving, it gets rid of calorie-hungry muscle tissue. Studies show that up to 70% of the weight lost while eating less comes from burning muscle—not body fat.[3]

41

Burning all this muscle means that starving ourselves leads to more body fat—not less—over the long term. As soon as we stop starving ourselves, we have all the calories we used to have but need less of them, thanks to all that missing muscle and our slowed-down metabolism. Now our fat metabolism system sees eating a normal amount as overeating and creates new body fat. In the *Journal of the American Medical Association*, researcher G.L. Thorpe tells us that eating less does not make us lose weight, "...by selective reduction of adipose deposits [body fat], but by wasting of all body tissues...therefore, any success obtained must be maintained by chronic under-nourishment." It is not practical or healthy to keep ourselves "chronically under-nourished," so we don't. Instead, we yo-yo diet. And that is why eating less is not an effective long-term fat loss approach.[4]

Why Eating Less Fails Long-Term 95% of the Time

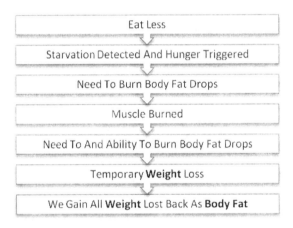

Imagine watching TV and seeing a commercial for a new medication. The ad tells you the medication slightly improves your vision as long as you keep yourself chronically sleep-deprived. At the end of the commercial, a quieter voice lists the medication's long-term side effects. One of them is that your vision will become much worse if you ever go back to sleeping a normal amount. Would you ever use that medication? Of course not. You cannot go through life tired. Its temporary benefit is not worth its long-term side effects.

Now imagine another commercial. This one is for a mail-order weight-loss meal program that slightly reduces your weight as long as you keep yourself chronically food-deprived. At the end of the commercial a quieter voice goes though the program's side effects.

The side effects include making you much heavier if you ever go back to eating a normal amount. Would you ever use that program? Of course not. You cannot go through life hungry. To escape the superstition of starvation, let's dive deeper into the science of its side effects.

> "...a general public health recommendation for weight reduction through dieting cannot be supported strongly with existing data."
>
> **D.S. WEIGLE, UNIVERSITY OF WASHINGTON**[5]

The Side Effects of Eating Less

My favorite experiment showing the side effects of eating less took place at the University of Geneva and involved three groups of rats all eating the same quality of food.

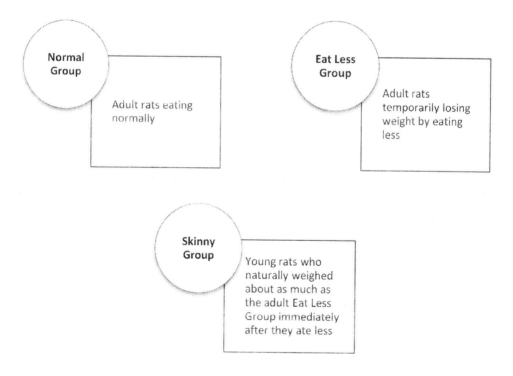

If the study were conducted on humans, the Normal Group would be typical thirty-five-year-old women. The Eat Less Group would be thirty-five-year-old women cutting calories until they fit into their high school jeans. And the Skinny Group would be high school girls who fit into size four jeans without trying.

For the first ten days of the study, the Eat Less Group ate 50% less than usual while the Normal Group ate normally. On the tenth day:

1. The Skinny Group showed up and ate normally.
2. The Eat Less Group stopped starving themselves and started eating normally.
3. The Normal Group kept eating normally.

This went on for twenty-five days and the study ended on day thirty-five.

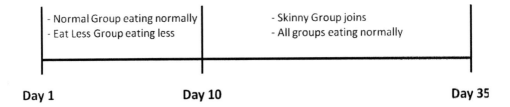

At the end of the thirty-five day study, the Normal Group had eaten normally for thirty-five days. The Eat Less Group had eaten less for ten days and then normally for twenty-five days. And the Skinny Group had eaten normally for twenty-five days.

Which group do you think weighed the most and had the highest body fat percentage at the end? The Skinny Group seems like an easy "no" since they are younger and naturally thinner than the other rats. Traditional fat loss theory would say the Eat Less Group is an easy "no" as well since they ate 50% less for ten days. So the Normal Group weighed the most and had the highest body fat percentage at the end of the study, right?

Nope.

The Eat Less Group weighed the most and had the highest percent body fat. Even though they ate less for ten days, they were significantly heavier than those who ate normally all the way through. Eating less led the rats to gain—not lose—body fat. MacLean at the University of Colorado describes this general metabolic behavior: "[When we eat less] metabolic adjustments occur...[which] contribute to a large potential energy imbalance that, when the forcible control of energy intake is relieved...results in an exceptionally high rate of weight regain."[6]

Here is the data:

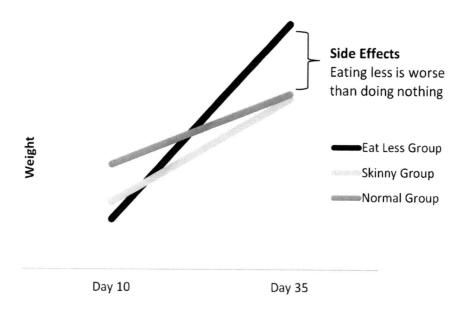

Side Effects
Eating less is worse
than doing nothing

━━ Eat Less Group

Skinny Group

Normal Group

Day 10   Day 35

Talk about side effects. Eating less was worse than doing nothing. Why? After our fat metabolism system is starved, its number one priority is restoring all the body fat it lost and then protecting us from starving in the future. Guess how it does that? By storing additional body fat. Researchers call this "fat super accumulation." From researcher E.A. Young at the University of Texas: "These and other studies...strongly suggest that fat super accumulation...after energy restriction is a major factor contributing to relapsing obesity, so often observed in humans."[7]

> **Fat Super Accumulation:** The unavoidable gaining of more body fat than we lose after we starve ourselves. The primary side effect of eating less. The main reason eating less is not an effective long-term fat loss technique.

The most disturbing aspect of fat super accumulation is that it does not require us to eat a lot. All we have to do is go back to eating a normal amount. The Eat Less Group in the study gained a massive amount of body fat quickly while eating *the same amount* as the Normal Group and the Skinny Group. The fat metabolism system was trying to make up for the past losses.

There is another reason: eating less slowed the metabolism. Put the same quantity and quality of food and exercise into a slowed-down fat metabolism system, and out comes more body fat. The University of Geneva researchers discovered that the Eat Less Group's fat metabolism systems were burning body fat over 500% less efficiently and had slowed down by 15% by the end of the study. They remarked: "These investigations provide direct evidence for the existence of a *specific metabolic component* that contributes to an elevated efficiency of energy utilization during refeeding after low food consumption," or once eating less stops. I call that "specific metabolic component" a clogged-up and slowed-down fat metabolism system. It results in a significant drop in our *need* and our *ability* to burn body fat.[8]

For another example of starvation's long-term side effects, consider Dr. Rudolph Leibel's study at Rockefeller University. A group of people weighing an average of 335 pounds starved themselves down to 220 pounds. After the starvation period was over, the researchers wanted to see what impact eating less had on the 220-pound dieters' need to burn body fat. To do this they brought in people who were the same age but naturally slim. This gave the researchers three groups of people to compare:

1. Non-starved 335-pound people
2. Formerly 335-pound people who weighed 220 pounds
3. Non-starved 138-pound people

Like a larger SUV should need more gasoline than a smaller motorcycle, the non-starved 335 pound people should need more calories than the non-starved 138-pound people, right?

Yes.

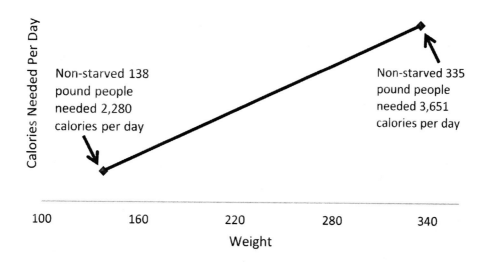

Non-starved 138 pound people needed 2,280 calories per day

Non-starved 335 pound people needed 3,651 calories per day

All things being equal, more body weight means more calories needed per day to maintain and move more mass. So after losing 115 pounds, you would think the 220-pound people must have slid down the graph and ended up here:

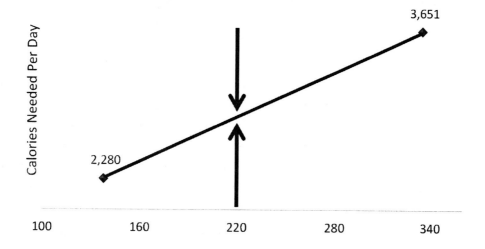

Right?

Not necessarily. It depends on how the 115 pounds were lost. After all, we know starvation burns calorie-hungry muscle while slowing down the fat metabolism system. So having starved away 115 pounds, how many calories did the 220-pound starvation dieters' need?

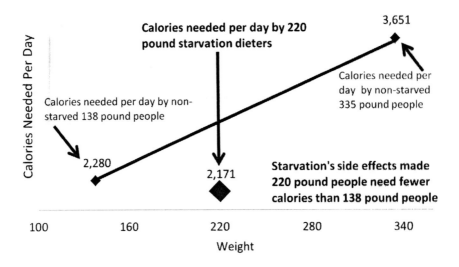

Thanks to starvation's side effects, the 220-pound people destroyed their need to burn body fat. The 220-pound starvation dieters ended-up needing 5% fewer calories per day than the non-starved 138 pound people, even though they had eighty-two more pounds of mass to move. That is a scary side effect. And that is why University of Wisconsin researcher R.E. Keesy said: "Disproportionately large declines in resting metabolism are seen in food-deprived men."[9]

Similar results were gained from a test done as far back as World War II. University of Minnesota researchers studied starvation to get a better understanding of how to help the hungry in war-torn Europe. The researchers recruited people in the United States and had them cut back to a 1,600 calories per day diet.[1] Their fat metabolism systems responded by slowing down by a whopping 40%. At the same time their strength fell by 28%, their endurance fell by 79%, and their rates of depression rose by 36%.[10]

Let's focus on the fat metabolism system slowing down by 40% for a moment. Say Jill needs and eats 2,000 calories per day. But now Jill wants to drop a few pounds for her vacation in two weeks, so she reads a magazine which tells her to starve herself, and she cuts back to 1,600 calories per day. According to this study, Jill's fat metabolism system would slow down by 40% and only need 1,200 calories per day. Before Jill ate less, she needed 2,000

---

1   1,600 calories per day is considered generous by today's "eat less" advocates.

calories per day and ate 2,000 per day. After eating less, Jill only needed 1,200 calories per day but ate 1,600 per day. When she stops eating less, she will eat 2,000 calories per day while only needing 1,200 per day. That's not helpful.

Back to the World War II study. In addition to completely destroying their need to burn body fat, as soon as subjects stopped eating less, they ate an average of 5,000 calories a day until they gained all the weight they lost back plus 5%. That is the good news. The bad news is that their body fat percentage was 52% higher than before they starved themselves. All the muscle they burned was replaced by body fat. They experienced fat super accumulation.[11]

The More We Starve Ourselves, the Worse Off We Are

The counterproductive nature of eating less is called yo-yo dieting for a reason. The continuous down-and-back-up cycle matters because the more often people yo-yo, the slower their fat metabolism system gets. In a University of Pennsylvania study, rats ate a fattening diet and gained weight, then ate less and lost weight, then went back on the fattening diet and gained weight, then went back to eating less and lost weight, and then went back on the fattening diet and gained weight. They yo-yo'ed up, down, back up, back down, and then back up.

The second time the rats tried to lose weight by eating less, they lost weight 100% slower and regained the weight 300% faster than the first time they ate less. After the rats stopped eating less for the second time, they "had a four-fold increase in food efficiency compared to obese animals of the same weight who had not cycled." Translation: The rats who yo-yoed the second time stored food as body fat 400% more efficiently than rats who constantly ate a fattening diet.[12]

Doing nothing is better than eating less. This study shows it is 400% better. Researcher D.M. Garner at Michigan State University had this to say about starvation dieting: "It is only the rate of weight regain, not the fact of weight regain, that appears open to debate."[13]

The Nail in the Eat-Less Coffin

We have heard the "eat less to weigh less" myth a lot, so we need a lot of evidence to break free from it. Even after all the evidence, there still may be a voice in the back of your head saying: "Now hold on. There has to be some truth in eating less means less body fat, because that's what everybody says." I felt the same way.

Harvard researchers provided one last study that freed my mind once and for all. They divided a massive sample of 67,272 people in five groups according to the quantity of calories they ate, and the researchers found that the *less* people ate, the *more* body fat they had. This finding is shown in the following chart, where "Body Mass Index" approximates "body fat."[14] [2]

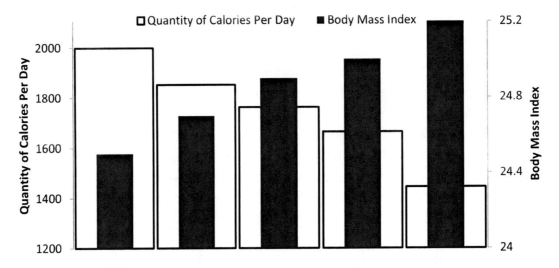

When you have a sampling that is so large, it makes sense to pay attention to the results. In my research, I found all sorts of studies like this. T. Mann at the University of California concluded: "[We] reviewed studies of the long-term outcomes of calorie-restricting diets to assess whether dieting is an effective treatment for obesity...In sum, there is little support for the notion that diets lead to lasting weight loss or health benefits."[15]

I also could provide studies showing that yo-yo dieting increases our risk of heart attack, stroke, diabetes, high blood pressure, cancer, immune system failure, eating disor-

2   From the Centers for Disease Control and Prevention: "Body Mass Index (BMI) is a number calculated from a person's weight and height. BMI provides a reliable indicator of body fatness for most people and is used to screen for weight categories that may lead to health problems." (Source: http://www.cdc.gov/healthyweight/assessing/bmi)

ders, impaired cognitive function, chronic fatigue, and depression. But that is beyond the scope of this book. For people who want to lose weight, the lesson is simple.[16]

Starvation does not make us thin. It makes us stocky, sick, and sad. It's bad for health and it's bad for fat loss. Your body just doesn't work that way.

The Philosophy of Long-Term Body Fat Loss

The 18th century German philosopher Immanuel Kant proposed a helpful theory when thinking about moral issues. He said we can tell whether an action is good or bad if it makes sense for everyone to do it all the time. For example, is it okay to lie? No, because if everyone always lied, society would fall apart.

His logic is even more useful in the fat-loss field. If any fat-loss program suggests you and I do something we cannot do over the long run, it is bad. We are trying to become slim for the rest of our lives. We do not want to lose body fat now only to gain it back later. So if we cannot follow a fat-loss program forever, forget it.

Whatever we do to lose body fat, we have to keep on doing it or we will gain all the body fat back. It is like pushing the accelerator pedal to make your car go sixty miles per hour. As soon as you stop pushing it, you will quickly slow down. Similarly, if you change the way you eat and exercise to burn body fat and then stop eating and exercising that way, you will quickly regain body fat. For instance, researcher P.C. Boyle reported in the *American Journal of Physiology* that as soon as rats stopped eating less, they gained weight twenty times faster than normal until they returned to at least their original weight.[17]

Nobody wants to gain body fat twenty times faster than normal, so before trying any diet or exercise program, be a philosopher and ask yourself, "Can I do this forever?" If the answer is yes, do it. If the answer is no, skip it.

CHAPTER 5

Exercising More Does *Not* Cause Long-Term Fat Loss

"My grandmother, she started walking five miles a day when she was sixty. She's ninety-seven today and we don't know where the hell she is."
ELLEN DEGENERES

We have seen that eating less is not effective. But what about exercising more? From the perspective of our fat metabolism system, there is no difference between the two. Eating 300 fewer calories is the same as burning 300 more calories. In both cases, our fat metabolism system reacts like this: "Oh no! Less nutrition! I am starving! Time to slow down, hang on to protective body fat, and burn calorie-hungry muscle." More calories out is the same as less calories in. Everything that makes the "eat less" principle fail makes "exercise more" fail too.[1]

That is not to say that all exercise is pointless. What is ineffective is traditional low-quality exercise. Exercising less—smarter—burns all sorts of body fat. You and I will cover that science in *Part 7—Solution: Exercise Less—Smarter*, but first we have to free our minds from the "exercise more to burn more" mythology.

In the same way that people drink more fluids when they exercise more, they also eat more when they exercise more. Researcher Hugo R. Rony found: "Consistently high or low energy expenditures result in consistently high or low levels of appetite. Thus men doing heavy physical work spontaneously eat more than men engaged in sedentary occupations." J.M. Friedman at Rockefeller University makes a similar point: "Exercise by itself has not been shown to be highly effective in treating obesity because the increased energy use from exercise is generally offset by increased caloric intake."[2]

Compounding the problem, many people who exercise more do not eat high-quality food. The majority of people get most of their calories from low-quality starches and sweeteners. Therefore, exercising more triggers the consumption of more low-quality food. More *low-quality* food means less need to burn body fat, more clogging, and a higher set-point. Far from burning body fat, we burn time and and build-up clogs.[3]

Pennington Biomedical Research Center researcher T.S. Church found, "After 18 months of exercise training and achieving 2,000 kcal [calories] per week of exercise, college-aged women had *no* weight loss." Church divided overweight women into four groups:

1. No change in exercise
2. Exercise more
3. Exercise even more
4. Exercise way more

After six months Church found: "The change in body fat was *not* statistically different across the...groups." He went on to note how more exercise did not cause more body fat to be burned because "a relatively high dose of exercise results in *compensatory* mechanisms that attenuate [offset] weight loss...Our findings are important because most exercise guidelines for weight loss recommend 200–300 minutes per week and we provide evidence that this amount of exercise induces compensation that results in *significantly less* weight loss than predicted."[4]

Here is one scenario for exercising more: Michelle goes for a 30-minute jog and burns 170 more calories than she would have burned by sitting at home and reading this book. She is trying hard to cut calories, so she does not drink any sugary sports drinks and fights through the hunger pangs after her jog. At dinner Michelle unconsciously drinks an extra glass of reduced-fat milk thanks to her increased thirst and hunger. The net result of her jog is thirteen more calories than if she had not exercised.

30 min. jog	-170 calories
12 oz. milk	+183 calories
Net	**+13 calories**

Much more commonly, people will have sweetened "power juice" while pounding it out on the treadmill. Afterward, they overeat low-quality food. The net result is more low-quality food and more clogging.

30 min. jog	-170 calories
24 oz. sports drink	+189 calories
Extra half serving of Fettuccine Alfredo	+390 calories
Net	**+409 calories**

The food industry is very well aware that exercising more encourages eating more low-quality food. That's why the following corporations serve on the executive board of the American Council on Fitness and Nutrition:[5]

- Coca-Cola Company
- PepsiCo
- Hershey Foods Corporation
- Sara Lee Corporation
- Kellogg Company
- Kraft Foods
- General Mills
- Campbell Soup Company
- ConAgra Foods
- Del Monte Foods
- Grocery Manufacturers Association
- H.J. Heinz Company
- Masterfoods USA
- National Restaurant Association
- Unilever United States
- American Association of Advertising Agencies
- American Beverage Association
- Association of National Advertisers

Are we told to exercise more because it is good for fat loss or because it is good for business? The National Soft Drink Association advises us to "consume at least eight glasses of fluids daily, *even more when you exercise.* A variety of beverages, *including soft drinks,* can contribute to proper hydration."[6]

But wait. If you exercise less, won't you gain body fat? As you'll see in chapter 6 and part 7, that depends on the type of exercise you do.

A Note About Sweeteners: When I talk about sweeteners, I am talking about sweeteners containing calories which are added to foods. Substances like sugar, high-fructose corn syrup, evaporated cane juice, etc. I am not talking about the sugars already found in natural foods like fruits and non-starchy vegetables. Those are fine. I am also not talking about calorie-free sweeteners like stevia, aspartame, sucralose, or saccharin. Those are fine in moderation. Studies show that calorie-free sweeteners *may* be harmful in ridiculously high amounts, while caloric added sweeteners are harmful in any amount. Researcher John Yudkin at the University of London tells us, "…think of what is already known that sugar can do, as distinct from what [sugar substitutes] might possibly do if taken in enormously unrealistic amounts…There is no doubt that people today are very worried about their food… but…most of them are worried about the wrong things." [7]

CHAPTER 6

Exercising Less Does *Not* Cause Long-Term Fat Gain

"It is reasonable to assume that persons with relatively high daily energy expenditures would be less likely to gain weight over time compared with those who have low energy expenditures. So far, data to support this hypothesis are not particularly compelling."
AMERICAN HEART ASSOCIATION[1]

The idea that we have an obesity epidemic because people are not exercising enough is another myth. Saffron A. Whitehead at St. George's University of London reported: "Most studies show that the obese do about the same physical activity as [the] lean."[2]

The only "weight versus activity" relationship that has been proven is that obesity leads to inactivity. Consider the conclusion of the 2004 University of Copenhagen study: "This study did *not* support that physical inactivity...is associated with the development of obesity, but...that obesity may lead to physical inactivity." More body fat leads to less exercise, not the other way around.[3]

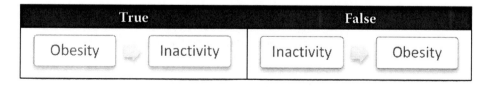

You might want to compare it to the idea that "partying less causes aging." People party less when they become older. They do not get older because they are partying less. With age comes deep metabolic changes that make partying until 3 am harder. The same holds true with exercise and obesity. People exercise less because they are obese. They do not become obese because they are exercising less. With obesity comes deep metabolic changes that make exercise harder.

Also, common sense tells us that if exercising less is the cause of our collective weight issues, we must be collectively exercising less. Are we?

Not even close.

The idea of aerobic exercise did not even exist in the mainstream until the 1968 publication of the book *Aerobics* by Dr. Kenneth H. Cooper. Dr. Entin, with the department of Biological Sciences at Northern Arizona University, explains the common view before then: "In the 1930's and 40's...high volume endurance training was thought to be bad for the heart. Through the '50's and even '60's, exercise was not thought to be useful...and endurance exercise was thought to be harmful to women." During that same period the percent of obese Americans was dramatically lower than today. Nowadays, Americans exercise more than anyone else in the world and are the sixth heaviest population in the world. How could doing too little of something that we did even less of before the problem existed cause the problem?[4]

> "...[Americans] are voluntarily exercising more than ever...While it seems perfectly clear that our lives are less physically demanding than they were in the 1950s, it's not necessarily the case that we are cumulatively burning fewer calories."
> ERIC J. OLIVER, UNIVERSITY OF CHICAGO[5]

Some experts say that we are getting heavier because we are using labor-saving devices. Yet that doesn't make sense. The vast majority of labor-saving devices became common in households decades before obesity shot up. Use of dishwashers, washing machines, vacuum cleaners, and all the major labor-saving devices increased most between 1945 and 1965. However, obesity increased little during that time period. Use of these devices increased very little between 1978 and 1998 while obesity rates shot up. So how could labor-saving devices be the cause of weight problems?

Reread the quote from the American Heart Association at the start of this chapter. Digging into the data and abandoning *assumptions* about our activity levels, researchers like New York University's Marion Nestle tell us, "...the activity levels of Americans appear to have changed little, if at all, from the 1970s to the 1990s."[6]

What about all the TV watching? That's got to be the cause, right? That too does not correspond with the facts. Tsinghua University professor Seth Roberts determined: "Time spent watching TV increased by 45% from 1965 to 1975, yet obesity increased little over that time; from 1975 to 1995, when obesity shot up, TV watching increased only a little."[7]

Finally, if general activity level determined weight, then the thinnest people in the world would be manual laborers, while the heaviest would be desk jockeys. People with manual labor jobs are "active" forty hours a week, every week, at their jobs. People with desk jobs are "inactive" forty hours a week. Are manual laborers slimmer than desk jockeys?

Let's look at the research. The Centers for Disease Control and Prevention collected data from over 68,000 adults and found that obesity rises as income falls and manual labor—i.e., work-related activity—rises. The data suggest that, on average, active manual laborers are heavier than inactive desk jockeys. Therefore, it seems that inactivity causes obesity as much as jackets cause cold weather.[8]

> *"A recent review of [319 studies] suggests that obese [peoples'] energy expenditure is higher than that of the [non-obese] population."*
> **JOHN E. BLUNDELL, UNIVERSITY OF LEEDS**[9]

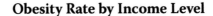

Obesity Rate by Income Level

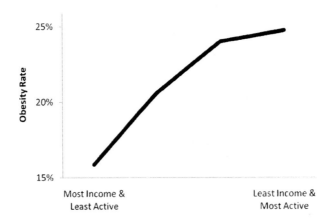

But wait a second. Aren't low-quality starches and sweets abundant in low-income areas (convenience stores, fast food, etc.), while high-quality non-starchy vegetables, seafood, lean meat, and fruits are scarce? Couldn't low-quality food be the cause of higher obesity rates in *more* active low-income areas?

Yes.

Eating lower-quality food creates the clog that causes chronic weight gain. People can be plenty active, but if they eat low-quality food, they will get clogged and gain body fat. Weight gain is determined by food and exercise quality, not quantity.

Still not convinced? Chapter 7 shows how you can eat more and burn more body fat—as long as you eat smarter.

CHAPTER 7

Eating More Does *Not* Cause Long-Term Fat Gain

"[We found] highly significant inverse correlations between food energy intake and adiposity [body fat]."
H. KEEN, KING'S COLLEGE LONDON[1]

Eating more low-quality food causes us to gain body fat. But that does not mean eating more food produces the same result. Interestingly enough, eating more high-quality food has been clinically proven to cause body fat to be burned. The research on this topic comes from all over:

- **J. Volek's Study at the University of Connecticut**: People in the eat-more-high-quality-food group ate 300 more calories per day and burned more body fat.[2]
- **F.F. Samaha's Study at the University of Pennsylvania**: People in the eat-more-high-quality-food group ate a total of 9,500 more calories and lost 200% more weight.[3]
- **P. Green's Study from *Obesity Research***: People in the eat-more-high-quality-food group ate a total of 25,000 more calories without gaining any additional weight.[4]
- **S. Sondike's Study from the *Journal of Adolescent Health***: People in the eat-more-high-quality-food group ate a total of 65,000 more calories and lost 141% more weight.[5]

How are these results possible? Research reveals two main reasons: First, a calorie is *not* a calorie. Second, an unclogged fat metabolism system burns excess calories instead of storing them. The next section will cover why a calorie is *not* a calorie, so let's turn first to how unclogging enables our body to burn—instead of store—excess calories.

Eat More, Burn More

Let's return to the idea of a clog. If you pour more water into an unclogged sink, then it will drain more water. You will only see water build up if you put more water into a *clogged* sink. Our fat metabolism system works the same way. If you put more food in an unclogged fat metabolism system, then it will burn more calories. Body fat will build up only if you put more food into a *clogged* fat metabolism system.

In a Mayo Clinic study, researchers fed people 1,000 extra calories per day for eight weeks. A thousand extra calories per day for eight weeks totals 56,000 extra calories. Everyone gained sixteen pounds—56,000 calories worth—of body fat, right?

Nope.

Nobody gained sixteen pounds. The most anyone gained was a little over half that. The least anyone gained was basically nothing—less than a pound. How could that be true? People are eating 56,000 extra calories and gaining basically no body fat? How can 56,000 extra calories add up to nothing?

That's because extra calories don't have to turn into body fat. They could turn into heat. They could be burned off automatically. Researcher D.M. Lyon in the medical journal *QJM* reported: "Food in excess of immediate requirements...can easily be disposed of, being burnt up and dissipated as heat. Did this capacity not exist, obesity would be almost universal."[6]

Eating more and gaining less is possible because an unclogged fat metabolism system has all sorts of underappreciated ways to process excess calories other than storing them as body fat. In the Mayo Clinic study, researchers measured three of them:

1. Increase the amount of calories burned daily.
2. Increase the amount of calories burned digesting food.
3. Increase the amount calories burned via unconscious activity.

Looking through the lens of the clog analogy, here is what they found:

Daily Response to 1,000 Extra Calories

	Clogged	Unclogged
Base Calories Burned Daily	Decreased by 100 calories ☹	Increased by 360 calories ☺
Calories Burned Digesting Food	Increased by 28 calories ☺	Increased by 256 calories ☺
Calories Burned Via Unconscious Activity	Decreased by 98 calories ☹	Increased by 692 calories ☺☺
Total Daily Response	**Burned 170 Fewer Calories** ☹	**Burned 1,308 More Calories** ☺☺☺

That is how some people ate 56,000 extra calories and gained essentially nothing. Instead of storing the excess calories as body fat, unclogged fat metabolism systems automatically increased the base amount of calories burned, the amount of calories burned digesting food, and the amount calories burned via unconscious activity.[7]

On the surface this study seems shocking, but we have all seen examples of "eat more, burn more" in our day-to-day lives. Think about naturally thin people you know who eat a lot, exercise a little, and stay slim. They eat more and burn more. Just as eating less causes the fat metabolism system to slow down, eating more causes an unclogged fat metabolism system to speed up.[8]

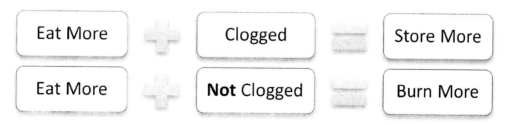

Eating less does *not* cause long-term fat loss. Exercising more does *not* cause long-term fat loss. Thinking in these terms won't help you. The issue is not calorie quantity, but poor calorie quality causing a hormonal clog that removes your fat metabolism system's need and ability to burn body fat. One more time, the issue is not calorie quantity, but poor calorie quality.

Unfortunately, the people teaching us about eating and exercise—the United States Department of Agriculture (USDA)—have not seen the science. Take this excerpt from chapter 3 of the USDA's *Dietary Guidelines for Americans*: "Since many adults gain weight slowly over time, even small decreases in calorie intake can help avoid weight gain."[9]

Here's the bureaucrats' basic misunderstanding: If "small decreases in calorie intake" lead to gradual weight loss, does that mean "small decreases in calorie intake" will eventually make us weigh nothing? Of course not. Why? Because our set-point automatically regulates our weight. But if that is true, then how can a small decrease in calorie intake help us avoid weight gain?

It can't.

The issue is not that our body wants us to weigh less, but that too many calories per day are blocking it. The issue is that our body does not want us to weigh less thanks to our elevated set-point. The same mechanism preventing "small decreases in calorie intake" from making you weigh nothing also prevents it from effectively causing your body to burn off excess fat right now.[10]

A more promising approach is to unclog and to lower your set-point. And you can do that easily by eating *more* high-quality calories. Remember the Harvard researchers who studied the massive sample of 67,272 people? They did another super-sized study. This one included 51,529 people divided into fifths according to the quantity and quality of calories they ate. This massive sample demonstrated two points:[11]

1. Eating more correlated with less body fat
2. Higher-quality food correlated with less body fat

Eating *More* Correlated With *Less* Body Fat

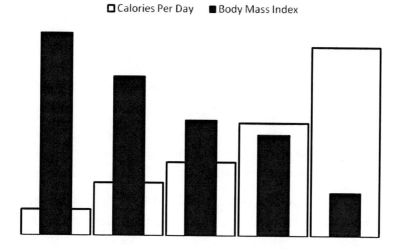

Higher-Quality Food Correlated With *Less* Body Fat

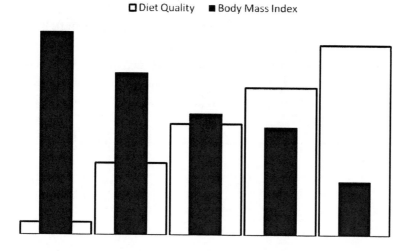

If you can escape the trap of old calorie quantity myths, you will never have to worry about your weight again. Part 2 shows how to increase the quality of your calories, lower your set-point, and get your body burning fat for you.

Doesn't the "Law of Thermodynamics" Prove Eating Less Burns Body Fat?

"The principle that weight gain [only depends on calorie quantity] would violate the second law of thermodynamics."
R.D. FEINMAN, STATE UNIVERSITY OF NEW YORK[12]

We know the traditional approach to fat loss fails 95% of the time, yet common sense seems to tell us: "If you eat less and exercise more, you must burn body fat. Anything else violates the law of thermodynamics."

There are four laws of thermodynamics. The two that apply to burning body fat do not prove that reducing the number of calories eaten makes the fat metabolism system burn *body fat*. They tell us energy cannot be created nor destroyed; energy can only change forms. When people eat less, the fat metabolism system must do *something*. That's it. The laws of thermodynamics prove nothing about *what* the fat metabolism system must do.[13]

Remember how it is easier for your metabolism to slow down than to burn body fat? And remember how it makes more sense to burn calorie-hungry muscle than it does to burn protective body fat? Put those two facts together, and instead of proving that eating less equals long-term fat loss, the applicable laws of thermodynamics prove that eating less makes the body slow down and burn muscle, which leads to long-term fat gain—not fat loss.[14]

PART 2

Myth: A Calorie Is a Calorie

"Attacking the obesity epidemic will involve giving up many old ideas that have not been productive. 'A calorie is a calorie' might be a good place to start."

R.D. Feinman, State University of New York[1]

CHAPTER 8

The Four Calorie Quality Factors

"That would be cool if you could eat a good food with a bad food and the good food would cover for the bad food when it got to your stomach. Like you eat a carrot with an onion ring and they would travel down to your stomach. Then they would get there and the carrot would say, 'It's cool, he's with me.'"
Mitch Hedberg

Beyond battling our basic biology, calorie balancing is bound to fail us because a calorie is *not* a calorie. The difference in calorie quality is really important. That's because the quality of the calories we eat influences our hormones. Those in turn determine our set-point. We can control our weight, just not the way you have been led to believe.[2]

Why Calorie *Quality* Is Important

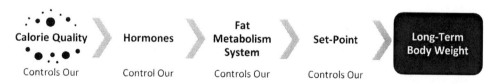

The *Calories In—Calories Out* theory of weight control depends on the assumption that our bodies work like balance scales. Balance scales do not measure quality. On a balance scale, a pound of feathers weighs the same as a pound of lead. Quality is irrelevant. So on a balance scale, 300 calories of vegetables is the same as 300 calories of pasta. The only problem is that the body is not a balance scale.

Body ≠ Balance Scale

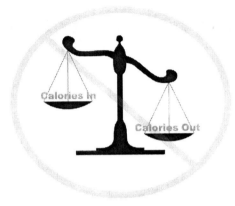

Let's look at the issue another way. Breathing in smoke-filled air for thirty years does something different to our respiratory system than breathing in the same quantity of fresh air. In the same fashion, putting 2,000 calories of low-quality food into our fat metabolism system does something different than putting in the same quantity of high-quality food. Quality counts. Our bodies do not work like balance scales.[3]

Marshall University conducted a childhood obesity study where researchers divided obese kids into two groups:

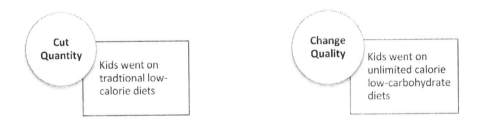

After two months, the Change Quality kids lost eleven pounds, but the Cut Quantity kids *gained* five pounds. We do not have to go on a low-carbohydrate diet, but it is a great example of how critical calorie quality is. People can eat and eat and eat and can still burn body fat because they have changed the quality of their calories.[4]

The quality of calories depends on four fascinating factors:
1. Satiety—How quickly calories fill us up and how long they keep us full
2. Aggression—How likely calories are to be stored as body fat
3. Nutrition—How many nutrients—aka protein, vitamins, minerals, essential fatty acids, etc.—calories provide
4. Efficiency—How many calories can be stored as body fat

The more Satisfying, unAggressive, Nutritious, and inEfficienct a calorie is, the higher its quality. The more SANE it is. The more body-fat-burning hormones it triggers. The more it clears our clog and prevents overeating. The more it restores our *ability* to burn body fat and maximizes our *need* to burn body fat.

The more unSatisfying, Aggressive, not Nutritious, and Efficient a calorie is, the lower its quality. The more inSANE it is. The more body-fat-storing hormones it triggers. The more it creates a clog and encourages overeating. The more it destroys our *ability* to burn body fat and removes our *need* to burn body fat.

The more we understand the four calorie-quality factors, the more clearly we will see how eating *more* high-quality SANE food is the only practical way to burn body fat long term. When you stay full of SANE food, you will not have any room for clog-causing inSANE calories. When we are totally full from a super-sized SANE supper, skipping the sundae after isn't a burden. It's a blessing in disguise. By staying full of SANE calories, we clear our clog, drop our set-point, and enable our fat metabolism system to burn body fat for us automatically.[5]

> *"...for the vast majority of people, being overweight is not caused by how much they eat but by what they eat. The idea that people get heavy because they consume a high volume of food is a myth. Eating large amounts of the right food is your key to success..."*
> JOEL FUHRMAN, DOCTOR AND AUTHOR[6]

Sound too good to be true? In all of the studies that follow, everyone ate the exact same quantity of calories, but one group's calories were of much higher quality (were much more SANE) than the other groups':

- University of Florida researcher J.W. Krieger analyzed eighty-seven studies and found that those people who ate SANE calories lost an average of twelve more pounds of body fat compared to those who ate an equal quantity of inSANE calories.[7]

- C.M. Young at Cornell University split people into three groups, each eating 1,800 calories per day, but at different levels of SANEity. The most SANE group lost 86.5% more body fat than the least SANE group.[8]

- In the *Annals of Internal Medicine*, F.L. Benoît compared a reduced-calorie inSANE diet to a reduced-calorie SANE diet. After ten days the SANE diet burned twice as much body fat.[9]

- Additional studies by researchers U. Rabast (1978,1981), P. Greene (2003), N.H. Baba (1999), A. Golay (1996), M.E. Lean (1997), C.M. Young (1971), and D.K. Layman (2003) all show that people who ate SANE calories lost an average of 22% more weight than those who ate the *exact* same quantity of inSANE calories.[10]

The science of SANE eating is surprising and encouraging. And keep in mind that you and I do not always have to eat SANEly. SANE eating does not require perfection. When you eat the SANE way, you will burn as little or as much body fat as you want to. Want to burn up to two pounds of body fat per week? Eat so much SANE food that you are too full for inSANE food. Want to burn up to two pounds of body fat per month? Eat less SANE food and some inSANE food. You make the decision. The more SANE food you eat, the slimmer you will be.

Let's look at each of the four factors of SANE eating. We'll start with Satiety. By the way, if the word seems oddly familiar, it comes from the same root as *satisfying*. You know what that means. Chapter 9 will reveal how to feel more satisfied while looking and feeling better.

CHAPTER 9

Calorie Quality Factor 1–Satiety

"Food intake occurs until signals arising largely from the gastrointestinal tract are interpreted by the central nervous system to produce...satiety"
D.S. WEIGLE, UNIVERSITY OF WASHINGTON[1]

A calorie is not a calorie when it comes to filling us up and keeping us full. Ever notice how a six-pack of beer makes people eat more pizza while five cans of tuna or thirty cups of broccoli—the same quantity of calories—would make them uncomfortably full? The capacity of calories to make us and keep us full is called Satiety. The fewer calories needed to fill us up and the longer those calories keep us full, the higher their Satiety.[2]

A study in the *Annals of Internal Medicine* showed that people who ate as much high-Satiety protein and natural fat as they wanted while avoiding low-Satiety starches and sweets, unconsciously avoided 1,000 low-quality calories per day. Even better, these folks felt as full as other people in the study who ate 1,000 more lower-Satiety calories.[3]

Why is eating 1,000 fewer low-quality calories per day a good thing? We have already proven how harmful starvation is. Yet there is a big difference between depriving our bodies of nutrition—starving ourselves—and being unable to fit as many calories into our stomach as we used to—by eating more high-Satiety foods. That's because high-Satiety foods contain dramatically more Nutrition than low-Satiety foods.

When we eat high-Satiety food, we get much more Nutrition and become full much more quickly. *More* food and *more* Nutrition is entirely different from less food and feeling hungry. The surplus of Nutrition from high-Satiety food takes starvation off our fat metabolism system's radar. After all, how could it think we are starving since we are taking in *more* Nutrition? Then it is free to burn body fat instead of slowing down or burning muscle.

In addition to keeping us too full for low-quality foods, high-Satiety foods have been shown to help clear our hormonal clog. That leads to long-term fat loss—not starvation.

How High-Satiety Eating Avoids Starvation's Side Effects

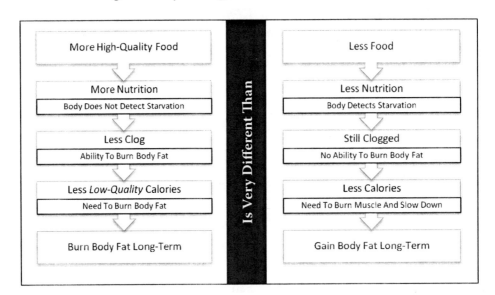

So we need to find the answers to two questions: What increases Satiety? And how do we eat more high-Satiety calories?

The water, fiber, and protein in food increase its Satiety. And we eat more high-Satiety calories by eating more water-, fiber-, and protein-rich foods such as non-starchy vegetables, seafood, lean meat, fat-free or low-fat cottage cheese, fat-free or low-fat *plain Greek* yogurt, eggs, legumes, and fruits.

Fiber: From the Mayo Clinic: "Dietary fiber, also known as roughage or bulk, includes all parts of plant foods that your body cannot digest or absorb. Unlike other food components such as fats, proteins or carbohydrates—which your body breaks down and absorbs—fiber isn't digested by your body." Taking up space in our digestive system until it "keeps us regular," fiber keeps us full for a long time. [4]

Non-Starchy Vegetables: The most SANE vegetables. Basically anything other than corn, potatoes, turnips, yams, parsnips, radishes, etc. Common non-starchy vegetables include: broccoli, carrots, cauliflower, celery, cucumber, eggplant, lettuce, mushrooms, onions, peas, peppers, spinach, squash, and zucchini. Generally speaking, vegetables which grow above ground—except corn...which is a starch—are super-SANE non-starchy vegetables.

We're going to get scientific for a second. We have two areas in our brain that tell us when we feel satisfied: the lateral hypothalamus and ventromedial hypothalamus. Think of them as our Satiety centers. They send their respective "you are hungry" or "you are satisfied" signals depending, basically, on three factors:[5]

1. How much do the calories we are eating stretch our digestive organs (our stomach, etc.)?
2. How much do the calories we are eating impact short-term Satiety hormones?
3. How much do the calories we are eating stimulate long-term Satiety hormones?

How much any given food stretches our stomach and other digestive organs is mostly determined by the amount of water and fiber in it. More water and fiber means bigger food. Bigger food means more stretch. More stretch means we get full faster and stay full longer.

That is why 200 calories of wet, fibrous celery is more filling than 200 calories of dry, fiber-free gummy bears. Calorie for calorie, celery is about thirty times the size of gummy bears, stretches our stomach and other digestive organs about thirty times more, and is therefore thirty times more satisfying.[6]

The amount of protein that food contains is also important. T.L. Halton at Harvard University concluded at the end of his study: "Protein, along with fiber and water, were significantly and positively correlated with satiety scores." The amount of protein in food impacts the other two factors influencing whether our brain is telling us we are hungry or full: short- and long-term Satiety hormones. More protein means more "full" signals being sent to our brains' Satiety centers via our hormones. More protein enables us to "full" ourselves into burning bunches of body fat.[7]

These scientific findings have been repeated in numerous other clinical trials:

- **University of Washington Study:** People ate an unlimited quantity of calories while having the percentage of protein in their diet increased from 15% to 30%. They responded by unconsciously avoiding 441 excess calories per day without feeling hungry.[8]
- **University of Sussex Study:** People ate either a high-protein or a low-protein meal. The high-protein people unconsciously ate 26% less than the low-protein people at their next meal without feeling hungry.[9]
- **University of Leeds Study:** People ate the exact same weight of food, but one group ate a higher percent from protein. The higher-protein group unconsciously ate at least 19% fewer calories than the lower-protein group without feeling hungry.[10]
- **Karolinska Hospital Study:** People ate more or less protein for lunch. The more-protein group got full on 12% fewer calories at dinner than the less-protein group.[11]

There is no lack of proof. Here is a summary of what researchers said in their studies:

- "Protein is more satiating than carbohydrate and fat in the short term...and in the long term."—M.S. Westerterp-Plantenga, Maastricht University[12]
- "An increase in dietary protein from 15% to 30% of energy at a constant carbohydrate intake produces a sustained decrease in...caloric intake."—D.S. Weigle, University of Washington[13]
- "Protein appears to be the macronutrient that suppresses energy intake to a greater extent than any of the other macronutrients."—John E. Blundell, University of Leeds[14]
- "Diets high in protein...resulted in greater weight losses than traditional low-fat diets...This effect is likely due to increased satiety caused by increased dietary protein."—D.A. Schoeller, University of Wisconsin-Madison[15]

In summary: More protein means more Satiety. More Satiety means we are too full for low-quality food. And less low quality food means less clogging, a lower set-point, and more burning of body fat.[16]

How to Eat More Satisfying Foods

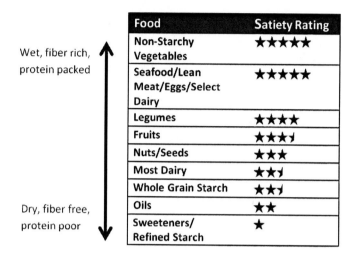

Food	Satiety Rating
Non-Starchy Vegetables	★★★★★
Seafood/Lean Meat/Eggs/Select Dairy	★★★★★
Legumes	★★★★
Fruits	★★★⬩
Nuts/Seeds	★★★
Most Dairy	★★⬩
Whole Grain Starch	★★⬩
Oils	★★
Sweeteners/Refined Starch	★

Wet, fiber rich, protein packed

Dry, fiber free, protein poor

Select Dairy: Dairy products which have more than 60% of their calories coming from protein and contain no added sweeteners. The most common examples are fat-free or low-fat cottage cheese and fat-free or low-fat *plain Greek* yogurt.

CHAPTER 10

Calorie Quality Factor 2–Aggression

"The crucial factor is not how much is eaten...or how much is expended, but how...those calories are utilized and made available when needed."
GARY TAUBES, IN *GOOD CALORIES, BAD CALORIES*[1]

A calorie is *not* a calorie when it comes to how likely it is to be stored as body fat. We can think about human biology like this: When we eat, a traffic cop tells calories where to go. How Aggressively calories approach this traffic cop determines their chances of being stored as body fat.

The traffic cop directs calories to repair, fuel, or fatten us—in that order. It first makes sure we have enough fuel to rebuild anything that has broken down. Next, it keeps us doing whatever we are doing. Last, it seeks to protect us from starving. As long as we have a calm and consistent flow of calories coming into our system, the cop does a great job directing them.

However, when calories approach the traffic cop Aggressively, it gets angry, throws its clipboard down, and sends those calories to fat cells. When we eat a plate of pasta and a breadstick, a massive wave of starch starts screaming all at once and the traffic cop says, "Oh, really. That's how you want to do it? To the fat cells...all of you." Like the rest of us, our body does not do its best work when dealing with a bunch of Aggressive requests all at once.

To keep calories out of our fat cells, we do not need to worry about eating less food. We need to worry about the *quality* of the food we are eating. Our body is fine with a lot of food. It is Aggressive food that aggravates it.[2]

Five hundred calm calories creeping into the bloodstream over many hours are less likely to be stored as body fat than five hundred Aggressive calories rushing in all at once. Any time the body has more calories available than it can deal with at one time, it stores them as body fat. That is why the *glycemic index* and *glycemic load* have become all the rage. They are handy measures of calories' Aggression.[3]

> **Glycemic Index:** A measure of foods' Aggression. The higher a food's glycemic index, the more Aggressive it is.
>
> **Glycemic Load:** A measure similar to glycemic index, which also considers quantity. The glycemic load measures a food's Aggression combined with the calories in a portion of it. [4]

To best understand calories' Aggression, glycemic index, and glycemic load, we first need to understand how our body fuels itself. It does not run on the food we eat. It runs primarily on glucose, a sugar our body creates from the food we eat. That may seem like a meaningless distinction, but it is not.

Storing body fat is not caused by eating a lot of food. Storing body fat is about a response to eating food that causes us to have more glucose in our bloodstream than we can use at one time. That is why calories' Aggression matters so much. The more Aggressive calories are, the faster they increase the levels of glucose in our bloodstream. The faster calories increase our glucose levels, the more likely we are to have more glucose than the body can deal with at one time. That's when it shuttles the excess into our fat cells.

Why the Distinction Between Food and Glucose Matters

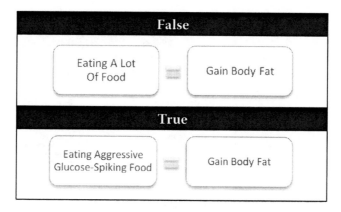

The distinction between "a lot of food" and "a lot of glucose right now" is important. We can eat all the food we want and never gain body fat if the glucose the food generates does not exceed the glucose level we can deal with right then. That is why the glycemic index, glycemic load, and low-glycemic diets like the *South Beach Diet* and the *Atkins' Diet* have gotten so much press. They are all tools which help people avoid Aggressive foods.

Fortunately, we do not need to worry about glycemic index or glycemic load because SANE foods prevent excess glucose from getting into our bloodstream. If we simply focus on increasing the amount of water-, fiber-, and protein-packed high-Satiety foods we are eating, we will automatically eat low-glycemic-index foods, ensure a low glycemic load, and store less body fat.[5]

Avoiding Aggressive calories has some terrific additional benefits. It lowers our risk of coronary heart disease, diabetes, unhealthy cholesterol levels, and heart disease. We do not get heavy and sick by eating a lot of food. We get that way by eating a lot of low-quality Aggressive food.[6]

How to Eat More (High-Satiety) UnAggressive Foods

Wet, fiber rich, protein packed, moderate fat

Food	unAggressive Rating
Non-Starchy Vegetables	★★★★★
Seafood/Lean Meat/ Eggs/Select Dairy	★★★★★
Nuts/Seeds	★★★★★
Oils[1] (Do not eat *a lot* of oils.)	★★★★★
Legumes	★★★
Fruits	★★★
Most Dairy	★★
Whole Grain Starch	↗
Sweeteners/ Refined Starch	

Dry, fiber free, protein poor, fat free

---

1   The fat in food is completely unAggressive. It does not increase the amount of glucose in the bloodstream at all. In fact, fat slows the release of glucose into the bloodstream. That is why foods containing fat are often less Aggressive than fat-free foods. That said, foods made-up of nothing but fat—oils, butter, cream etc.—are not particularly SANE because they are not especially Satisfying, Nutritious, or inEfficient. They are fine in moderation, but don't go crazy with them.

CHAPTER 11

Calorie Quality Factor 3–Nutrition

"Low energy density [high Nutrition] is not an inevitable characteristic of low-fat diets; as many of the low-fat foods presently being promoted in our commercial food supply are based on sugar or highly refined carbohydrates."
W.C. WILLETT, HARVARD UNIVERSITY[1]

Two hundred and fifty calories of Twinkies are not the same as 250 calories of broccoli. Clearly a calorie is *not* a calorie when we are discussing the Nutrition we need to burn body fat and be healthy. So what is nutritious? Like everything else, the key to Nutrition is *quality*, but all we are ever told about is quantity—aka the Nutrition facts labels on food.

The information found on food labels tells us half of what determines Nutrition: the quantity of nutrients in the food. The other half is the quality of the calories we are getting along with those nutrients.

Talking merely about the quantity of nutrients in food leads to a very fattening view of Nutrition. Consider the American Heart Association's endorsement logos on boxes of sugar-stuffed cereal because the cereal was "enriched." A high quantity of nutrients combined with low-quality calories is not nutritious.[2]

Most people already know that thinking about the *quantity* of nutrients in food is not sufficient. We know that ten doughnuts are not ten times as nutritious as one doughnut. We have to consider nutrients relative to calories, or Nutrition *quality*.

Determining Nutrition quality is simple. We take the nutrient quantity information provided on Nutrition labels and divide it by the number of calories in a serving of the food. This provides the food's Nutrition *per calorie*. Many nutrients per calorie—provided by non-starchy vegetables, seafood, lean meats, select dairy, and fruits—means high Nutrition. Few nutrients per calorie—see starches and sweets—means low Nutrition.

For example, here's how one cup of enriched wheat flour compares to one cup of spinach in terms of nutrient *quantity*. I've shaded the cell of the food with more of the given nutrient when we measure by the cup.

Nutrient *Quantity* of Enriched Wheat Flour vs. Spinach
(Nutrients Per Cup)

Nutrients (% DV)[1]	Enriched Wheat Flour	Spinach
Vitamin A	0%	56%
Vitamin C	0%	14%
Vitamin E	3%	3%
Vitamin K	1%	181%
Thiamin	74%	2%
Riboflavin	41%	3%
Niacin	52%	1%
Vitamin B6	3%	3%
Folate	63%	15%
Calcium	2%	3%
Iron	34%	5%
Magnesium	9%	6%
Phosphorus	13%	1%
Potassium	4%	5%
Zinc	8%	1%

1 DV: Recommended Daily Value based on a 2,000 calorie diet.

Looking at quantity, enriched wheat flour seems more nutritious than spinach. Here's why that's misleading. One cup of enriched wheat flour contains 495 calories. One cup of spinach contains 7 calories. Looking at quality—nutrients *per calorie*—we see something much different—and more useful.

Nutrient *Quality* of Enriched Wheat Flour vs. Spinach
(Nutrients Per 250 Calories)

Nutrients (% DV)	Enriched Wheat Flour	Spinach
Vitamin A	0%	2000%
Vitamin C	0%	500%
Vitamin E	2%	107%
Vitamin K	1%	6464%
Thiamin	37%	71%
Riboflavin	21%	107%
Niacin	26%	36%
Vitamin B6	2%	107%
Folate	32%	536%
Calcium	1%	107%
Iron	17%	179%
Magnesium	5%	214%
Phosphorus	7%	36%
Potassium	2%	179%
Zinc	4%	36%

When we make a fair comparison—comparing 250 calories of enriched wheat flour against 250 calories of spinach, instead of comparing 495 calories of enriched wheat flour against 7 calories of spinach—we see that spinach is dramatically more nutritious than enriched wheat flour.[3]

Looking at Nutrition this way is useful for two reasons:

1. It gives us a more accurate view of which foods are nutritious.
2. It helps us burn body fat instead of slowing down or burning muscle.

Like Satiety and Aggression, a food's Nutrition depends on water, fiber, and protein. Water and fiber have no calories, and protein calories do not "count" as much as carbohydrate or fat calories (more on this in chapter 12). Since a food's Nutrition is found by dividing the number of nutrients by the number of calories, more water, fiber, and protein reduce the relative number of calories in the food and therefore increase its Nutrition.[4]

$$\frac{\text{Nutrients}}{\downarrow \text{Calories}} = \uparrow \text{Nutrition}$$

Viewing Nutrition in terms of water, fiber, and protein gives us a dramatically different view of which foods are nutritious. Consider cereal, bread, or "healthy" whole grain starches. They are all dry and contain little protein, so they are starting out zero for two. Fiber is their only hope.

The companies selling starchy products say we get a great deal of fiber from their whole-grain products, but is that actually true? Well, the four grams of fiber in 250 calories of whole-grain cereal is 100% more fiber than the two grams of fiber in 250 calories of refined-grain cereal, but that is only comparing grains. You have to ask if grains are a good source of Nutrition relative to more water and protein-packed foods we could be eating. So are whole grains good sources of Nutrition relative to non-starches?

Not even close.

Sure, whole grains are better than processed grains, but that is like saying one broken leg is better than two. It does not make either option good. Look at the fiber *per calorie* in whole grains compared to more water and protein-packed foods:

Grams of Fiber in 250 Calories[5]

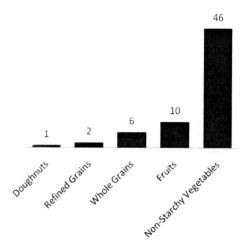

Whole grains do have six times more fiber than doughnuts, but non-starchy vegetables have nearly fifty times more fiber. Whole grain toast is better than a doughnut, but that is not saying much considering the other foods we could be eating. For example, if we eat 250 calories worth of non-starchy vegetables, we will get about forty-six grams of fiber. To get the same amount of fiber from whole grains, we would have to eat a whopping 1,917 calories worth of whole grains.

Number of Calories Needed to Get the Same Amount of Fiber

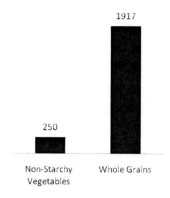

Starch is an excellent example of how careful you have to be when trying to judge Nutrition—comparing nutrients per calorie. We could be eating all sorts of whole-grain starches thinking we are at the top of the Nutrition mountain, while we are actually sitting at the bottom getting buried with low-quality calories. A little Nutrition plus a lot of unSatisfying and Aggressive calories is not a happy combination.

Fortunately for us, we do not need to do all sorts of math with Nutrition labels to maximize the Nutrition of our diets. Researchers at Colorado State University did the math for us. They analyzed the Nutrition quality of the most common foods and found that if we maximize the Satiety and minimize the Aggression of our diet—by eating more water-, fiber-, and protein-packed foods—we will get the most Nutrition per calorie automatically.

Nutrition Quality Per Calorie[6]

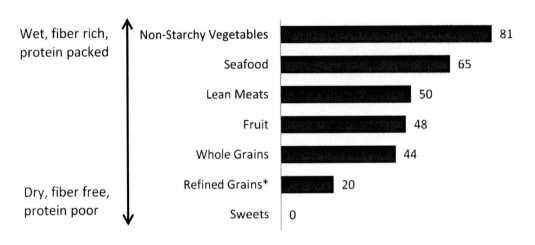

(*Data on refined grains is an estimate)

If you would like to calculate calorie quality for yourself, the math is easy and informative. For example, carefully check the foods people call "good sources of protein," such as beans, milk, and nuts. Are these foods good sources of protein per calorie? Divide the grams of protein in a serving by the number of calories.

Grams of Protein in a 250 Calorie Serving[7]

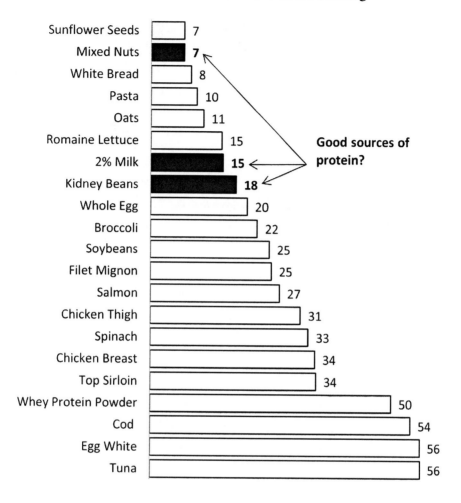

Nutrition quality also affects the need to burn body fat instead of the need to slow down and burn muscle. When we eat more water-, fiber-, and protein-packed food, we get more Nutrition while avoiding overeating—or overwhelming the body with glucose. Combine *more* nutrients with less glucose, and we burn body fat without the negative side effects of eating less. After all, our fat metabolism system has more Nutrition than ever before. A surplus of Nutrition is the opposite of starvation.[8]

How to Eat More Nutritious Foods

Food	Nutrition Rating
Non-Starchy Vegetables	★★★★★
Seafood/Lean Meat/Eggs/Select Dairy	★★★★
Fruits	★★★★
Legumes	★★★
Nuts/Seeds	★★★
Most Dairy	★★
Whole Grain Starch	★
Oils	
Sweeteners/Refined Starch	

Water, Fiber, and Protein Rich

Water, Fiber, and Protein Poor

CHAPTER 12

Calorie Quality Factor 4–Efficiency

"Efficiency...is dependent on...the nature of the fuel and the processes enlisted by the organism. A simple example is the inefficiency of low-test gasoline...If a 'calorie is a calorie'...were true, [then gasoline is gasoline and] nobody would pay extra for high test gasoline."

R.D. FEINMAN, STATE UNIVERSITY OF NEW YORK DOWNSTATE MEDICAL CENTER[1]

Last but far from least, a calorie is *not* a calorie when it comes to how Efficiently our fat metabolism system converts it into body fat. If Satiety measures how quickly calories fill us up, and Aggression shows how likely calories are to be stored as body fat, and Nutrition determines how many nutrients calories provide, then Efficiency is concerned with how easily calories are stored as body fat. The more inEfficient calories are at being stored as body fat, the better. Keeping the science of SANE eating simple, fiber and protein are entirely inEfficient.[2]

Explaining the inEfficiency of fiber is easy. Fiber is not digested, and therefore can never be stored as body fat. The body tries and tries to digest fiber, but then after burning a bunch of calories trying to break down and absorb fiber, it gives up and passes fiber through the digestive system. That is why fiber helps keep us regular.

Explaining the inEfficiency of protein is a bit more involved. To start with let's talk about the calories we burn digesting food. Our body digests fat and carbohydrate Efficiently. However, it takes our body five to ten times more energy to digest protein. In fact, about 30% of the calories we get from protein are burned digesting it. Protein's inEfficiency doesn't stop there.[3]

Even after we burn 30% of protein calories during initial digestion, the road from chicken breast to love handles is far from over. Correction: there is no road from chicken breast to love handles. Protein cannot be stored as body fat. However, there is a super-highway shuttling glucose to our fat cells. So when we have excess protein lying around, excess protein is sent to the liver to be converted into glucose.

The process of converting protein into glucose is called *gluconeogenesis* (*gluco* = sugar, *neo* = new, *genesis* = creation). This process burns another 33% of the original protein calories eaten. Combine the third of protein calories burned during digestion with the third of those remaining calories burned during *gluconeogenesis*, and you and I are left with a measly 47% of the original protein calories. What started off as 300 calories of juicy protein is reduced to 140 calories of glucose in the bloodstream. But wait, there's more.[4]

Converting that newly formed glucose into body fat consumes another 25% of the glucose calories. So when everything is said and done, even if we never move a muscle, only 35% of the calories we get from protein can be stored as body fat. You read that correctly. Over two-thirds of calories from protein are burned converting protein into a compound which can be stored as body fat.[5]

The InEfficient Path from Protein to Glucose to Body Fat

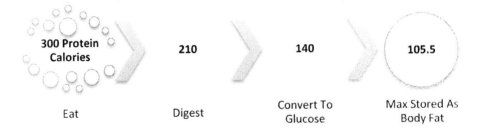

| 300 Protein Calories | 210 | 140 | 105.5 |
| Eat | Digest | Convert To Glucose | Max Stored As Body Fat |

If we followed the same digestion process for starch, we would find that 211 of 300 starch calories can be stored as body fat. That means 70% of calories from starch can be stored as body fat. In other words, calories from starch are twice as Efficient at becoming body fat as calories from protein.

	Calories from Protein	Calories from Starch
Eaten	300	300
Digested	210	282
Converted into Glucose	140	282
Converted into Body Fat	105.5	211
105.5 x 2 = 211 **Calories from starch are twice as Efficient at being converted into body fat as calories from protein**		

Demonstrating the difference an inEfficient diet can make on a daily basis, consider the maximum daily calories we could ever convert into body fat if we got 0%, 25%, 50%, 75%, or 100% of a 2,400 calorie diet from protein.[6]

Max Calories Ever Converted Into Body Fat In A 2,400 Calorie Diet[7]

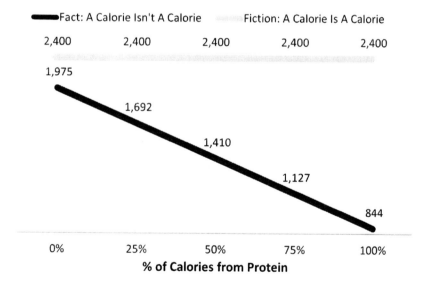

This graph does not mean we should eat 100% protein. Yet we can eat more and burn more by eating more protein-packed (and fiber-packed) food. And keeping long-term fat loss simple, the same techniques we are using to increase Satiety, decrease Aggression, and increase Nutrition, also decrease the Efficiency of our calories.

How to Eat More InEfficient Foods

↑ More fiber- and protein-packed per calorie

Food	inEfficiencyRating
Seafood/Lean Meat/Eggs/Select Dairy	★★★★★
Non-StarchyVegetables	★★★★★
Legumes	★★★
Nuts/Seeds	★★½
Most Dairy	★★½
Fruits	★★
Whole Grain Starch	★
Sweeteners/ Refined Starch	½
Oils	

↓ Less fiber- and protein-packed per calorie

How Body Fat Is Created

With all this talk of calories being more or less Efficient at being stored as body fat, it is worth quickly covering how body fat gets created. The process of creating new body fat is called *lipogenesis* (*lipo* = fat and *genesis* = creation). And with genesis in mind, in the beginning there was food, and food was classified by its dominant macronutrient.

The Three Macronutrients and Their Common Sources

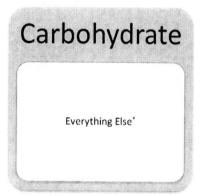

Protein	Fat
Seafood	Whole Eggs
Lean Meat	Tofu
Egg Whites	Oils
Whey Protein Powder	Nuts And Milled Flax Seeds
Fat-Free/Low-Fat Cottage Cheese	Fatty Meat
Fat-Free/Low-Fat *Plain Greek* Yogurt	Whole-Fat Dairy

Carbohydrate

Everything Else*

*Vegetables, fruit, most dairy, beans, and everything else is a carbohydrate.
They are not proteins or fats, so what else could they be?

As soon as our fat metabolism system gets its hands on protein, fat, or carbohydrate, it turns them into amino acids, fatty acids, or glucose, respectively.

The First Step from Food to Body Fat

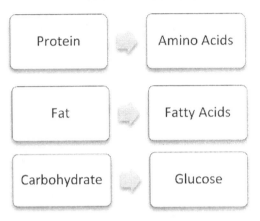

This first step is important because it is another example of why a calorie is *not* a calorie. Once fat is converted to fatty acids, if there are more fatty acids around than we currently need, all of them are sent off to be stored as body fat. The glucose we get from carbohydrates does not work that way. Glucose cannot be stored as body fat without the hormone insulin. And then there are the inEfficient amino acids from protein. Amino acids must first be converted into glucose. Once they become glucose, they need insulin or they cannot be stored as body fat.

Now let's assume the hormone insulin is making its rounds and we have glucose on its way to fat cells. At that point all remaining glucose is converted into fatty acids and we are one step away from new body fat. During the last step in the process all those fatty acids combine with a glycerol molecule to form triglyceride—aka body fat. This is called esterification and it is not possible without a substance called glycerol-3-phosphate.[8]

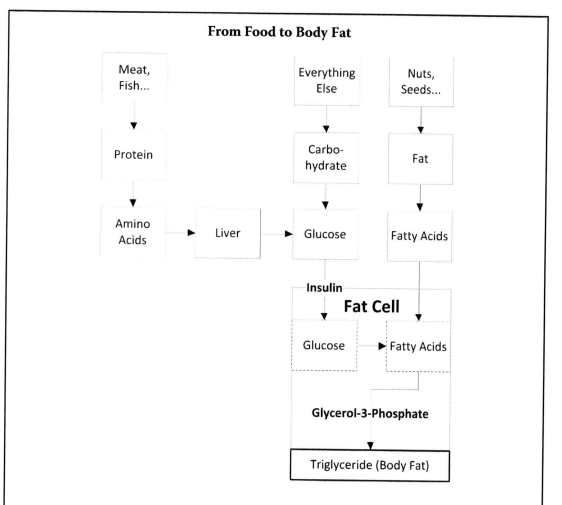

From Food to Body Fat

How is this scientific knowledge useful? Three ways:

1. A calorie is not a calorie, considering that protein is five calorie-burning steps away from body fat—convert into amino acids, convert to glucose, meet up with insulin, transform to fatty acids, and hook up with glycerol-3-phospate—while fat is only two calorie-burning steps away—convert into fatty acids and hook up with glycerol-3-phospate.
2. It is impossible to store glucose as body fat without enough insulin. The more Aggressive a calorie is, the more insulin it triggers. That is one of the reasons we do not like Aggressive calories.
3. No body fat gets stored without glycerol-3-phospate. Guess where we get the most glycerol-3-phospate? InSANE starches and sweets. Carbohydrates are not bad.

Non-starchy vegetables are carbohydrates and they are the most SANE foods around. It is just that inSANE carbohydrate from starches and sweets fuel body fat formation.[9]

Put this all together and it gets clearer why eating more—smarter—works while eating less does not. When people eat less, they are still overeating since their metabolism slows down. Additionally, they have plenty of insulin and glycerol-3-phospate thanks to the inSANE low-quality starches and sweets they continue eating. Overeating plus insulin and glycerol-3-phospate means new body fat.

On the other hand, when we eat more—smarter:

1. We avoid overeating thanks to high-Satiety.
2. We get calories into our bloodstream slowly and they trigger little insulin thanks to low-Aggression.
3. We maximize the number of nutrients we get from those calories thanks to high-Nutrition.
4. We burn a lot of calories during digestion thanks to low-Efficiency.

Eating all this SANE food makes us too full for inSANE starches and sweets. By avoiding starches and sweets, we do not have enough insulin or glycerol-3-phospate to fuel body fat formation. Free from excess insulin and glycerol-3-phospate, we eat more food and store less body fat.[10]

CHAPTER 13

A More SANE Approach to Calories

"We found marked improvement of glucose tolerance [unclogging] after advice to eat a...diet, based on lean meat, seafood, fruits, vegetables, root vegetables, eggs and nuts as staple foods, while avoiding cereals, dairy products, refined fat, sugar and salt. Control subjects, who were advised to follow a (Mediterranean-like) diet based on whole grains...did not significantly improve their glucose tolerance [unclog themselves]."

S. LINDEBERG, UNIVERSITY OF LUND[1]

Now that we have covered the four calorie quality factors, burning more by eating more makes better sense. Let's bring all the factors together.

Our body fat level is controlled by our set-point and fat metabolism system. Our set-point and fat metabolism system are controlled by hormones. Our hormones are controlled by the quality of our diet. The quality of our diet is controlled by the quality of our calories. The quality of our calories is controlled by their Satiety, Aggression, Nutrition, and Efficiency. SANE high-quality calories trigger body-fat-burning hormones. InSANE low-quality calories trigger body-fat-storing hormones. SANE calories are packed with water, fiber, and protein. They enable us to feel full so we can easily avoid dry, fiber-free, and protein-poor calories.

When we raise the quality of our diet, our hormones heal, the clog in our fat metabolism system clears, and our set-point falls. We create both the need and the ability to burn body fat. Then our bodies behave like the bodies of naturally thin people. We burn body fat all day automatically.[2]

You and I can start leveraging this science today by applying two principles:

Stay Too Full for Starch and Sweets

Eat so many SANE foods that you are too full for inSANE starches and sweets. When eating out, avoid pasta and rice dishes, or ask your server to "hold the starch, double the vegetables." At home, skip the rolls and enjoy larger helpings of the main course (seafood/lean meat) and extra helpings of non-starchy vegetables.[1]

The More Natural It Is, the More SANE It Is

The closer a food is to a plant we could gather or an animal we could hunt, the more SANE it is. On the contrary, the further a food is from a plant or animal, the less SANE it is. This point has nothing to do with eating organic versus non-organic food. Until someone discovers a Cheerios tree, a pasta plant, or a bread bush, non-organic oranges are more SANE than organic Cheerios, pasta, or bread. And added sweeteners like sugar and high-fructose corn syrup are the most inSANE "foods" in the world. Eating added sweeteners is like stuffing paper towels down a drain. It is not a question of whether it will cause a clog. It is a question of how much damage the clog will cause.

Summarizing, let's:
- Feast: On as many non-starchy vegetables as we possibly can. Broccoli, carrots, cauliflower, celery, cucumber, eggplant, lettuce, mushrooms, onions, peas, peppers, spinach, squash, and zucchini, are the most common options. Deeply-colored leafy vegetables are the best options.
- Feast: On lean protein at least five times a day. Seafood, lean meat, egg whites, whey protein powder, fat-free or low-fat cottage cheese, and fat-free or low-fat *plain Greek* yogurt are the most practical ways to do this.

---

1 Starchy Vegetables—the type of vegetables we should not feast on—include any form of corn and potato, as well as turnips, yams, parsnips, radishes, etc. Corn and non-sweet potatoes should be avoided completely. Everything else can be enjoyed in moderation.

> **Whey Protein Powder:** Whey comes from milk. And yes, the nursery rhyme "Little Miss Muffet sat on a tuffet eating her curds and whey..." is referring to the same whey we are talking about here. Remove the fat and water from whey and you are left with a SANE and convenient whey protein powder drink mix.

[3]

- Eat: Plenty of fruit. Focus on berries—blueberries, strawberries, etc.—and citrus fruits—grapefruit, oranges, etc. Bananas, grapes, and apples are not bad. However, they are not the best options for body fat loss because they have relatively low Nutrition compared to berries and citrus fruits.
- Eat: Plenty of nuts and seeds. Focus on milled flax seeds. At least a quarter cup of milled flax and a handful of nuts every day.

> **Milled Flax Seeds:** These can be found in the health foods sections of most grocery stores and are extremely SANE. In addition to filling us up, they provide an incredible amount of nutrients—such as omega-3 fatty acids—which are otherwise hard to get. Make sure to get *milled* flax seeds—flax seeds ground into a flour-like powder. Whole flax seeds are not digestible.

- Eat: As many beans and dairy products other than fat-free or low-fat cottage cheese and *plain Greek* yogurt as you need to stay happy. They are great for variety, but not necessary to burn body fat or to optimize health. *Note: Try to completely avoid dairy that has more than ten grams of sugar per serving—i.e. most yogurt, flavored milk, ice cream, etc.*
- Avoid: Oil, whole grains, and any form of starch given their inSANEity. Anything good that starch—even whole-grain starch—does nutritionally, non-starchy vegetables and fruit do better.
- Avoid: All sweets and added sweeteners. Sweets and added sweeteners are the least SANE "foods" in the world.

A SANE Approach to Lowering Your Set-Point

Type of Food	SANEity Rating	How Much to Eat
Non-Starchy Vegetables	★★★★★	As much as you possibly can 10+ servings per day
Seafood/Lean Meat/Egg Whites/Whey Protein Powder/Select Dairy	★★★★★	More than most people currently do 6 servings per day
Nuts & Milled Flax Seeds	★★★⌁	More than most people currently do 4 servings per day
Fruits	★★★	More than most people currently do 4 servings per day
Legumes	★★★	As needed 0-2 servings per day
Most Dairy	★★⌁	As needed 0-2 servings per day
Oils	★★★	As little as possible
Whole Grain Starch	★⌁	As little as possible
Processed Starch	⌁	None
Sweeteners		None

Before we dig deeper into the specifics of eating more—smarter—there are two more important areas to explore. First, the science of how calorie quality influences the hormones which control our set-point. Second, the source of all this calorie quantity confusion. Part 3 disproves the old myth that calories are all that matter. Part 4 reveals the origins of the calorie quantity myths.

PART 3

Myth: Calories Are All That Matter

"The 'classical theory' that fat is deposited in the adipose tissue [body fat] only when given in excess of the caloric requirement is finally disproved."
E. WERTHEIMER, IN *PHYSIOLOGICAL REVIEWS*[1]

CHAPTER 14

Understanding Hormones, Especially Insulin

"Insulin has profound metabolic effects in the determination of body weight..."
B. DOKKEN, UNIVERSITY OF ARIZONA[2]

"...obesity is impossible in the absence of adequate tissue concentrations of insulin."
M. GOLDBERG, IN *JOURNAL OF THE AMERICAN MEDICAL ASSOCIATION*[3]

The critical effect hormones have on body fat has been well known in scientific circles for a long time. Especially the hormone insulin. Most of us know insulin only in reference to diabetics. They need insulin shots. Yet a true understanding of how hormones generally—and insulin specifically—work in relation to body fat reveals the cause of, and solution to, weight gain and related diseases such as diabetes.[4]

At the risk of being gross, one way scientists discovered the important relationship between hormones and weight is through the procedure known as parabiosis. Parabiosis occurs when researchers cut two live animals open and then join them so they share the same blood supply and hormones. In other words, researchers create Siamese twins.

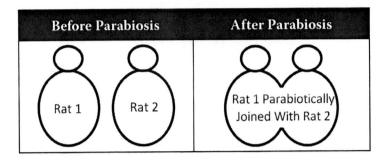

Why would researchers create a Franken-rat with one set of hormones but twice as much of everything else? Because it allows them to conduct studies showing the impact hormones have on body fat. For example, when researchers join an obese rat to a lean rat, the lean rat gets leaner regardless of the quantity of calories it eats. How is that possible? Think back to how the set-point works.

The obese rat's fat metabolism system is producing a massive amount of body-fat-burning hormones in an effort to get the obese rat back to normal automatically. But because the obese rat is clogged and cannot respond to the body-fat-burning hormones effectively, it stays heavy. However, the lean rat is not clogged. The clog-free rat *is* able to respond to all of those body-fat-burning hormones. Lots of body-fat-burning hormones plus the ability to respond to them equals burning body fat despite eating the same quantity of calories.

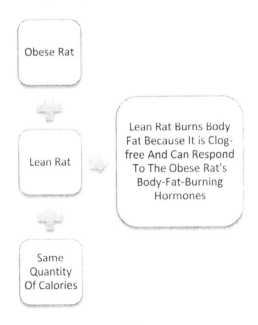

In a similar manner, when researchers stitch a normal rat and a starved rat together, the starved rat's body-fat-storing hormones make the normal rat get fatter regardless of the quantity of calories the normal rat eats. The starved rat is producing body-fat-storing hormones in an effort to get back to its set-point. These body-fat-storing hormones enter the normal rat, and its unclogged fat metabolism system does exactly what the hormones tell it to do: the normal rat stores body fat without eating any more or exercising any less.[5]

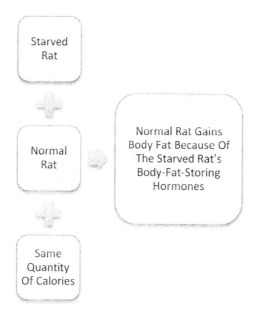

Besides the horror of joining living animals together, these studies powerfully demonstrate the massive impact hormones have on body fat. And that is only the tip of the investigative iceberg.

Researchers at the Gladstone Institute of Cardiovascular Disease made two sets of mice overeat and watched as mice with less of "a key enzyme in mammalian triglyceride synthesis [in body fat creation]" were "protected against diet-induced obesity."[6]

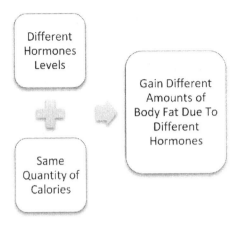

Researchers at the Veterans Affairs Palo Alto Health Care System then went one step further and genetically altered mice so they would no longer have a primary enzyme responsible for storing body fat. These rats ate more and gained 70% less than normal mice. In the researchers' words, completely independent of calories, altering mice's hormones caused "a drastic reduction in lipogenesis [body fat creation]."[7]

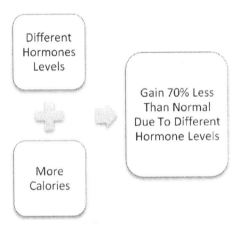

Two more: Researchers at the University of Basel genetically altered mice's hormone levels such that the mice stayed lean, "...in spite of reduced physical activity," and were "unaffected [by] caloric intake." And P.J. Havel from the University of California tells us that, "...mice which are unable to produce ASP [a specific hormone], consume 30% more food than wild-type mice, yet have reduced adipose [body fat] mass and are resistant to weight gain."[8]

These and hundreds of other experiments clearly show that hormone levels strongly influence weight gain or loss. In the journal *Neuroscience & Biobehavioral Reviews,* J. Le Magnen captures the importance of healing our hormones before we are free of body fat: "humans that become obese gain weight because they are no longer able to lose weight." Le Magnen's statement is brilliant. Gaining body fat because we lost the ability to burn body fat thanks to a hormonal clog is totally different than gaining body fat because we eat too much or exercise too little. And if we are gaining body fat because we lost the ability to burn body fat, then what good is eating less or exercising more?[9]

How Hormones Help Store or Burn Body Fat

Researcher P.J. Havel from the University of California presents the scientific explanation of how hormones handle our love handles: "Short-term [hormonal] signals are primarily from the GI tract [digestive system]…and are involved in promoting sensations of satiety…. The long-term [hormonal] signals insulin and leptin are produced and circulate in proportion to recent energy intake and body adiposity [body fat]. Together, the short- and long-term [hormonal] signals interact to regulate energy balance…" In other words, our digestive system, muscle tissue, and fat tissue are constantly communicating with our nervous system and brain via hormones. They are talking about how much fuel they think we need to keep us at our set-point. If they think we are at risk of rising above our set-point, they automatically decrease our calories in and increase our calories out, and vice versa.[10]

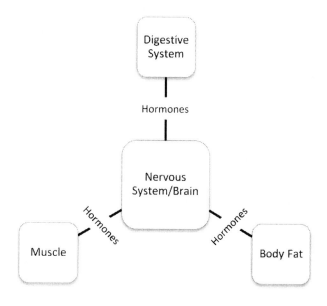

When we eat SANE high-quality calories, this conversation goes well. The right amount of hormones are used and the right message gets across: "Burn body fat." When our hormones are able to do their job, we have the ability to burn body fat, and away our body fat goes.

However, when we eat inSANE low-quality calories, communication breaks down. Our fat metabolism system doesn't have a good idea of how much fuel we need, hormones go bonkers, and our fat metabolism system demands more food since it does not know what is going on and errs on the side of not starving. Thanks to this communication break-down, we end up overeating, hormonally clogged, and heavier.[11]

To gain a deeper understanding of this communication breakdown, let's look at a specific hormone—insulin—and its role in this process. Insulin is a good choice because it is known in scientific circles as, "...the most important hormonal factor influencing lipo-genesis [body fat creation]."[12]

Up Close and Personal with the Hormone Insulin

Insulin's job is to get energy into cells. For example, after we eat lunch, our body digests it and then releases insulin to carry those freshly digested calories into our cells. Since insulin is activated only when we need to get fuel into our cells, our fat metabolism system "hears" insulin in the bloodstream "communicating" that we have energy on its way to our cells and therefore do not need to use any stored energy—aka burn body fat. So the hormone insulin—not the calories we ate—blocks the burning of body fat. That point is extremely important.

Our fat metabolism system does not decide to burn or store body fat based on calories. It makes these decisions based on the hormones those calories trigger. That is why the quality of calories matters so much. As we have already seen, higher-quality calories trigger body-fat-burning hormones while low-quality calories trigger body-fat-storing hormones.[13]

You can cut calories all day and will not burn body fat if you are eating low-quality calories which trigger excess body-fat-storing hormones such as insulin. Why? Hormones like insulin remove our *ability* to burn body fat regardless of whether or not we *need* to according to calorie quantity. That is why scientists refer to the hormone insulin as the "principal regulator of fat metabolism."[14]

Here is the sad part. Calories from inSANE starch and sweets trigger the release of ridiculous amounts of insulin. All that insulin gets those inSANE starch and sweets' calories into our cells, but then we still have insulin left over in our bloodstream. That excess insulin clogs us up and removes our *ability* to burn body fat.[15]

Where the Average American Gets Calories[16]

(Insulin-spiking starch and sweeteners make up 43% of what we eat)

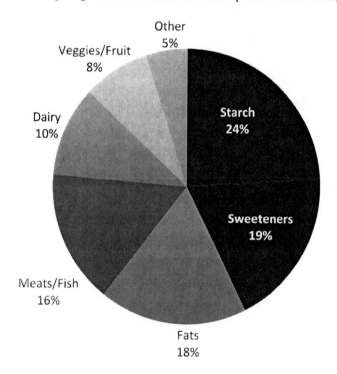

Things go from bad to worse if this inSANEity keeps up for too long. Not only does all the excess insulin destroy our ability to burn body fat, it makes the fat metabolism system resistant to insulin. How does this process work? Compare becoming resistant to the effects of insulin with becoming resistant to the effects of alcohol. When people drink alcohol in moderation, everything is fine. It takes relatively little alcohol to generate the desired effect, so people don't drink too much of it. However, if people drink too much alcohol, they become resistant to alcohol's effects. Then they have to drink more alcohol to get the desired effect. This volume of alcohol eventually destroys their liver and makes them gain body fat. This leaves heavy drinkers in an unfortunate place where they have become resistant to alcohol and have to drink an unhealthy amount of it to get the desired effect.

Similarly, when people eat mostly SANE foods and just a little inSANE starch and sweets, everything is fine. It takes little insulin to get energy into cells, so the body doesn't produce too much of it. However, if people eat mostly starch and sweets, their bodies become resistant to insulin's effects. Then their body has to produce more insulin to get energy into cells. This volume of insulin eventually destroys their pancreas and makes them gain body fat.

Even more unfortunate, at least one in four Americans are insulin resistant. All this excess insulin forms the backbone of our clog. Not only does it crush our ability to burn body fat, it also increases the rate at which we store body fat because excess insulin preferentially puts calories into our fat tissue. This happens because no matter how resistant other tissues become to insulin, our fat tissue is always receptive. And while that is technically good because it keeps insulin resistance from killing us, it can crush any dreams of losing weight. We end up with more body fat and no ability to burn it.[17]

inSANE Body Fat Gain

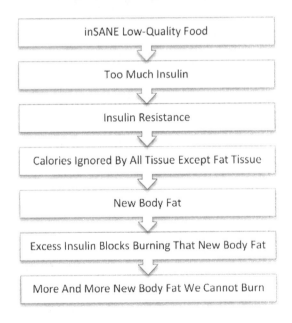

inSANE Low-Quality Food

Too Much Insulin

Insulin Resistance

Calories Ignored By All Tissue Except Fat Tissue

New Body Fat

Excess Insulin Blocks Burning That New Body Fat

More And More New Body Fat We Cannot Burn

Once most of the calories we eat are being stored in fat cells because insulin cannot get them into other cells, *internal starvation* has set in. We eat plenty of food but starve on the inside because insulin cannot effectively get that energy into any cells other than our fat cells. With excess insulin shuttling most calories into fat tissue and eliminating our ability to burn body fat, the fat metabolism system has no choice but to slow down, burn muscle tissue, and demand more food. It does what it always does when it senses starvation.

Consider Terri. She is internally starving and needs 500 calories of energy. Terri is also a yo-yo dieter and has already slowed down her metabolism and burned as much muscle as she can. Needing some calories, Terri eats 500 calories. Instead of those 500 calories getting into the cells needing it, only 250 make it in while the other 250 are ignored—thanks to insulin resistance—and stored as new body fat. Terri still needs 250 calories. She cannot slow down anymore. She cannot burn any more muscle. And thanks to all the excess insulin floating around, she does not have the ability to burn body fat. What is her only option? Overeat. Specifically, eat 250 extra calories.

So Terri snacks on 250 extra calories to keep her cells from starving. But now only a fraction of the 250 make it to the cells needing it while the rest is stored as body fat. Again, she must overeat even more. This process of overeating to keep a clogged fat metabolism system running repeats itself until Terri eats 1,000 calories to meet her need for 500 calories. Terri's fat metabolism system is leaking calories into her fat cells and has to compensate by taking in extra calories.

Continue this "overeat to compensate for the clog" cycle day after day and Terri gains body fat. And on the surface it looks like she is gaining body fat because she is eating too many calories. But eating too many calories is not the *cause* of her new body fat. It is a *symptom* of a deeper problem: her hormonal clog. Terri's high consumption of calories is not the *cause* of her weight gain. It is a *symptom* of the hormonal clog caused by inSANE low-quality calories.[18]

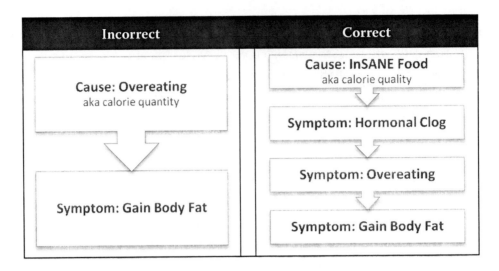

Even the American Heart Association, which champions calorie quantity, acknowledged that calorie quantity does not *cause* obesity when they remarked: "One can argue that people become obese because they consume more calories than they expend, but this doesn't tell us why the imbalance exists or the best way to correct it." Put differently: "People become obese because they overeat, but that doesn't tell us the *cause* of their overeating or how to fix it."[19]

Obesity is not *caused* by eating too many calories, and it is not cured by eating fewer calories. Hilde Burch at Baylor University concludes: "Though [overeating] is observed with great regularity, it is not the cause of obesity; it is a symptom of an underlying disturbance.... The changes in weight regulation and fat storage are the essential disturbances."[20]

Problems are not solved by treating symptoms. That is why the calorie-quantity-based approach to fat loss, eating less and exercising more, fails 95% of the time long-term. It is only treating symptoms. It is based on the myth that gaining body fat is *caused* by calorie quantity, and that is wrong.

Know what else is wrong? How our government started and keeps fueling this fat-loss fiction to fund the food, fitness, and pharmaceutical industries. You can't believe everything you hear. These companies are seeking profits. You have to seek something far more dear: your health.

What Is Type 2 Diabetes?

"Just twenty years ago, the best information available suggested that 30 million people had diabetes. A bleaker picture has now emerged. Diabetes is fast becoming the epidemic of the 21st century."
PRESIDENT PIERRE LEFÈBVRE, INTERNATIONAL DIABETES FEDERATION[21]

If left untreated, insulin resistance turns into type 2 diabetes. To quickly understand type 2 diabetes, let's go back to the example of the clogged sink. Type 2 diabetes is like running water into a clogged sink for so long that water overflows all over the place and the faucet breaks down. Once so much insulin is produced that it is overflowing our bloodstream while our ability to produce insulin has broken down, we have type 2 diabetes.

This build-up and breakdown causes potentially lethal havoc on the body. The Center for Disease Control and Prevention estimates people diagnosed with diabetes by the age of forty die twelve years sooner if they are male, and fourteen years sooner if they are female.[22]

Type 2 diabetes is terrible. What is even worse is its disturbing growth. In the late 1800s, one in every 4,000 people was diabetic; today one in every four people is diabetic or pre-diabetic. That is a 100,000% increase in one century, and researchers estimate that we are on our way to a third of men and nearly a half of women in the U.S. becoming type 2 diabetic. That is insane. That is caused by inSANE calories.[23]

Estimated Cases of Diabetes (in Millions)[24]

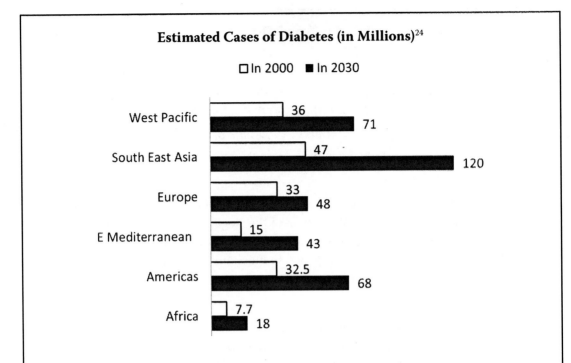

How do we avoid this? Eat more. Exercise less. Smarter. Studies show 80% of type 2 diabetics can reduce or completely eliminate their need for medication by eating a more SANE diet, while reversing more than a third of a lifetime's worth of insulin resistance after only a few months by exercising smarter.[25]

PART 4

Source: Government Guidelines and Graphics

"Dietary guidelines necessarily are political compromises between what science tells us about nutrition and health and what is good for the food industry."

MARION NESTLE, NEW YORK UNIVERSITY[1]

CHAPTER 15

Where the Calorie-Quantity Confusion Came From

"The USDA-sponsored Dietary Guidelines for Americans and its Food Guide Pyramid are nutritionally and biochemically unsound...They radically changed the food habits of tens of millions of Americans in a massive human experiment that has gone awry.... Today, there is little doubt that there is a clear temporal association between the 'heart healthy' diet and the current, growing epidemics of cardiovascular disease, obesity, and type-2 diabetes."

A. OTTOBONI, IN THE *JOURNAL OF THE AMERICAN PHYSICIANS AND SURGEONS*[2]

One way to clear up all the confusion about calorie-quantity is to start from the very beginning. Let's look at the history of eating using a scale of one day. Say 12:00am last night was the dawn of our first ancestors, and right now it's one second before midnight. Up until 11:57pm our ancestors stayed healthy and fit, eating only what could be hunted or gathered—vegetables, seafood, meat, eggs, fruit, nuts, and seeds. At 11:57pm, people started farming, became "civilized," and began eating starch and a small amount of sweets. Two seconds ago, people started eating processed starches and sweets. Only right now—one second before midnight—did people start getting most of their calories from manufactured starch- and sweetener-based food products.[3]

That means the diet recommended by the government's *Dietary Guidelines* was not possible for 99.8% of our history. Our ancestors did not hunt or gather pasta, rice, cereal, or bread. They did not eat whole grains. They ate no grains. They did not cut back on added sweeteners. They did not know what added sweeteners are. Emory University researcher S.B. Eaton tells us: "During the late Paleolithic [the vast majority of human history], the great majority of carbohydrates was derived from vegetables and fruit, very little from cereal grains and none from refined flours."[4]

This idea is interesting to think about when it comes to our health. Obesity, diabetes, heart disease, and cardiovascular disease are called "diseases of civilization." They did not become issues until agriculture enabled production of starches and sweets about 12,000 years ago. And they did not reach epidemic status until starches and sweets made up most of our diet.[5]

Of course, some people might object: "Back then, people did not live as long as we do now." That is an excellent point. I felt the same way until I read research revealing three facts about hunter-gatherers:

1. They are few and far between today, but hunter-gatherer tribes are still around, and scientists have studied them intensively. The studies show that they are free from obesity, diabetes, heart disease, and cardiovascular disease.[6]
2. While their *average* age of death is lower than ours, many ancient hunter-gatherers lived beyond the age of sixty. Emory University researcher S. Boyd tells us: "Occasionally one hears the claim that primitive people all died too young to get degenerative diseases. This claim is simply false—many lived well into and through the age of vulnerability for such disorders, yet didn't get them."[7]
3. Let's take old age out of the equation entirely. Obese and type 2 diabetic "civilized" children are running around all over the place. The children of hunter-gatherers were obesity and diabetes free.[8]

The lowering in the quality of our diet and the lowering in the quality of our health are not coincidences. Could it be possible that we are not designed to digest the food that makes up the majority of the modern diet?

The Chair of the Department of Nutrition at Harvard School of Public Health states un-equivocally: "The USDA Pyramid is wrong. It was built on shaky scientific ground...[and] has been steadily eroded by new research from all parts of the globe.... At best, [it] offers wishy-washy, scientifically unfounded advice." Here's what the *Journal of the American College of Cardiovascular Exerciselogy* has to say: "The low-fat-high-carbohydrate diet, promulgated [publicized] vigorously by the...food pyramid, may well have played an un-intended role in the current epidemics of obesity...diabetes, and metabolic syndromes." The Co-Founder of the Center for Science in the Public Interest chimes in: "Good advice about nutrition conflicts with the interests of many big industries, each of which has more lobbying power than all the public-interest groups combined."[9]

We are not getting bigger and sicker because we are putting too much fuel into our fat metabolism systems. We are getting clogged from putting the wrong quality of fuel into our fat metabolism system. The further the quality of our calories has gotten from the high-quality SANE food we ate for 99.8% of our evolutionary history, the bigger and sicker we have become.[10]

The Source of Our Weight Problems

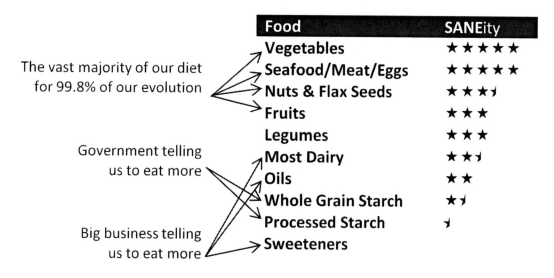

Food	SANEity
Vegetables	★ ★ ★ ★ ★
Seafood/Meat/Eggs	★ ★ ★ ★ ★
Nuts & Flax Seeds	★ ★ ★ ★↲
Fruits	★ ★ ★
Legumes	★ ★ ★
Most Dairy	★ ★↲
Oils	★ ★
Whole Grain Starch	★↲
Processed Starch	↲
Sweeteners	

The vast majority of our diet for 99.8% of our evolution

Government telling us to eat more

Big business telling us to eat more

Decades of advanced dietary research have taken place alongside spiking obesity and disease rates. This research recommends a diet much different than any version of the government's *Dietary Guidelines.* For example, Marion Nestle at New York University notes how the scientific community has long criticized the USDA's *Food Guide Pyramid*'s failure to "recognize the biochemical equivalency of sugars and starches in the body." More simply, starch has the same impact on our body as sugar. Why don't the government's guidelines reflect this research? Who needs science when a constant barrage of food, fitness, and pharmaceutical industry marketing bullies us into believing that the government's recommendations are healthy?[11]

A great deal of money is being made from our nutritional confusion.

The Source of Our Problem

Even worse, the government created these guidelines in much the same way it creates laws: by listening to lobbyists and by making compromises. The history of the USDA guidelines and graphics is nothing short of shocking.

CHAPTER 16

Politicians Playing Physicians

"The low-fat, high-carbohydrate diet recommended by the...USDA Food Guide Pyramid may be among the worst eating strategies for someone who is overweight.... People on low-fat diets generally lose about two to four pounds after several weeks, but then gain that weight back even while continuing with the diet. Randomized trials of weight loss usually show little net weight changes after a year."
W.C. WILLETT, HARVARD UNIVERSITY[1]

Detailing the disturbing history of the government's role in our diet would take an entire book. If you would like to find out the whole story, you can read an excellent book called *Good Calories, Bad Calories* by Gary Taubes. Here I will provide the short version.

The original release of the government's *Dietary Guidelines*—and subsequent Food Guide Pyramid and MyPlate graphics—came about because certain politicians were playing physicians. The Chair of the Department of Nutrition at Harvard School of Public Health notes: "Some recommendations on diet and nutrition are misguided because they are based on inadequate or incomplete information. That hasn't been the case for the USDA's pyramids. They are wrong because they brush aside evidence on healthful eating that has been carefully assembled over the past forty years." In the *Journal of the American Physicians and Surgeons*, researcher A. Ottoboni adds: "There is considerable concern today

123

that the diet the Pyramid illustrates is responsible for the current epidemic of cardiovascular disease. The concurrent epidemics of obesity and type-2 diabetes are unintended consequences that can also be attributed to this diet."[2]

How did the government come up with these *Dietary Guidelines*? J.B. German from the University of California has written: "At the time the 1980 guidelines were established, there was no solid basis for understanding what the consequences of such overall dietary changes would be for most persons." The *Dietary Guidelines* and graphics were not drawn up by nutrition scholars. They were derived from a political document released in 1976 called *Dietary Goals for the United States*.[1] The *Dietary Goals* was designed by the Senate Nutrition Committee to do two things. The first was to "increase carbohydrate consumption to account for 55% to 60% of calorie intake." The second was to, "reduce overall fat consumption from 40% to about 30% of calorie intake."[3]

These goals and the rest of the document are more speculative than scientific. For example, T.A. Sanders at King's College London, notes, "The scientific basis for a reduction in the proportion of energy from fat below 30% is *not* supported by experimental evidence." A.S. Truswell from the University of Sydney tells us: "The first edition of *Dietary Goals...* took nutritionists by surprise...was written by a group of politically interested activists with small knowledge of nutrition.... The collected objections can be summarized very briefly: Too soon, more research needed, relationships not proved; politically motivated." Here is what the American Medical Association had to say when *Dietary Goals* was released: "There is a potential for harmful effects for a radical long term dietary change as would occur through adoption of the proposed national goals." More blunt criticism was delivered by University of Wisconsin-Madison researcher A.E. Harper: "The dietary goals report is not scientifically sound: it is a political and moralistic document." And finally, my favorite comes from the president of the National Academy of Sciences in his testimony to the Senate in regards to *Dietary Goals:* "What right has the federal government to propose that the American people conduct a vast nutritional experiment, with themselves as subjects, on the strength of so very little evidence that it will do them any good?"[4]

---

1   First there was Dietary Goals (1976), then came the Dietary Guidelines (1980), the Food Guide Pyramid (1992), MyPyramid (2005) and finally MyPlate (2011). Additionally, since the release of the original Dietary Guidelines, the government has re-released the same basic guidance every five years.

But despite being unproven and controversial among the scientific community, the government declared *Dietary Goals* "the truth" on these grounds: "We [the government] live in the present and cannot afford to await the ultimate proof before correcting trends we believe to be detrimental." With that uneducated guess, a low-fat, low-protein, high-starch diet was declared "healthy." Sadly, the results have been anything but.[5]

Percent of Americans at Least Overweight [6]

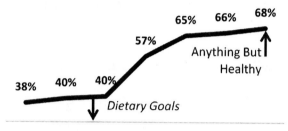

Millions of Americans with Diabetes

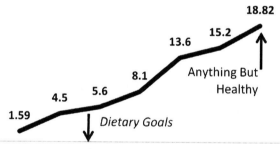

Millions of Hospital Discharges for Cardiovascular Diseases in the U.S.

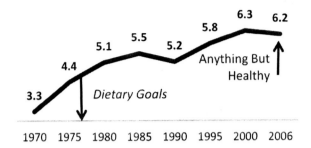

Millions of Non-Fatal Heart Disease Incidents in the U.S.

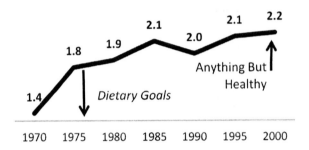

To understand why the Senate Nutrition Committee gave us these *Dietary Goals* in the first place, we have to go back a few more decades. One man single-handedly convinced the country that natural foods are deadly.[7]

Fat Fiction

In the 1950s, Ancel Keys examined diet and heart disease trends in twenty-two countries. He was apparently more interested in headlines than science because he then published a study that included data from only the six countries that showed a scary link between diet and heart disease. Keys garnered a massive amount of press and then went on tour preaching that eating fat is deadly.[8]

Heart Disease Deaths per 1,000 Men [9]
(Japan, Italy, England, Australia, Canada, and USA)

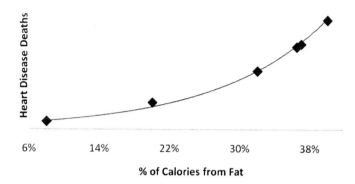

Here are the facts: When the data from *all twenty-two* countries in Keys' study is examined, they show *no* relationship between fat intake and heart disease deaths. Keys selectively picked data and designed a headline-worthy conclusion. In the words of a fellow researcher, "No information is given by Keys on how or why the six countries were selected."[10]

Further exposing the sketchiness of Keys' methods, those same researchers revealed that by selectively choosing six different countries from Keys' data, they could create a graph suggesting that eating *more* fat *decreases* the risk of dying from heart disease.

Heart Disease Deaths per 1,000 Men
(Finland, Australia, Ireland, Switzerland, Germany, and the Netherlands)

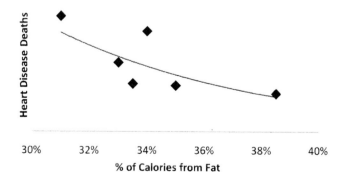

Finally, looking at Keys' data a few years later, they concluded, "The examination of *all* available basic data...show that the association [between fat and heart disease] lacks validity." They also discovered a "a strong *negative* association...for both animal protein and fat with mortality from non-cardiac diseases." Even the American Medical Association spoke up in protest: "The anti-fat, anti-cholesterol fad is not just foolish and futile...it also carries some risk."[11]

No matter. The "fat is evil" myth started a nationwide campaign to replace natural foods containing fat with fat-free products and climaxed with the government's *Dietary Guidelines*, Food Guide Pyramid, MyPyramid, and MyPlate diets. Those diets are high in starch because starch is low in fat. Unfortunately, over a billion dollars' worth of studies have failed to prove that the government's guidelines are good for anything other than profits.[12]

From the Harvard Medical School: "Few public health messages are as powerful and as persistent as this one: Fat is bad...The average American has substantially reduced the percentage of calories that she or he gets from fat over the past three decades...But we are not any healthier for all of this effort. In fact, we are worse off for it."[13]

Numerous studies have found no link between dietary fat and heart disease. When P.W. Siri-Tarino of the Children's Hospital & Research Center in Oakland examined 21 studies which included a total of 347,747 people, he found: "There is *no* significant evidence for concluding that dietary saturated fat is associated with an increased risk of heart disease or cardiovascular disease."[14]

The National Heart, Lung, and Blood Institute funded an enormous trial designed to link the consumption of foods containing fat to heart disease. The $115 million Multiple Risk Factor Intervention Trial took 12,866 men with high cholesterol, split them into two groups, and fed one group the government guidelines' diet for seven years with the hopes of lowering the incidence of heart disease. The government's diet resulted in a 7.1% *increase* in heart disease deaths.[15]

The Women's Health Initiative of the National Institutes of Health completed a $700 million study to test the fat hypothesis. A whopping 48,835 women ate their normal diet or the government diet for about eight years. At the end of the study, the regular- and government-diet women weighed the same and no differences were found in their health. The researchers concluded: "Dietary intervention that reduced total fat intake did not significantly reduce the risk of coronary heart disease, stroke, or cardiovascular disease." As reported in the study: "[This] trial is the largest long-term randomized trial of a dietary intervention ever conducted to our knowledge, and it achieved an 8.2% reduction... in total fat intake...*No* significant effects on incidence of coronary heart disease or stroke were observed." The *New York Times* ran the headline: *Low-Fat Diet Does Not Cut Health Risks, Study Finds.*[16]

A massive study named MONICA involved 113 groups of scientists and doctors in twenty-seven countries studying everything they thought could contribute to heart disease. They found little if any association between the average cholesterol level and heart-related mortality.[17]

In The Western Electric Study—known in academic circles as one of "the most informative prospective studies to date"—researchers concluded: "Although the focus of dietary recommendations is usually a reduction of saturated fat intake, *no* relation between saturated fat intake and risk of coronary heart disease was observed [in their study]."[18]

There's no shortage of data. In the Malmö Diet and Cancer Study, 28,098 men and women were split into four groups according to their intake of foods containing fat. After six years of observation, researchers found: "Individuals receiving more than 30% of their total daily energy from fat and more than 10% from saturated fat, did *not* have increased mortality. Current dietary guidelines concerning fat intake are thus generally *not* supported by our observational results [data]." Additionally: "With our results added to the pool of evidence from large-scale prospective cohort studies on dietary fat, disease and mortality, traditional dietary guidelines concerning fat intake are thus generally *not* strongly supported." And the icing on the cake: "*No* deteriorating effects of high saturated fat intake were observed for either sex for any cause of death."[19]

I'll briefly point out three more studies: the Nurses' Health Study, the Health Professionals Follow-Up Study, and the Nurses' Health Study 2. Together these studies tracked 300,000 people. None of these studies showed total fat intake increasing the risk of heart disease. The only conclusive finding was that eating *more* plant fats—such as the fats in flax seeds and nuts—*lowers* the risk of heart disease. The researchers involved reported: "Intake of linolenic acid [unsaturated fat] was inversely associated with risk of myocardial infarction [heart attacks]...These data do *not* support the strong association between intake of saturated fat and risk of coronary heart disease suggested by international comparisons."[20]

> *"It is now increasingly recognized that the low-fat campaign has been based on little scientific evidence and may have caused unintended health consequences."*
> **F.B. Hu, Harvard University**[21]

The government was trying to help with the guidelines, but sadly, it failed. Even worse, it keeps on failing. Scientists know it, and the data show it. Chapter 17 exposes why we haven't been told about it.[22]

CHAPTER 17

Focused on the Wrong Target

"The idea that you become fat by eating fat is just as silly as to say that you become green by eating green vegetables."
UFFE RAVNSKOV, MD, PH.D.[1]

Sugar-laden muffins, nutritionally neutered toast, and insulin-exploding juice are touted as part of a balanced, nutritious breakfast because they are low in fat. We look at food and ask ourselves, "Is this low in fat?" If the answer is yes, we think it is healthy. Yet foods that contain fat are not necessarily unhealthy. Researcher M. Leosdottir from Lund University stated: "Most researchers today agree on total fat intake *not* being a risk factor for cardiovascular disease or cancer."[2]

In addition to not killing us, foods containing fat do not make us fat. We think so because a gram of fat contains more calories than a gram of carbohydrate or protein. Fat has nine calories per gram while protein and carbohydrate only have four. The problem is that fat's higher quantity of calories does not mean eating it causes us to store body fat. That thinking is rooted in the *Calories In—Calories Out* theory of fat loss, which we now know is wrong.

According to the National Academy of Sciences, "Obesity itself has *not* been found to be associated with dietary fat in either inter- or intra- population studies." Harvard researcher

W.C. Willett adds, "There is *no* good evidence linking dietary fat with excess weight. In fact, there is plenty of evidence showing that the percentage of calories from fat is *not* the culprit leading to excess weight." There is even evidence that *lower* fat intake correlates with *higher* obesity rates. Willett continues, "In country-to-country surveys across Europe, women with the lowest fat intake are the most likely to be obese, while those with the highest fat intake are the least likely."[3]

A fellow researcher at Harvard, F.B. Hu, makes a similar point: "Although reduction in percentage of calories from dietary fat intake is commonly recommended for weight loss, long-term clinical trials have provided no good evidence that reducing dietary fat *per se* can lead to weight loss."[4]

This data seems counterintuitive because we've been led to believe that eating fat encourages overeating. We've been misinformed.

Think back to Satiety. Water, fiber, and protein play the biggest role in the Satiety of food, and Satiety determines how many calories we eat. Notice how there is no mention of fat there. Many water-, fiber-, and protein-packed foods contain fat. For example, seafood, meat, nuts, and flax seeds all contain fat. But when we focus on eating less fat, we replace these high-Satiety foods with low-Satiety starches and sweets. Since low-Satiety foods require more calories to fill us up, this swap causes us to eat more—not less—calories. So, far from discouraging overeating, avoiding SANE foods that contain fat *encourages* overeating.[5]

The last four decades of data tell the same story. We were told to avoid eating fat, so we reduced our relative intake of fat, increased our intake of starches and sweets, increased our total caloric intake, and ended up heavier and diabetic as a result.

Less Natural Foods Containing Fat, More Overeating [6]

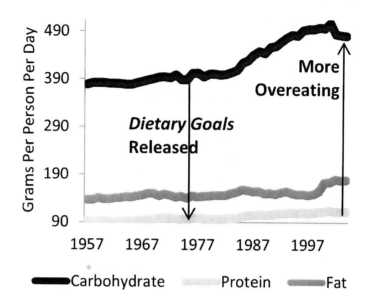

Less Natural Foods Containing Fat, More Body Fat [7]

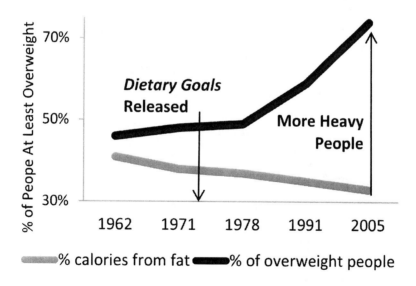

How We Eat vs. Our Incidence of Weight Gain [8]

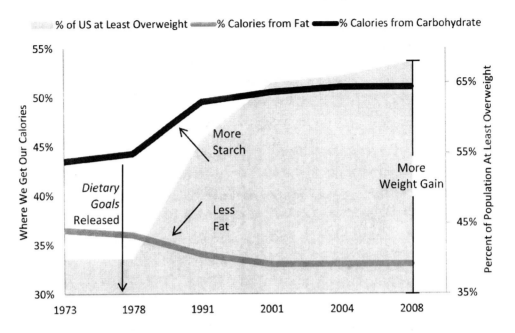

How We Eat vs. Our Incidence of Diabetes [9]

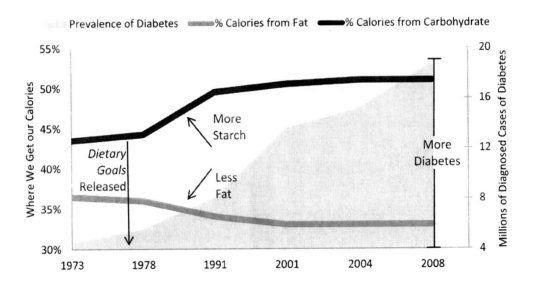

The government knows this too. The Centers for Disease Control and Prevention (CDC) reported: "During 1971-2000, a statistically significant increase in average energy intake occurred...The increase in energy intake is attributable primarily to an increase in carbohydrate intake." Even the authors of the government's guidelines—the U.S. Department of Agriculture—have gone on record stating that since the 1970s the major dietary trend has been a "greatly increased consumption of carbohydrates." They found that starch consumption had increased by nearly sixty pounds per person per year, and sweetener consumption had increased by nearly thirty pounds. That is ninety additional pounds of low-quality low-Satiety food—every year.[10]

The emphasis on low fat leads to inSANEity and misses an important point. Long-term health and fat loss does not result from diets low in fat, carbohydrate, or protein. Fat is not evil. Carbohydrates are not bad. And protein is not dangerous. The best way to burn body fat is to be balanced and SANE.

However, when you look at the government's pyramid and plate, balance is nowhere to be found:[11]

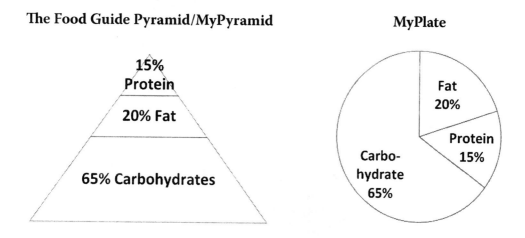

The Food Guide Pyramid/MyPyramid

15%
Protein
20% Fat
65% Carbohydrates

MyPlate

Fat 20%
Protein 15%
Carbohydrate 65%

How are these balanced diets? They are high in carbohydrates and low in everything else. Consider the high-fat *Atkins* diet. It is called "high-fat" because it advises individuals to get 65% of their calories from fat. Look at the USDA's pyramid and plate diets that advise us to get 65% of our calories from carbohydrate. Doesn't that make them high-carbohydrate diets? This could be why the January 13, 2011, edition of *USA Today* poked fun at the 72% of Americans who claimed to eat a balanced diet. The implication: "How could 70% of you be overweight if you ate a balanced diet?" We could easily be overweight if the "balanced" diet we are told to eat by the government is actually out of balance.[12]

This imbalance exists in other guidelines as well. The American Heart Association Nutrition Committee calls a 40% carbohydrate, 30% fat, and 30% protein diet a "low-carbohydrate/very-high-protein diet." Since when does 40:30:30 indicate that anything is very high?[13]

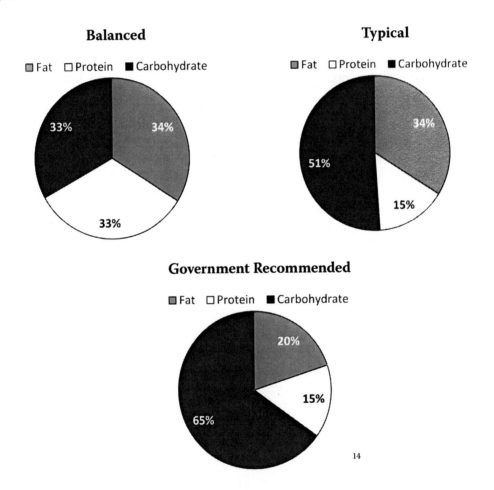

What could be the reason for this confusion? The answer lies in another myth that has been proven false: eating foods that contain fat leads to unhealthy cholesterol levels.[15]

CHAPTER 18

Eating Fat Will *Not* Hurt Your Cholesterol

"Although low-fat high-carbohydrate diets are recommended...in an effort to reduce the risk of coronary artery disease, the results of short-term studies have shown that these diets can lead to...an increased risk of coronary artery disease."
THE AMERICAN DIABETES ASSOCIATION[1]

As with other popular misconceptions about how our bodies work, confusion runs rampant about the word "cholesterol." Ancel Keys played a key role in creating this problem. Along with his other claims, he needed a scientific sounding explanation for how foods containing fat kill us. Looking at his data, Keys noticed that people eating more foods that contain fat generally had higher total cholesterol. While there was—and still is—no proof that high *total* cholesterol causes cardiovascular issues, Keys called it the cause of their heart problems.[2]

Even while Keys was touting his new findings, the Federal Register (the official log of the federal government of the U.S.) was on record with the true scientific data at that time: "The role of cholesterol in heart disease has *not* been established. A causal relationship between blood cholesterol levels and these diseases has *not* been proved. The advisability of making extensive changes in the nature of the dietary fat intake of the people of this country has *not* been demonstrated."[3]

Likewise, to this day, no studies have proven high *total* cholesterol causes heart disease. In the *American Journal of Medicine* T. Gordon reported, "*Total* cholesterol *per se* is *not* a risk factor for coronary heart disease at all." Dr. Uffe Ravnskov analyzed 26 randomized and controlled trials which were designed to lower *total* cholesterol and, theoretically, the risk of cardiovascular disease and death. Ravnskov's analysis put people into two groups:[4]

1. **Treatment Group**: People who ate less food that contain fat and/or took cholesterol-lowering drugs.
2. **Control Group**: People who did not eat less food that contain fat and did not take cholesterol-lowering drugs.

Across the studies, the total number of heart attack deaths was equal between the groups, and *more* people died overall in the group who ate *less* fat and/or took cholesterol-lowering drugs. Ravnskov concluded: "Lowering serum cholesterol concentrations does not reduce mortality and is unlikely to prevent coronary heart disease."[5]

Average Outcomes Across the 26 Studies

	Treatment Groups	Control Groups
Fatal Heart Attacks	2.9%	2.9%
Total Death Rate	6.1%	5.8%

For foods that contain fat and cholesterol to be killers, three points must be proven:

1. Eating natural foods that contain fat leads to risky levels of cholesterol.
2. These levels of cholesterol *cause* cardiovascular disease.
3. The diet outlined by government's guidelines improves these cholesterol levels.

None of these things have been proven.

University of California's J.B. German summarizes the state of cholesterol research: "The approach of many mainstream investigators…has been narrowly focused to produce and evaluate evidence in support of the hypothesis that dietary saturated fat elevates LDL cholesterol and thus the risk of coronary artery disease. The evidence is *not* strong, and, overall, dietary intervention by lowering saturated fat intake does *not* lower the incidence of nonfatal coronary artery disease; *nor* does such dietary intervention lower coronary disease or total mortality."[6]

Eating SANE foods containing fat has never been proven to lead to risky levels of cholesterol. The effect of natural dietary fat on cholesterol has never been proven to cause cardiovascular disease. In fact, studies have shown the opposite. The high-starch, low-fat, and low-protein diet promoted by the government's guidelines has been proven to *worsen* the type of cholesterol that decreases the risk of heart disease (HDL cholesterol).

Here is where the confusion about cholesterol comes up. There are different types of cholesterol, and most of them are helpful or neutral. The two most commonly discussed are LDL (low-density lipoprotein) and HDL (high-density lipoprotein). They are required to produce new cells and hormones. Because of this critical role, even if we never ate any cholesterol, our liver or intestines would produce it.

When it comes to predicting heart health, the American Heart Association, International Diabetes Federation, and World Health Organization agree that *low* HDL cholesterol—not *high* LDL cholesterol—is what matters. Looking at disease and death rates at various levels of LDL and HDL cholesterol, researchers have found that people with *low* HDL run a much greater risk of heart disease.[7]

Relative Risk of Heart Disease[8]

(Total Cholesterol in Parenthesis)

	100 mg/dl LDL	160 mg/dl LDL	220 mg/dl LDL
85 mg/dl HDL	Very Low (185)	Very Low (245)	Very Low (305)
65 mg/dl HDL	Low (165)	Low (225)	Moderate (285)
45 mg/dl HDL	Low (145)	Moderate (205)	High (265)
25 mg/dl HDL	Moderate (125)	High (185)	Very High (245)

There are two things to note. First, *total* cholesterol is irrelevant. If someone tells you their *total* cholesterol is 185, what is their risk of heart disease? Looking at the preceding table, it is either very low or high, depending on how much of that 185 consists of HDL cholesterol. Similarly, if someone tells you their *total* cholesterol is 245, they either have a herculean heart or a hemorrhaging heart, depending on their HDL levels.

Second, note how increasing HDL cholesterol is more important for heart health than decreasing LDL cholesterol. High HDL cholesterol protects us from heart problems more than dropping our LDL levels ever could. Heart-healthy diets are not about lowering *total* cholesterol. They are about raising HDL cholesterol.[9]

> *"There is a wealth of...evidence that increasing the concentration of HDL cholesterol through diet will lower the risk of coronary artery disease."*
> **R.P. MENSINK, MAASTRICHT UNIVERSITY**[10]

> *"...low HDL-cholesterol levels increase coronary heart disease risk...[programs] resulting in an increase in HDL-cholesterol levels could decrease the incidence of ischemic heart disease."*
> **J.P. DESPRES, LAVAL UNIVERSITY** [11]

The most effective way to raise our HDL levels is to eat more fat and less starch. Fat raises HDL. Starch lowers HDL.[12]

The Impact of Fat and Starch on Cholesterol and Health

	HDL	LDL	Health Impact
Unsaturated Fats (plants, seafood, white meat)	↑	↓	☺
Saturated Fats (dark/red meat)	↑	↑	😐
Starch (grains, corn, potatoes)	↓	↓	☹

Since lower HDL does more harm than lower LDL does good, any diet which tells us to replace SANE sources of fat with inSANE starch worsens our cholesterol. This is why D. Mozaffarian at Harvard University wrote: "[Focusing] on effects of total and saturated fat on...total and low-density lipoprotein [LDL] cholesterol may have failed to reduce coronary heart disease risk and inadvertently worsened...insulin resistance, and weight gain." Researcher A. Garg wrote the following in the *Journal of the American Medical Association*: "High-carbohydrate diets...caused persistent deterioration of glycemic control and accentuation of hyperinsulinemia [caused clogs], as well as increased...very-low-density lipoprotein [bad] cholesterol levels."[13]

Regrettably, under the government's guidelines, we are supposed to replace natural foods containing fat with low-fat-high-starch products to lower our *total* cholesterol. Why? Lower *total* cholesterol is meaningless, and lower HDL cholesterol is terrible for us. Researchers have demonstrated this for decades.[14]

The February 1989 issue of the *Diabetes Care* journal put out by the American Diabetes Association contained a study comparing the government's diet with a more SANE way of eating. The study concluded, "VLDL [bad] cholesterol was significantly *increased*... High-density lipoprotein [good] cholesterol concentrations were significantly *decreased* after consumption of the 60% carbohydrate diet."[15]

Comparable results were found with the equally imbalanced U.K. dietary guidelines. In the words of University of Glasgow researcher S.R. Arefhosseini, "Following the U.K. dietary guidelines resulted in changes...more likely to favor an *increased* risk of coronary heart disease."[16]

Even saturated fats, about which so much has been said, are not cholesterol criminals. The American Heart Association found: "No adequately designed randomized controlled study in the general population has shown that...decreasing saturated fat...intake significantly decreases coronary heart disease mortality." Saturated fats aren't bad; they're just not the best type of fat. Unsaturated fats are better. Studies show a specific type of unsaturated fat—polyunsaturated fats, especially omega-3 fatty acids—protect our heart and help us burn body fat.[17]

Good Sources of Polyunsaturated Omega-3 Fatty Acids[18]

(Milligrams in 250 Calories)

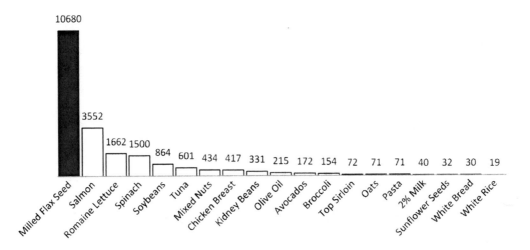

What is the bottom line? Studies show that any diet telling you to replace SANE sources of fat with inSANE starches is unhealthy and fattening. M.L. McCullough at Harvard University made this point: "Limiting unsaturated fats, which is usually done by increasing carbohydrates...is detrimental.... Low-fat, high-carbohydrate diets provide a higher glycemic load, aggravate hyperinsulinemia [clogging], and may thus increase the risk of diabetes and coronary artery disease."[19]

Sadly, the government's diet tells us to do exactly what science says we should avoid.[20]

If you think this is troubling, wait until you see what happened when big business jumped on the government bandwagon.

Today's Typical Diet: Almost Completely inSANE

"'Give us this day our daily bread,' says the Lord's Prayer, and 2,000 years ago food derived from cereal grains [starches] were the staples of most peoples' diets. But in relation to our long human existence, dependence on bread is a very late phenomenon."
S. BOYD, EMORY UNIVERSITY[21]

Loren Cordain from Colorado State University found that a whopping 72% of what we eat today was not eaten for at least 99.8% of our evolutionary history.[22]

How Much of Today's Typical Diet Is Not Natural

Food	% Calories
Starches	**24%**
Whole Grains	4%
Refined Grains	20%
Added Sweeteners	**19%**
Sucrose	8%
High-Fructose Corn Syrup	8%
Glucose	3%
Refined Oils	**18%**
Salad, Cooking Oils	9%
Shortening	7%
Margarine	2%
Alcohol	**1%**
Dairy	**11%**
Milk	4%
Cheese	3%
Butter	1%
Other	3%
Total	**72%**

The diet we evolved to eat has been flipped on its head. Is it any wonder our health and fitness have been flipped on their heads as well? Over 70% of our diet is comprised of unnatural food. Over 70% of us have unhealthy and inflated waistlines. Coincidence or common sense? How can the government and food manufacturers invert the diet our ancestors ate for millions of years and expect good things to happen?

PART 5

Source: Big People, Big Profits

"Why has the scientific evidence from long-standing obesity research not found its way into the minds of the public...? Perhaps it is because these views are shaped by a constant barrage of advertisements from the diet industry which has a multi-billion dollar interest in promoting the view that weight can be controlled through volition [willpower] alone."

J.M. FRIEDMAN, ROCKEFELLER UNIVERSITY[1]

CHAPTER 19

How Health Is Bad for Business

"There is a lot of money being made...feeding both oversized stomachs and feeding those enterprises selling fixes for oversized stomachs...And both industries—those selling junk food and those selling fat cures—depend for their future on the prevalence of obesity."
W. WEIS, IN THE *ACADEMY OF HEALTH CARE MANAGEMENT JOURNAL*[2]

Everyone knows that Washington, DC is the home of lobbyists. We lament that they have too much influence over our elected officials. Yet it never occurs to many of us that some of the largest lobbying efforts in the country are made by firms representing the food industry. The days of the nice farming family growing their crops are long gone. Today our food is grown by huge agribusiness concerns. According to a 2007 report by Mary Hendrickson and William Heffernan at the University of Missouri, 83.5% of beef, 80% of soybeans, and 55% of flour are produced by the top four firms in those industries. A single company supplies the seeds for 90% of genetically modified corn and soybeans.[3]

Or consider the dairy industry. How did dairy products end up with their own food group while becoming a "required" part of a "balanced" diet? The $1.4 billion dollars spent on agribusiness lobbying may have played a part.[4]

That's why we need to watch where we get our nutrition information. Is the source driven by science or profits? When the answer is profits, we hear things like this from the Grocery Manufacturers of America—the people responsible for ensuring grocery stores are as profitable as possible: "Policies that declare foods 'good' or 'bad' are counterproductive." The Sugar Association agrees: "All foods have a place in a balanced diet." A similar platitude is offered by the National Soft Drink Association: "As refreshing sources of needed liquids and energy, soft drinks represent a positive addition to a well-balanced diet."[5]

None of these statements are backed by science. We will not become clogged if we treat ourselves to starch and soda occasionally. But does that mean starch and sweets should be *recommended* as part of a balanced diet? Food corporations know better than anyone what the facts are, but they are not going to condemn themselves. Quite the opposite. Food companies aggressively fight any scientific information that threatens their bottom line.

Sadly, the crowding out of sound science by money doesn't stop there. Nearly two-thirds, or 64 percent, of the members of national committees on nutrition and food receive compensation from food companies. David Willman at the *Los Angeles Times* reported: "At least 530 government scientists at the National Institutes of Health, the nation's preeminent agency for medical research, have taken fees, stock, or stock options from biomedical companies in the last five years." Both the food industry and our government are paid to keep profits high, not to teach us about nutritional science. A famous quote puts it plainly: "It is hard to get someone to believe one thing when they are paid to believe another."[6]

Marion Nestle, Michele Simon, and Michael Pollan have all written excellent books detailing how the food industry harms our health. I highly recommend reviewing their work. In the meantime, one short example is all we need to show how wellness stacks up against profits for the food industry.

Science, millions of years of evolution, and common sense tell us that mother's milk beats out formula as the best food for babies. Basic human decency tells us that it would be wrong to persuade mothers who cannot afford sufficient quantities of formula to buy it anyway. Neither of these stopped the food industry from marketing infant formula to mothers in developing countries. This led to formula being diluted and contaminated, and, tragically, increased infant mortality. No matter. The food industry continued their promotional campaign, which included an advertisement distributed in Africa that depicted an African baby holding a container of formula with the caption: "The very best milk for your baby." Dr. Cecily Williams, a pediatrician who spent years working with African infants, reported: "Statistics have been collected to show that the death rate among artificially fed babies is much greater than that among breast-fed babies. And this is a death rate that shows a very marked class prejudice.... Misguided propaganda on infant feeding should be punished as the most criminal form of sedition...these deaths should be regarded as murder."[7]

In a world with more socially responsible corporations, we would have dietary guidelines focused on health instead of profits. They would look something like this:

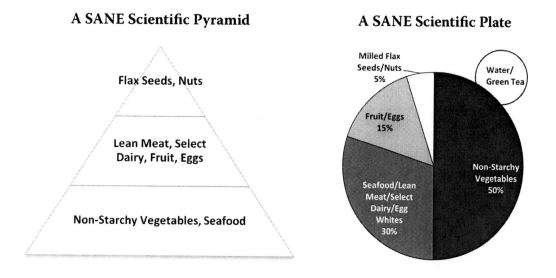

A SANE Scientific Pyramid

Flax Seeds, Nuts

Lean Meat, Select Dairy, Fruit, Eggs

Non-Starchy Vegetables, Seafood

A SANE Scientific Plate

Milled Flax Seeds/Nuts 5%

Water/Green Tea

Fruit/Eggs 15%

Non-Starchy Vegetables 50%

Seafood/Lean Meat/Select Dairy/Egg Whites 30%

Why has the food industry moved so slowly to answer the concerns of many nutritional scientists? At the risk of being repetitive, it's because the people generating the guidelines the industry adheres to—the USDA—are not responsible for nutrition. They are responsible for a profitable food industry. That is why they are called the Department of Agriculture instead of the Department of Health, Nutrition, and Fat Loss. Dr. Marion Nestle, author of *Food Politics*, tells us: "The USDA is in the position of being responsible to the agriculture business. That is their job. Nutrition is not their job."[8]

Lest you think I am engaging in conspiracy theory, take a look at this chart. Note how the worse we do health-wise, the better the food industry does money-wise:

Food Quality/SANEity vs. Profitability[9]

Type of Food	Quality/SANEity	Profitability
Sweeteners		★ ★ ★ ★ ★
Processed Starch	⌐	★ ★ ★ ★ ★
Whole Grain Starch	★⌐	★ ★ ★ ★
Oils	★ ★	★ ★ ★ ★
Dairy	★ ★⌐	★ ★ ★
Legumes	★ ★ ★	★
Fruits	★ ★ ★	★
Nuts, Flax Seeds	★ ★ ★⌐	★
Seafood/Lean Meat/Eggs	★ ★ ★ ★ ★	★
Non-Starchy Vegetables	★ ★ ★ ★ ★	★

CHAPTER 20

Sweeteners: More Profitable, Common, and Dangerous than Ever

"If only a small fraction of what is already known about the effects of sugar were to be revealed in relation to any other material used as a food additive, that material would promptly be banned."
JOHN YUDKIN, UNIVERSITY OF LONDON[1]

The most common and powerful weapon in the food industry's arsenal is added sweeteners. Researcher Michael F. Jacobson, with the Center for Science in the Public Interest, said, "Carbonated soft drinks are the single most-consumed food in the American diet." The problem has gotten so bad that at the turn of the millennium the average American ate over 150 pounds of sweeteners per year because food companies add them to at least the following products:[2]

- baked or processed foods
- most anything not refrigerated
- low-calorie snacks

- "weight loss" products
- beverages
- "protein" bars

- low-fat salad dressing
- dairy products
- cough syrups

Thanks to this sweet saturation, the average American is eating a little under a half-pound of added sweeteners *per day*. That is a cup of clog every day. Two centuries ago, people ate about one-tenth of that. During the previous 99.8% of our evolution, our ancestors ate none.[3]

Sweeteners vs. Obesity [4]

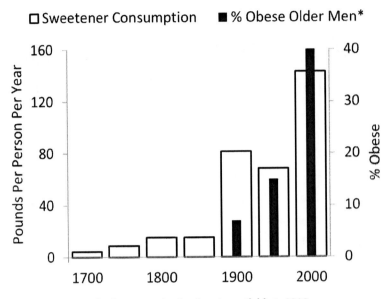

☐ Sweetener Consumption ■ % Obese Older Men*

*The first year obesity data is available is 1900

Why is this such a problem? Barry Popkin of the University of North Carolina at Chapel Hill pointed out that as early as the 1950s, research "showed that the link between sugar consumption and coronary heart disease...was stronger than the link between heart disease and the consumption of saturated fats from animal foods." This work, however, was ignored.[5]

How did this inSANEity happen? Food that has all of its fat processed out tastes bad. It is hard to sell bad-tasting food. So food companies add sweeteners when they remove fat. Combine the government's "food containing fat is evil" guidelines with $36 billion of "we have yummy low-fat food" marketing, and the result is that nearly a fifth of the average American's total calories come from sweeteners.[6]

The worst part is that we have no practical choice under the *Dietary Guidelines* regime. If foods that contain fat are off the table, then almost everything else has been stuffed with sweeteners. As a general rule, if it is not coming directly from a plant or an animal, then it has been sweetened. Even if it does not taste sweet, it has been altered with at least one of the following:

- Agave Nectar
- Barley Malt
- Beet Sugar
- Brown Sugar
- Buttered Syrup
- Cane Crystals
- Cane Juice Crystals
- Cane Sugar
- Caramel
- Carob Syrup
- Castor Sugar
- Confectioner's Sugar
- Corn Sweetener
- Corn Syrup
- Corn Syrup Solids
- Crystalline Fructose
- Date Sugar
- Demerara Sugar
- Dextran
- Dextrose
- Diastatic Malt
- Diatase
- Ethyl Maltol
- Evaporated Cane Juice
- Fructose
- Fruit Juice
- Fruit Juice Concentrates
- Galactose
- Glucose
- Glucose Solids
- Golden Sugar
- Golden Syrup
- Granulated Sugar
- Grape Sugar
- High-Fructose Corn Syrup
- Honey
- Icing Sugar
- Invert Sugar
- Lactose
- Malt Syrup
- Maltodextrin
- Maltose
- Maple Syrup
- Molasses
- Muscovado Sugar
- Panocha
- Raw Sugar
- Refiner's Syrup
- Rice Syrup
- Sorbitol
- Sorghum Syrup
- Sucrose
- Sugar
- Syrup
- Treacle
- Turbinado Sugar
- Yellow Sugar

Memorizing this list isn't necessary. However, it is important to know that *any* form of caloric sweetener causes clogs. Put differently, our fat metabolism system does not care where caloric sweeteners come from. To our metabolism, apple juice is basically the same as soda, since they both contain about thirty grams of sugar. A "weight loss" bar with thirty grams of sweeteners in it causes the same clog as a candy bar with thirty grams of sugar in it. "Heart smart" cereal is worse than breakfast pastries because they are both full of sweeteners, but folks feel bad eating more than two pastries while they will happily fill bowl after bowl with "enriched" sweetened cereal for breakfast.

It's also important to understand that the sweetener high-fructose corn syrup is especially common and fattening. This substance's high sweetness and low cost makes it one of the most ubiquitous ingredients in low-calorie and low-fat products. Combine this with the guidance to avoid calories and foods containing fat, and we end up unintentionally eating 10,475% more high-fructose corn syrup than we did in 1970.[7]

Grams of High-Fructose Corn Syrup Eaten Per Person Per Day [8]

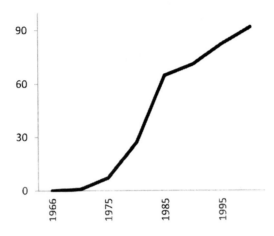

High-Fructose Corn Syrup (HFCS) Is Becoming More Common [9]

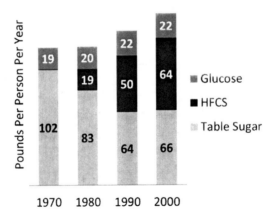

Eating all that high-fructose corn syrup is particularly harmful. To use the example of a clogged drain, think of eating high-fructose corn syrup as pouring quick-drying cement down your drain. Rats fed high-fructose corn syrup consistently get fatter and sicker than rats fed the exact same amount of sugar. The problem gets worse. Beyond leaving us hungry, clogged, and overweight, high-fructose corn syrup makes other food fill us up less. High-fructose corn syrup does not have low Satiety. It has *negative* Satiety. It leaves us hungrier than if we did not eat it. It alters our baseline levels of Satiety hormones and drives us to eat more and more over time.[10]

As if this wasn't enough, studies at Princeton University show: "Laboratory rats given a high-sugar diet and then withdrawn from sugar experience changes in both behavior and brain chemistry similar to those seen during withdrawal from morphine or nicotine." Related research reports: "We have clearly shown sugar addiction in rats...causing brain and behavioral effects analogous to a little dose of amphetamine [stimulants]." In short, added sweeteners are addictive.[11]

When you switch to a SANE diet, you will experience the effects of sweetener addiction for the first couple of weeks. You feel like you are going through withdrawal because, well, you are. It takes the body a couple of weeks to overcome the chemical dependence caused by the sea of sweeteners we have been led to eat. But the switch is worth the effort. After all, who wants to be an addict?

Sweeteners: The New Cigarettes?

In 1998 Coca-Cola offered schools $10,000 to advertise Coke discount cards to their students. Deeply in need of the funds, Greenbrier High School in Augusta, Georgia, invited Coke employees to lecture in classes and added the analysis of Coca-Cola to its chemistry curriculum. The school went on to make all 1,230 students dress in red or white shirts and to spell-out "Coke" while they snapped photos to send to Coke execs.[12]

Considering how harmful and addictive sweeteners are, why was the Coke stunt considered harmless fun while it would be illegal to do the same thing with other harmful and addictive substances?

Sweeteners and tobacco are both harmful and addictive. Yet the promotion of the former is encouraged while the promotion of the latter is highly regulated. The rationale cannot be that tobacco is so much more harmful. Tobacco only kills 8 percent more people. Both industries are even run by the same companies.[13]

Annual Deaths Caused by...[14]

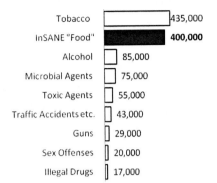

Tobacco	435,000
InSANE "Food"	**400,000**
Alcohol	85,000
Microbial Agents	75,000
Toxic Agents	55,000
Traffic Accidents etc.	43,000
Guns	29,000
Sex Offenses	20,000
Illegal Drugs	17,000

A Brief History of Big Tobacco Taking Over the "Food" Industry

- 1970—Philip Morris buys Miller Brewing
- 1978—Philip Morris buys 97% of Seven-Up
- 1985—R.J. Reynolds buys Nabisco Foods
- 1985—Philip Morris buys General Foods
- 1988—Philip Morris buys Kraft, Inc.
- 1990—Philip Morris acquires Jacobs Suchard
- 1993—Philip Morris buys Nabisco cereals
- 2000—Philip Morris buys Nabisco Holdings

Sweeteners and tobacco are even rationalized the same way by industry insiders. Here is how both describe the safety of their products:

Tobacco	InSANE Food Products
"I believe nicotine is not addictive." **Philip Morris Tobacco Company president**[15]	"Soft drinks do not cause pediatric obesity, do not reduce nutrient intake, and do not cause dental cavities" **National Soft Drink Association**[16]

They share the same marketing tactics:

Tobacco	InSANE Food Products
"The base of our business is the high school student." **Lorillard Tobacco Company**[17]	"We always, always have kid related programs." **Vice President, McDonald's**[18]

And finally, on health:

Tobacco	InSANE Food Products
"We believe the products we make are not injurious to health." **Tobacco Industry Research Committee**[19]	"Actually, our product is quite healthy. Fluid replenishment is a key to health…Coca-Cola does a great service because it encourages people to take in more and more liquids." **Coke's CEO**[21]
"We accept an interest in people's health as a basic responsibility, paramount to every other consideration in our business." **Tobacco Industry Research Committee**[20]	"The soft drink industry has a long commitment to promoting a healthy lifestyle for individuals—especially children." **The National Soft Drink Association**[22]

With so much in common, it seems odd that one of these is treated like the plague while it is fine for the food industry to spend hundreds of millions of dollars per year advertising sweets to children. Particularly when psychologists have shown that before the age of eight, children do not see commercials as marketing, they see them as fact.[23]

Consider the study from the *Journal of Marketing* that showed 70% of six-through-eight-year olds believe fast foods are healthier than food prepared at home. Researcher Kelly Brownell at Yale reports: "A study of Australian children ages nine to ten indicated that more than half believe that Ronald McDonald knows best what children should eat." He went on to report: "The average American child sees 10,000 food advertisements each year, just on television. Children watching Saturday morning cartoons see a food commercial every five minutes. The vast majority are for sugared cereals, fast foods, soft drinks, sugary and salty snacks, and candy…Between 1976 and 1987, the ratio of high- to low-sugar ads increased from 5:1 to 12.5:1."[24]

What's the moral of the story? Food companies are not going to stop with sweeteners. Nor can we rely on our government for help. They are the very source of the guidelines that leave us no practical choice other than to be slathered with sweeteners. It is up to us to end this inSANEity.

Chapter 21 shows how we can get our SANEity back.

It's All About Results—A Pragmatism Primer

"The efficacy of any treatment of obesity can be appraised only by the permanence of the result."
– H. BURCH, BAYLOR UNIVERSITY[25]

Pragmatists are results-oriented—they believe something is right or wrong based on its results. People can try anything they want and the true worth of the program is revealed by its results. If it works, it is right. If it fails, it is wrong. Consider Communism, for example. A pragmatist asks how Communism worked out in the real world and lets that settle the argument about its merits.

When it comes to fat loss, the pragmatic view is: "Does the fat-loss program cause you to lose body fat and keep it off forever without compromising the rest of your life? If so, then it is right. If not, then it is wrong." Unfortunately, this commonsense approach is not common practice. Despite the decades of data and tens of millions of heavy diabetic people that prove traditional weight-loss programs wrong, those people have been brainwashed into thinking that they failed because they didn't lose any weight, not that the traditional weight-loss programs failed them.

If a program fails, it is the program's fault. Programs are designed to deliver results. If it failed to deliver results, the program failed, not the person.

Think about software programs. If you cannot figure out how to use a software program, it is not because you failed. It is because the software program failed. Good software is easy to use. That is what makes it good software. It delivers excellent results for you. What good is any software program if it does not serve you?

Similarly, if you cannot stick to a fat-loss program forever, it is not because you are a failure. Good fat-loss programs are easy to use. That is what makes them good. They deliver excellent results for you.

Consider Oprah. She is one of the strongest and smartest women ever. Now look at Oprah's weight-loss efforts. Thinking pragmatically, thinking about results, what do we know about the weight-loss programs Oprah tried? If they were right, Oprah would be thinner and spend less time and money trying to burn body fat. She is far from a failure at anything. The programs failed her.

If Oprah hires someone to design her house and the house collapses, we would not blame Oprah. And if Oprah hires someone to design a piece of software and she cannot figure it out, the software designer is at fault. So, if Oprah hires someone to design a weight-loss program and she does not lose weight, the program failed—Oprah did not.

Results are all that matter. People do not fail fat-loss programs. Fat-loss programs fail people.

How Humanity Can Get Its SANEity Back

"We found marked improvement...after advice to follow a Paleolithic [SANE] diet compared with a healthy Western diet...The study adds to the notion that healthy diets based on whole-grain cereals and low-fat dairy products are only the second best choice in the prevention and treatment of type 2 diabetes."

S. LINDEBERG, UNIVERSITY OF LUND[1]

How do we avoid this inSANEity? We need to be pragmatic and ask: Is there any way of eating that is proven to keep folks free from obesity, diabetes, heart disease, and cardiovascular disease—aka the "diseases of civilization?"

Yes. We can eat the way we did before civilization. We can eat so much SANE food that we are too full for inSANE food.[2]

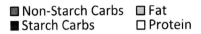

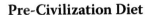

Pre-Civilization Diet

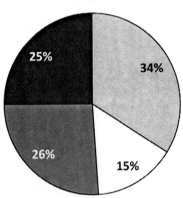

Today's Typical Diet

Government Recommended Diet

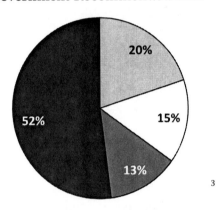

Unless our fat metabolism system completely transformed itself in the last 0.02% of our evolutionary history—the 12,000 years since we first started farming, filling it with food that it is not designed to digest will cause a clog. University of London researcher John Yudkin notes: "For a fairly considerable [evolutionary] alteration to occur in a population, something between 1,000 and 10,000 generations [25,000 to 250,000 years] are needed.... If there have been great changes in man's environment that occurred in a much shorter time...there are likely to be signs that man has not fully adapted, and this will probably show itself as the presence of disease." More simply: We did not change, but the quality of our diet did. It is making us heavy, diabetic, and sick.[4]

A study from the University of Texas Southwestern Medical Center at Dallas showed that our modern diet increases nearly all the risk factors for the diseases of civilization when compared to a pre-starch and sweetener diet. Similar work at the Haimoto Clinic and Duke University Medical Center has shown a more natural diet to be the best diet available for clog clearing. In a University of Melbourne study, middle-aged Australian hunter-gatherers started out lean and free from type 2 diabetes, then switched to a diet inspired by the government's guidelines and became overweight and type 2 diabetic. Then they reverted back to their natural diet. In only seven weeks, the tribesmen lost an average of 16.5 pounds.[5]

The list of clinical studies proving the same results goes on. But the bottom line is, as S. Boyd from Emory University tells us: "Following a diet comparable to the one that humans were genetically adapted to should postpone, mitigate, and in many cases prevent altogether, a host of diseases that debilitate us."[6]

Let's turn now to how we can do that. Part 6 and part 7 show you how to eat more and exercise less—smarter.

PART 6

Solution: Eat More–Smarter™

"Treating obesity will come not from repetition of anachronistic preconceptions [outdated theories] but rather from the rigorous scientific approach."
J.M. FRIEDMAN, ROCKEFELLER UNIVERSITY[1]

CHAPTER 22

How to Eat More–Smarter

"Good news: The FDA has approved pills that help you lose weight by making you feel full. The recommended dosage is five thousand pills a day."
CONAN O'BRIEN

You and I already know that we can eat more—smarter—by consuming more, higher-quality calories. But we first need to know what the highest-quality calories are, where we can get them, and why eating *more* of them helps us to burn body fat. Fortunately, we already know the answers to all of these questions.

We know that four factors determine calorie quality:

1. **S**atiety—How well calories prevent overeating
2. **A**ggression—How likely calories are to be stored as body fat
3. **N**utrition—How many nutrients are provided per calorie
4. **E**fficiency—How many calories can be converted into body fat

We know SANE calories come from the water-, fiber-, and protein-packed foods found in nature. That makes sense. Why would anything or anyone "design" us to run on a low-fat-low-protein-high-starch diet which was not possible for 99.8% of our evolutionary history?

Finally, you and I know we want to eat *more* SANE natural food because that's the easiest way to avoid inSANE unnatural starches and sweets. Now for the day-to-day details.

First and foremost: Do not diet. Dieting is restricting yourself abnormally for a short period of time. As D.S. Weigle at the University of Washington tells us, "energy-restricted diets are a physiologically unsound means to achieve weight reduction." You're better off switching over to eating more of the right foods. As E.C. Westman of Duke University reminds us, "The persistence of an epidemic of obesity and type 2 diabetes suggests that new nutritional strategies are needed if the epidemic is to be overcome." Your "new nutritional strategy" is neither abnormal nor short-term. You'll simply eat the way our ancestors ate for 99.8% of our history. You'll get back to normal eating so that your biological processes can get back to functioning normally.[2]

Still, when people see you dropping pounds of body fat while eating more, they will ask what diet you are on. If you have to give an answer, say you are on the *Natural Balanced Diet*. Natural because you are eating the food you evolved to eat—food that comes directly from the earth. Balanced because natural food automatically provides a perfect ratio of protein, fats, and carbohydrate—about a third of each.

Protein, Carbohydrate, and Fat in Common "Diets"[3]

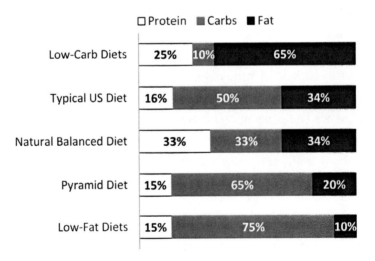

Consistent with the principle of not dieting, you will not be counting calories or using rigid meal plans. You will eat non-starchy vegetables, seafood, lean meat, fat-free or low-fat cottage cheese, fat-free or low-fat *plain Greek* yogurt, eggs, berries, citrus fruits, milled flax seeds, and nuts—in basically that order—and make your plate look like this:[4]

What a Natural Balanced Plate Looks Like

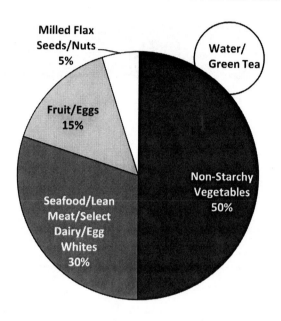

Rigid step-by-step plans do not work in the real world. Imagine trying to learn addition by memorizing every possible combination of numbers. Beyond being ridiculous, it's useless in real life. You and I learned addition by understanding the general rules and thinking logically from there. Permanent reduction of body fat is no different. Let's learn the general rules of eating more—smarter—and take it from there.

Here is the general idea for the types of food we should be eating relative to common diets:

Types of Food to Eat Relative to Common Diets

	Vegetables & Fruits	Seafood, Meat, & Eggs	Milled Flax Seeds & Nuts	Dairy & Beans	Oils	Starch	Added Sweeteners
Low-Carb Diet	Low	High	High	Low[1]	High	None	None
Typical U.S. Diet	Low	Medium	Low	Medium	High	High	High
Natural Balanced Eating	**Very High**	High	Medium	Medium	Low	None	None
Pyramid Scheme	Medium	Low	Low	Medium	Low	**Very High**	Low
Low-Fat Diet	Medium	Low	Low	Medium	None	**Very High**	Low

Here are the nutrients we will get relative to the typical U.S. diet:

A Natural Balanced Diet vs. the Typical U.S. Diet[5]

	Natural Balanced	Typical U.S.
Carbohydrate	Less	More
Sugar and Starch	Much less	Much more
Fruits	More	Less
Non-Starchy Vegetables	Much more	Much less
Protein	More	Less
Fat	Equal	Equal
Unnatural Trans-Fats[2]	Much less	More
Natural Unsaturated Fat	More	Less
Natural Saturated Fat	Equal	Equal
Antioxidants	Much more	Much less
Fiber	Much more	Much less
Vitamins & Minerals	Much more	Much less
Body Fat Stored	Much less	More
Food Eaten	More	Less

1 Except for cheese. Low-carbohydrate diets generally encourage relatively high intakes of cheese.

2 Unnatural fats engineered by food product manufacturers to decrease costs and increase shelf-life. These are like the high-fructose corn syrup of fats, and should be avoided.

Review the last row of the last table. I am not saying eat *more* for shock value. Researchers estimate that prior to the advent of starch and sweeteners, our ancestors ate about five pounds of food per day. Thanks to all the water, fiber, and protein, SANE foods are literally larger than inSANE foods. Our shopping carts, refrigerators, and plates will be much fuller when we replace inSANE foods with SANE foods.[6]

No more tiny, sweet, starchy breakfasts. You can have luscious omelets overflowing with non-starchy vegetables and lean meat or generous protein-packed smoothies. No more flaccid sandwiches for lunch and soggy starch for dinner. Enjoy a triple serving of delightful seafood or succulent lean meat accompanied by a mountain of non-starchy vegetables. Let's add milled flax seeds to everything we can and enjoy nuts and fruits—focusing on berries and citrus fruits—as wonderful on-the-go snacks. Add some fat-free or low-fat cottage cheese or some fat-free or low-fat *plain Greek* yogurt as needed, and you will be satisfied and slim.

That is all there is to it from the eating side of things. It is not complicated. It cannot be complicated. How could it be? Staying healthy and fit is the most basic ability anyone could ever have.

There are specific tips and tricks later in the book to help you get back to normal eating in today's abnormal world, but for now eat more—smarter—by eating:

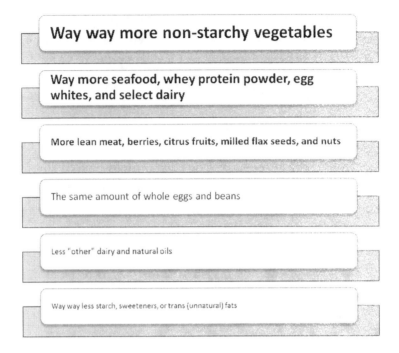

Way way more non-starchy vegetables

Way more seafood, whey protein powder, egg whites, and select dairy

More lean meat, berries, citrus fruits, milled flax seeds, and nuts

The same amount of whole eggs and beans

Less "other" dairy and natural oils

Way way less starch, sweeteners, or trans (unnatural) fats

Freed from the myths and marketing at the heart of the obesity epidemic, the solution is simple: Return to normal. Eat as much as you want, whenever you want, as long as the food is coming from SANE sources so that you get a natural, balanced amount of carbohydrate, protein, and fat, while staying satisfied.

CHAPTER 23

A Natural Balanced Amount of Carbohydrates

"Diets should be moderate in carbohydrate, moderate in fat, and protein should contribute 25% to 30% of energy intake."
D.A. SCHOELLER, UNIVERSITY OF WISCONSIN-MADISON[1]

No matter how misinformed they are, people will say you are on a low-carbohydrate diet when they see you taking in a natural balanced amount of carbohydrates. Eating a large amount of non-starchy vegetables is the single most important aspect of eating more—smarter. These types of vegetables *are* carbohydrates. Therefore, eating more—smarter—is not a low-carb diet. People make this mistake because they do not realize that the vast majority of the foods making up their "balanced" diet are carbohydrates.

Defining carbohydrates as foods with most of their calories coming from carbohydrate, fats as foods with most of their calories coming from fat, and protein as foods with most of their calories coming from protein, we end up with:

Common Proteins, Fats, and Carbohydrates

Proteins
Seafood
Lean Meat
Egg Whites
Whey Protein Powder
Fat-Free/Low-Fat Cottage Cheese
Fat-Free/Low-Fat *Plain Greek* Yogurt

Fats
Whole Eggs
Tofu
Oils
Nuts & Milled Flax Seeds
Fatty Meat
Whole-Fat Dairy

Carbohydrates
Everything Else

For example, the calories in whole milk come from 30% carbohydrate, 21% protein, and 49% fat. Whole milk is mostly fat, so it is a fat. The calories in skim milk come from 53% carbohydrate, 42% protein, and 5% fat. Skim milk is mostly carbohydrate, so it is a carbohydrate. How about the so called "good source of protein" beans? They are 76% carbohydrate, 21% protein, and 3% fat. Beans are a carbohydrate. Broccoli is a carbohydrate with 71% of its calories coming from carbohydrate. So are bananas—93% carbohydrate. The point is that grains, potatoes, rice, breads, pasta, beans, fruits, vegetables, and most dairy products are carbohydrates. That does not leave much to put in the non-carbohydrate bucket other than seafood, meat, eggs, tofu, oils, nuts, whey protein powder, milled flax seeds, fat-free or low-fat cottage cheese, and fat-free or low-fat *plain Greek* yogurt.

With the vast majority of foods being carbohydrates, most people eat diets very high in carbohydrate and then call anything that is not very high in carbohydrate a high-protein or a high-fat diet. That is a mistake. Avoiding a diet very high in carbohydrate is not the same as going on a low-carbohydrate diet. No low-carbohydrate dieting for us. Just a natural and balanced intake of carbohydrate.

Also, try to avoid the complex differentiation between simple carbohydrate and complex carbohydrate. This distinction only causes confusion. For example, SANE fruits contain simple carbohydrates, while inSANE starches contain complex carbohydrates. The key to long-term fat loss and health is eating more water-, fiber-, and protein-rich SANE foods. The only water-, fiber-, and protein-rich SANE carbohydrates are non-starchy vegetables and fruits.

◆ ◆ ◆

While non-starchy vegetables and fruits made up a substantial proportion of our ancestors' diet, protein was also vital for them. Perhaps they did not take down a woolly mammoth every time they needed some protein, but they found other sources. You too can use those sources in your natural balanced diet.

CHAPTER 24

A Natural Balanced Amount of Protein

"Exchange of protein for carbohydrates has been shown to improve blood lipids.... Higher protein diets have been associated with lower blood pressure and reduced risk of coronary heart disease."
T.L. HALTON, HARVARD UNIVERSITY[1]

Eating a natural amount of protein—at least one gram of protein per pound of body weight per day—is critical to getting our biological functions back to normal.[1] Why? First, high-Satiety protein fills us up and keeps us full, so we have no room for low-quality food. Second, our fat metabolism system will burn body fat instead of muscle. As researcher D.K. Layman from the University of Illinois tells us: "Use of higher protein diets reduces lean tissue loss to less than 15% and when combined with exercise can halt loss of lean tissue during weight loss."[2]

Some people say that eating at least a gram of protein per pound of body weight hurts the kidneys and liver. This is not borne out, however, in clinical testing. For instance, A.H. Manninen at the University of Oulu concluded: "Simply stated, there is no scientific evidence whatsoever that high-protein intake has adverse effects on liver function."

---

1   If you are very heavy, then eat a gram of protein per pound of two-thirds to three-quarters of your body weight. For example, a 350 pound woman should eat between 225 and 263 grams of protein per day. Generally speaking, if you weigh less than 200 pounds, do not exceed 250 grams of protein per day.

T.L. Halton at Harvard University addresses the other part of the argument: "There is little evidence that high protein diets pose a serious risk to kidney function in healthy populations."[3]

On the other hand, guess how many studies show positive health benefits and body-fat loss stemming from a more balanced intake of protein? Dozens. A typical report comes from Loren Cordain at Colorado State University: "There is now a large body of experimental evidence increasingly demonstrating that a higher intake of lean animal protein reduces the risk for cardiovascular disease, hypertension, dyslipidemia, obesity, insulin resistance, and osteoporosis while not impairing kidney function." That's because researchers have shown that humans evolved to get about a third of our calories from protein. Dr. Cordain goes on: "So called ...'very high protein diets' (30%—40% total energy) actually represent the norm which conditioned the present day human genome... The evolutionary template would predict that human health and well-being will suffer when dietary intakes fall outside this range."[4]

How could a basic part of human evolution harm rather than help us? Emory University researchers S.B. Eaton and M. Konner made the point well when they noted, "It would be paradoxical if humans...should now somehow be harmed as a result of protein intake habitually tolerated or even required by their near relatives."[5]

> "...the Nurses' Health Study is the only large prospective study to have examined the link between dietary protein and cardiovascular disease....The group of women who ate the most protein...were 25% less likely to have had a heart attack or to have died of heart disease...eating a lot of protein doesn't harm the heart."
> **W.C. WILLETT, HARVARD UNIVERSITY**[6]

> "Seafood and poultry have been associated with lower rates of coronary heart disease and cancer...."
> **M.L. MCCULLOUGH, AMERICAN CANCER SOCIETY**[7]

How did the myth that protein is bad for us get started in the first place? The myth came out of studies where animals that were fed extreme amounts of protein experienced problems. However, rather than proving more protein is harmful, these studies prove that until we exceed two grams of protein per pound of body weight per day, we will get only healthier and slimmer by upping our protein intake.[8]

To put two grams of protein per pound of body weight into perspective, an inactive 150-pound person would not enter the protein danger zone until they ate eleven chicken breasts per day, every day. That would total two grams of protein per pound of body weight, and would mean that 60% of their total calories ware coming from protein. That is a terribly imbalanced diet and an unnatural amount of protein.[9]

Bad things happen if we eat too much of anything. Luckily, it is nearly impossible to eat too much high-Satiety protein. Additionally, a natural increase in our protein intake will improve our cholesterol, triglycerides, and insulin regulation, while lowering our risk of cardiovascular disease. And it does not matter if the protein comes from lean meat. In fact, low levels of animal protein have been associated with an *increased* risk of strokes.[10]

Let's focus on meat for a moment. There is nothing wrong with eating high-quality meat. Besides the fact that meat was a cornerstone of our diet for most of our evolutionary history, there is no clinical data showing that meat is unhealthy. The *Journal of the American Medical Association* reviewed 147 studies on the impact of diet on health. They found zero correlation between meat consumption and cardiovascular disease. Separately, researchers found that people in England have eaten about the same amount of animal fat—the source of most of the concern with meat—since 1910. Meanwhile, the number of heart attacks increased 1,000% between 1930 and 1970. It looks like animal fat is not causing the climb.[11]

Similarly, during basically the same period of time in the U.S., a similar increase in heart attacks occurred while the amount of animal fats being consumed dropped. Meat is not unhealthy. It is a fantastic source of protein and therefore a key part of a natural balanced diet. J.H. O'Keefe at the Mid America Heart Institute listed all of the advantages: "Diets high in lean protein can improve lipid profiles and overall health...Lean animal protein eaten at regular intervals improves satiety levels, increases thermogenesis [calorie burning], improves insulin sensitivity [clears clogs], and thereby facilitates weight loss while providing many essential nutrients."[12]

Last but not least, at some point one of your more annoying coworkers will bring up some misguided magazine article arguing that protein promotes osteoporosis. This myth comes from the fact that digesting protein requires more calcium than the digestion of fat or carbohydrates. Certain individuals claim this finding shows that eating a lot of protein will suck calcium from our bones. That is inaccurate.

First, you will not be eating *a lot* of protein. You will be eating the amount humans evolved to eat. Second, you will have no need to grab calcium from your bones since a natural balanced diet provides at least 150% more calcium than the typical U.S. diet. Third, protein digestion does not negatively impact bones if intake of the mineral phosphorus is increased, and a natural balanced diet does that. Finally, while more protein increases the need for calcium, it also increases the body's ability to absorb calcium. When more protein is taken in, the body automatically makes better use of calcium. Studies show that a natural level of protein *increases* bone density by raising levels of the protein IGF-1.[13]

> "With respect to adverse effects, no protein-induced effects are observed on net bone balance or on calcium balance in young adults and elderly persons. Dietary protein even increases bone mineral mass and reduces incidence of osteoporotic fracture."
> **M.S. WESTERTERP-PLANTENGA, MAASTRICHT UNIVERSITY**[14]

Good Sources of Protein

The only drawback with protein is the misinformation about good sources of protein. For our purpose, we will define good sources of protein as common foods with more calories coming from protein than from fat or carbohydrates. In this category there are only six good sources of protein.

The Six Good Sources of Protein

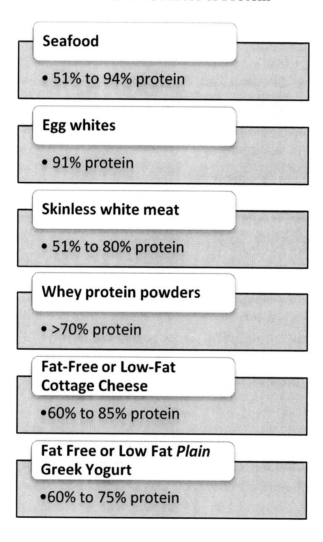

Seafood

• 51% to 94% protein

Egg whites

• 91% protein

Skinless white meat

• 51% to 80% protein

Whey protein powders

• >70% protein

Fat-Free or Low-Fat Cottage Cheese

•60% to 85% protein

Fat Free or Low Fat *Plain* Greek Yogurt

•60% to 75% protein

Beyond that are three other pretty good sources of protein. They are given that designation because quite a few of their calories come from fat. Which is fine. Natural fats are good for us. We should be getting about a third of our calories from fat. But let's call a spade a spade. If 43% of the calories in soybeans—aka tofu—come from fat and 33% come from protein, we are eating mostly fat when we eat soybeans. Again, that is fine. Soybeans are SANE. But it does not make sense to call something that is mostly fat or carbohydrate a good source of protein. Pretty good is reasonable though.

The Three Pretty Good Sources of Protein

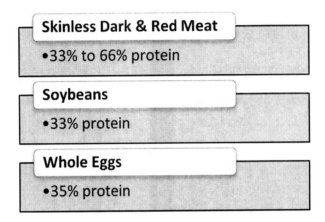

Skinless Dark & Red Meat
- 33% to 66% protein

Soybeans
- 33% protein

Whole Eggs
- 35% protein

Everything else is not even close to being a good source of protein. Dairy products other than the cottage cheese and *plain Greek* yogurt are mostly fat and sugar. Beans are mostly carbohydrate. Nuts are mostly fat. Again, being mostly fat or carbohydrate does not necessarily make these foods inSANE. However, they cannot be called good sources of protein.[16]

What is the other part of a natural, balanced protein plan? Is it the word dreaded by all people wishing to banish body fat? Yes, the remaining part of the diet which kept our ancestors healthy and slim for millions of years is fat. Chapter 25 recaps the facts.

CHAPTER 25

A Natural Balanced Amount of Fat

"Simply lowering the percentage of energy from total fat in the diet is unlikely to...reduce coronary heart disease incidence."
F.B. Hu, Harvard University[1]

Overcoming the fear of eating fat is critical to eating a natural, balanced ratio of nutrients. We should never again skip SANE sirloin steak and non-starchy vegetables in favor of inSANE whole wheat spaghetti with whole wheat garlic bread. Fat is delicious, Satisfying, unAggressive, and impossible to overeat unless combined with starch or sweeteners. That is why most people end up losing weight on low-carbohydrate, high-fat diets like *Atkins*. Basically, any diet that discourages dietary fat encourages weight gain.[2]

You and I have already reviewed the research disproving that foods that contain fat are fattening, but let's quickly recap. If we set aside the myths we've been told for the past forty years, there is no reason to think that fat is bad for us. Natural foods contain fat. Natural foods were the only thing our ancestors ate for 99.8% of our evolution. How could the only foods available to us for 99.8% of our evolution harm us? If anything, we must have evolved to thrive on foods that contain fats. Furthermore, the *theory* that fat is fattening has never been proven, despite over a billion dollars worth of research attempting to do so. Ironically, researchers *have* proven that unsaturated fats help burn body fat.

Finally, a decline in the proportion of fat in our diet has been accompanied by the largest spike in obesity and disease rates in history.[3]

A great many scientific studies show that worrying about eating fat is at best a distraction, and at worst harmful and fattening. Consider the research done just at Harvard Medical School:[4]

- "The emphasis on total fat reduction has been a serious distraction in efforts to control obesity and improve health in general."
- "Within the United States, a substantial decline in the percentage of energy from fat during the last two decades has corresponded with a massive increase in the prevalence of obesity. Diets high in fat do not appear to be the primary cause of the high prevalence of excess body fat in our society, and reductions in fat will not be a solution."
- "Among European countries, no association was observed between the national percentage of energy from fat and median body mass index in men...a clear inverse relation was observed in women."
- "Limiting unsaturated fats, which is usually done by increasing carbohydrate... is detrimental. This is consistent with metabolic studies indicating that replacing unsaturated fats with carbohydrate increases triacylglycerol and decreases HDL cholesterol. Furthermore, low-fat, high-carbohydrate diets provide a higher glycemic load, aggravate hyperinsulinemia [clogging], and may thus increase the risk of diabetes and coronary artery disease."
- "Studies and...trials have provided strong evidence that a higher intake of [omega-3] fatty acids from fish or plant sources lowers risk of coronary heart disease."

Chapter 26 shows you how to eat SANE, natural, not necessarily fat-free foods, while feeling more satisfied and energized than ever.

Five Steps to Eating More–Smarter

"Moderate replacement of dietary carbohydrate with low-fat, high-protein foods in a diet containing a conventional level of fat significantly improved...cardiovascular risk profiles in healthy...subjects."
B.M. WOLFE, UNIVERSITY OF WESTERN ONTARIO[1]

Acommon assumption is that switching over to a healthier lifestyle means spending a lot more money and time on food. That's not true, at least not the way the eat more—smarter—program works. It focuses on enabling you to eat more SANE food while spending as little time and money as possible. While growing your own vegetables and buying organic food is great, I am going to assume that spending any more than twenty minutes and $10 on food per day is not practical. Eating more—smarter—is based on general principles that work in real life.

Also keep in mind that obesity has been linked to a long list of ailments:[2]

- Depression
- Discrimination
- Osteoarthritis
- Rheumatoid Arthritis
- Birth Defects
- Breast Cancer
- Cancer of the Esophagus
- Colorectal Cancer
- Renal Cell Cancer
- Cardiovascular Disease
- Impaired Respiratory Function
- Carpal Tunnel Syndrome
- Chronic Venous Insufficiency
- Daytime Sleepiness
- Deep Vein Thrombosis
- Type 2 Diabetes
- Gallbladder Disease
- Gout
- Heart Disorders
- Hypertension
- Impaired Immune Response
- Infections
- Infertility
- Liver Disease
- Low Back Pain
- Obstetric and Gynecologic Complications
- Chronic Pain
- Pancreatitis
- Sleep Apnea
- Stroke
- Surgical Complications
- Urinary Stress Incontinence

Philip A. Wood at the University of Alabama at Birmingham states plainly "that obesity increases risks of disease as much as 20 years of aging does." With excess body fat linked to such major problems, there's no need to worry about minor dietary issues before we've switched from inSANE food to SANE food. As researcher John Yudkin from the University of London puts it: "There is no point in worrying about imaginary dangers. If you do, you will be likely to go on overlooking the real dangers."[3]

A good example of this principle is artificial sweeteners. Has a typical intake of artificial sweeteners been proven to be fattening? No. Has a typical intake of sugar and high-fructose corn syrup been proven to be fattening? Yes. If you crave sweets, do not worry about replacing sugar and high-fructose corn syrup with artificial sweeteners. Of course, eliminating all sweeteners would be ideal. But there is no need to worry about the *possible* negative effects of artificial sweeteners before you've freed yourself from the *proven* negative effects of actual sweeteners.

The Five Steps to Eating More—Smarter

These steps are designed to help you develop excellent health along with a world-class physique. If your goals are more modest, then you don't need to follow these rules precisely. Do what works for you. The key is letting the scientific facts guide you to make sure that you accomplish your goals as efficiently as possible.

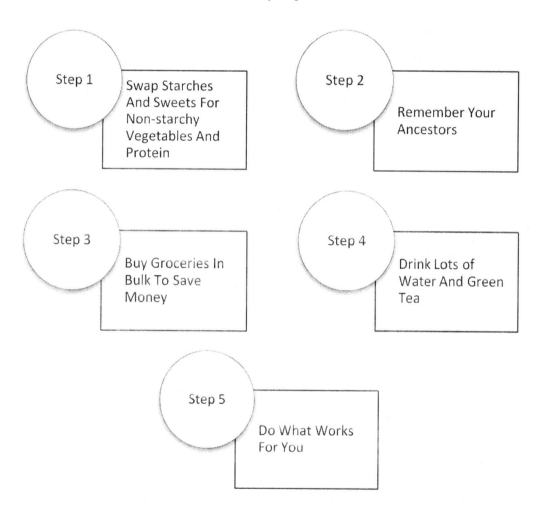

Step 1 — Swap Starches And Sweets For Non-starchy Vegetables And Protein

Step 2 — Remember Your Ancestors

Step 3 — Buy Groceries In Bulk To Save Money

Step 4 — Drink Lots of Water And Green Tea

Step 5 — Do What Works For You

Step 1: Eat So Many Non-Starchy Vegetables and So Much Protein That You Are Too Full for Starches and Sweets

If it is a non-starchy vegetable, overeat it. I am talking ten or more servings of non-starchy vegetables per day (lists of non-starchy vegetables, protein, fruits, nuts, and seeds are coming up in a few pages).

While it is absolutely not required, eating ten or more servings of non-starchy vegetables per day is easier if you use a blender to make vegetable and fruit smoothies. Don't use a juicer. It removes fiber and healthy nutrients. Use a blender and mix a lot of any green vegetable with fresh or frozen berries or oranges. Add some vanilla-flavored whey protein powder, cinnamon, and vanilla extract, and the smoothie is quite tasty.

If fresh non-starchy vegetables are not available, frozen ones are fine. Wheat grass and other powdered green "super foods" are convenient but taste bad. If you can tolerate wheat-grass-like powders, I recommend buying them in bulk online (I use znaturalfoods.com). The finer the consistency of the powder, the easier it is to mix and drink. Get the finest powder you can find.

Avoid canned vegetables and canned fruits if at all possible. Focus on fresh or frozen, deeply colored, non-starchy vegetables that grow above ground. When it comes to fruits, focus on berries and citrus. They are the most SANE options.

When it comes to protein, the most effective (body fat-burning) way to eat enough protein is to divide your protein intake into at least five 30-gram servings evenly spaced throughout the day. Fortunately, this is easy. Here is one way to do it.

- **Step 1.** Add eight egg whites to breakfast. Scramble them. Microwave them. Whatever. This shot of pure protein jump starts your fat metabolism system and sets you up to burn body fat all day. A whey protein shake also works. Make sure the shake has less than ten grams of sugar in it, and at least thirty grams of protein in it. Prep time: five minutes.

- **Step 2:** Drink a whey protein shake between breakfast and lunch. Same sugar and protein recommendation as above. Prep time: five minutes.

- **Step 3:** Eat a double portion of protein along with a triple serving of non-starchy vegetables for lunch. Prep time: no additional time. You have to do something for lunch anyway.

- **Step 4:** Drink another whey protein shake between lunch and dinner. Same sugar and protein recommendation as above. Prep time: five minutes.

- **Step 5:** Eat a double portion of protein along with a triple serving of non-starchy vegetables for dinner. Prep time: no additional time. You have to do something for dinner anyway.

Total Prep Time = Fifteen minutes
Total Positive Impact = Dramatic

If you enjoy the convenience of whey protein powders, I recommend getting sample packets online or at a local supplement store until you find one that you like. Good supplement stores give out sample packets of whey protein for free. If they do not, they are likely shady and I recommend going to a different supplement store. When you find one you like, buy it in bulk online. I use vitaglo.com, Amazon.com, or supplementwarehouse.com.

Other inexpensive and convenient forms of protein are canned tuna, canned salmon, egg whites, frozen salmon burgers, frozen turkey burgers, fat-free or low-fat cottage cheese, fat-free or low-fat *plain Greek* yogurt, and canned chicken. When it comes to seafood and meat, canned is fine. I am not a fan of what canning does to the taste of the food, but it is less expensive and more convenient.

Putting these recommendations all together, the first step to eating more—smarter—is as simple as doubling the amount of seafood, lean meat, eggs (eat three egg whites for every whole egg), fat-free or low-fat cottage cheese, or fat-free or low-fat *plain Greek* yogurt, and tripling the amount of non-starchy vegetables that you would typically eat at each meal. This guarantees you will be too full for starch or sweets while never leaving the table feeling deprived.

When eating a double serving of protein and a triple serving of non-starchy vegetables is not practical, mix a scoop or two of whey protein and some milled flax seeds with water and drink it before the meal. Blend it with some ice if it is convenient.

Of course nobody can do this all the time, but the more non-starchy vegetables and protein that you eat in place of starches and sweets, the healthier you will be and the more body fat you will burn.

"Cutting back on carbohydrates [specifically starches and sweets] and replacing those calories with protein lowers the levels of triglycerides that increase the risk of heart disease and also boosts HDL, the protective form of cholesterol."
W.C. WILLETT, HARVARD UNIVERSITY[4]

"Diets with increased protein have now been shown to improve adult health with benefits for treatment or prevention of obesity, osteoporosis, type 2 diabetes, Metabolic Syndrome, heart disease."
D.K. LAYMAN, UNIVERSITY OF ILLINOIS[5]

Step 2: Remember Your Ancestors

Unless hunters and gatherers hunted or gathered it, we are not designed to digest it and it will create a clog. If anything other than cooking or blending is required between the plant or animal and your stomach, then it does not belong in your stomach to begin with.

Here is a quick quiz to illustrate this rule. Circle how we get the foods listed. The answers are in the next footnote.

The "Is It Actually Natural" Quiz[1]

Food	How Humans Get It		
Fruit	Process/Manufacture	Gather	Hunt
Bread	Process/Manufacture	Gather	Hunt
Rice	Process/Manufacture	Gather	Hunt
Vegetables	Process/Manufacture	Gather	Hunt
Seafood	Process/Manufacture	Gather	Hunt
Meat	Process/Manufacture	Gather	Hunt
Nuts	Process/Manufacture	Gather	Hunt
Flax Seeds	Process/Manufacture	Gather	Hunt
Pasta	Process/Manufacture	Gather	Hunt
Sweets	Process/Manufacture	Gather	Hunt
Cereal	Process/Manufacture	Gather	Hunt
Eggs	Process/Manufacture	Gather	Hunt

The exceptions to this rule are whey protein powder, fat-free or low-fat cottage cheese, fat-free or low-fat *plain Greek* yogurt, and starchy vegetables. Whey and select dairy are SANE, so enjoy them even though they were not available to our hunter-gatherer ancestors. On the other hand, even though starchy "vegetables" such as potatoes and corn were available to our ancestors, these foods should be avoided.[2]

One more note about "processing." The only kinds of "processing" which do not cause clogs are freezing, cooking, canning (for meat and seafood only), and grinding/blending. There is nothing wrong with frozen vegetables, frozen fruit, canned tuna, salmon, or chicken, and ground meats. Pre-cooked and canned seafood and meat are also fine, but precooked or canned vegetables and fruits should be avoided unless they are your only option.

When in doubt, look at the ingredient list. If it is more than three items long—excluding spices—or contains anything that could not be hunted or gathered, then it is inSANE.

---

1 Fruit—Gather. Bread—Process/Manufacture. Rice—Process/Manufacture. Vegetables—Gather. Seafood—Hunt. Meat—Hunt. Nuts—Gather. Flax Seeds—Gather. Pasta—Process/Manufacture. Sweets—Process/Manufacture. Cereal—Process/Manufacture. Eggs—Gather.

2 One or two servings of sweet potatoes per week is fine.

For instance, Costco sells these wonderful frozen salmon and turkey burgers. The ingredients are basically salmon or turkey along with some seasoning. That is good food. I grill a bunch every few days and take them to work since they are excellent "desk food." Costco also sells fish sticks and chicken nuggets with ingredient lists about as long as this paragraph and chocked full of unnatural substances. Those are not good.

Step 3: Buy Groceries in Bulk to Save Money

A great way to affordably eat a lot of high-quality food is to buy it at bulk wholesalers like Costco or Sam's Club whenever possible. By buying in bulk, you will be able to eat more higher-quality food while spending about $10 per day on food. That is a great deal.

Here is the actual grocery list my wife and I take to Costco every *other* week. That is the other nice thing about buying in bulk. It dramatically reduces the amount of time you have to spend grocery shopping.

Non-Starchy Vegetables
- 2 bulk packages of mushrooms
- 3 bulk packages of red peppers
- 1 bulk package of all natural tomato sauce
- 5 bulk packages of romaine lettuce
- 5 bulk packages of spinach
- 2 bulk packages of frozen mixed vegetables
- 2 bulk packages of frozen green beans
- 1 bulk package of celery
- 2 bulk packages of sugar snap peas
- 1 bulk package of carrots

Seafood
- 2 bulk packages of salmon
- 1 bulk package of canned tuna
- 1 bulk package of salmon burgers

Meat/Eggs
- 1 rotisserie chicken
- 1 bulk package of eggs
- 1 bulk package of ham steaks
- 1 bulk package of turkey burgers
- 1 bulk package of ground turkey

Fruit
- 1 bulk package of grapefruit
- 1 bulk package of oranges
- 3 bulk packages of frozen blueberries
- 3 bulk packages of frozen mixed berries
- 1 bulk package of frozen strawberries

Nuts/Seeds
- 1 bulk package of mixed nuts
- 1 bulk tub of natural peanut butter
- 1 bulk tub of soy nuts
- 2 pounds of milled flax seeds (ordered online)

Other
- 1 bulk package of 2% fat cottage cheese
- 1 bulk package of unsweetened cocoa powder
- 1 bulk package of black beans
- 1 bulk package of fat-free or low-fat *plain* Greek yogurt

This is a lot of food. Fortunately, it only costs about $10 per person, per day, and we do not need to buy all of it every time we go to the store.

Step 4: Drink Lots of Water and Green Tea

Studies show that the more water we drink, the more body fat we burn. More water decreases the concentration of various substances in our blood, which consequently increases our *ability* to burn body fat. Additionally, more cold water increases our *need* to burn body fat. Studies show we burn about two calories for every ounce of cold water we drink.[6]

> *"...increases in drinking water were associated with significant loss of body weight and fat over time..."*
> **J.D. Stookey, Children's Hospital Oakland Research Institute** [7]

Water is all good. Eight glasses of water a day is required to burn body fat effectively. More is better. If your urine is not clear, if you are ever thirsty, or if you have room to drink things other than water—or green tea—then you could be slimmer and healthier by drinking more water.

The easiest way to drink an optimal amount of water is to fill up a gallon jug in the morning and to make sure it is empty two hours before you go to bed. Another great way to boost your water intake is to fall in love with green tea—the only beverage as beneficial as water.

Green tea comes from the same plant as black tea (the tea most common in the U.S. and Europe) but it is processed differently. Its unique processing leaves green tea with a large amount of a substance called polyphenols—especially ECGC (*epigallocatechin gallate*). From a health perspective, the polyphenols in green tea have been shown to help prevent:

- Weight Gain
- Cancer
- Hypertension
- Cardiovascular Disease
- Dental Issues
- Insulin Resistance

- Virus Infections
- Bone Issues
- Parkinson's Disease
- Alzheimer's Disease
- Kidney Stones
- Eye Issues

- Atherosclerosis
- Low HDL Cholesterol
- Inflammatory Bowel Disease
- Diabetes
- Liver Disease
- Bacterial Issues[8]

The body fat burned by green tea well outweighs the body-fat-burning effects of the small amount of caffeine in it (which is one-fifth the caffeine in a cup of coffee). Researchers suspect green tea's unique body fat burning effect has to do with the interaction of green tea's polyphenols, caffeine, and the hormone noradrenaline. To maximize all the benefits green tea has to offer, drink *ten* bags worth of it per day.[9]

Now you may be thinking, "Ten bags of green tea on top of all that water? I am going to spend all day in the bathroom, be really jittery, and will not have any money left. Isn't that too much fluid, too much caffeine, and too much money?" Luckily, this is not an either/or proposition:

- **Hydration**: All the green tea we drink counts toward our water goals. If you drink ten eight-ounce cups of green tea, that counts as ten eight-ounce cups of water. Also, you can brew a lot of green tea in a little water. For example, I brew eight bags of green tea at a time in eight ounces of water. I let it sit for a few minutes, add ice, and drink it through a straw—key for keeping teeth white. Do that once in the morning and once in the afternoon, and you are good to go.
- **Caffeine**: Decaf green tea is as healthy and helpful as regular green tea. If you crave caffeine like me, a bag of regular green tea only contains 30 milligrams of caffeine, and up to 300 milligrams of caffeine per day is harmless. Ten bags of green tea per day gives us 300 milligrams of caffeine per day.[10]

8 oz. Unless Otherwise Noted	Caffeine (mg)
1 Max Strength Nodoz Pill	200
Brewed Coffee	150
One Bag Black Tea	80
Monster Energy Drink	80
Rockstar Energy Drink	80
1.5 oz. Espresso	77
Red Bull Energy Drink	76
Full Throttle Energy Drink	72
One Bag Green Tea	30
Decaffeinated Coffee	7
One Bag Decaf Green Tea	3

11

- **Overspending**: It is cheap and easy to buy regular or decaf green tea in bulk. I have Amazon.com ship a bulk container of green tea to me automatically every month for $0.08 per bag—including shipping and handling.[3] That is less than a dollar a day to get all the benefits green tea has to offer. The monthly delivery part is also good because the fresher the green tea, the better it is for us.[12]

Also keep in mind that there is a big difference between drinking tea for enjoyment and drinking green tea for health. Tea is like wine. Just as there is $5 wine and $500 wine, there is $0.08 green tea and $8.00 green tea. If you already enjoy more expensive tea, keep it up and add drinking at least ten bags of less expensive green tea to your day.

If you do not like green tea hot, add ice and drink it cold. If you do not like caffeine, drink decaf. If you do not want to stain your teeth, drink it through a straw. If you do not like the taste, add some lemon juice or drink it with something SANE you do like. And stick to sipping green tea instead of swallowing green tea supplements. Studies show that most green tea supplements are not as good for us as natural green tea.[13]

---

3 Search Amazon for "Bigelow Decaffeinated Green Tea, 40-Count Boxes (Pack of 6)" and sign-up for their "Subscribe & Save" service.

Finally, drinking more water and green tea makes it easier to avoid drinking inSANE calories. The easiest way to create a clog is to drink inSANE calories. If it is not water, green tea, or something else calorie-free—aka coffee without cream or sugar—or something you personally blended from SANE foods—drinking it will destroy the fat metabolism system fast and furiously.[14]

Calories Drank Per Person Per Day in the USA[15]

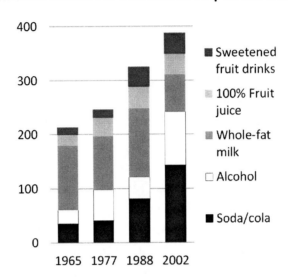

"*The average American today gets more than 450 calories a day from beverages...beverages provide twice as many calories today as they did in 1965....*"

ROBERT PAARLBERG, HARVARD UNIVERSITY[16]

Step 5: Do What Works for You

It is perfectly reasonable to reach this point and say, "I cannot do *all* of that" or "I do not want to do *all* of that." No problem. Eating smarter does not mean being perfect. You merely need to be armed with the information necessary to look and feel good. You can apply as much or a little of it as you like, depending on how much body fat you want to lose and how much better you want to feel.

What most people find is that they start doing the basics outlined here—swap as many starches and sweets as possible for non-starchy vegetables and protein—love the results, and then want to go further.

Here is a handy table to guide you to your specific fat loss goal.

How to Achieve Your Fat Loss Goal[17]

How to Become Obese	• Only eat at least thirty grams of protein with dinner • Eat mostly starch and sweets • Eat dessert all the time • Eat unlimited low-quality food all the time Which amounts to eating this daily: • 10+ servings of starch or sweets • 0-1 thirty gram servings of protein • 0-1 servings of non-starchy vegetables • 0 servings of berries or citrus fruits Do not exercise.
How to Become Overweight	• Eat at least thirty grams of protein with lunch and dinner • Trade starch and sweets for protein and non-starchy vegetables at most dinners • Get too full for dessert sometimes • Eat unlimited low-quality food twice a week Which amounts to eating this daily: • 8 servings of starch or sweets • 2 thirty gram servings of protein • 2 servings of non-starchy vegetables • 1 serving of berries or citrus fruits Do not exercise.
How to Become Typical	• Eat at least thirty grams of protein with breakfast, lunch, and dinner • Trade starch and sweets for protein and non-starchy vegetables at dinner • Get too full for dessert at more than half of your meals • Eat unlimited low-quality food twice a week Which amounts to eating this daily: • 4 servings of starch or sweets • 3 thirty gram servings of protein • 4 servings of non-starchy vegetables • 2 servings of berries or citrus fruits Exercise traditionally.

How to Become Fit	• Eat at least thirty grams of protein with breakfast, lunch, dinner, and two hours before dinner • Trade starch and sweets for protein and non-starchy vegetables at lunch and dinner • Get too full for dessert most of the time • Eat unlimited low-quality food once a week Which amounts to eating this daily: • 2 servings of starch or sweets • 4 thirty gram servings of protein • 7 servings of non-starchy vegetables • 3 servings of berries or citrus fruits • 1 quarter cup of milled flax seeds Exercise less—smarter.
How to Become Hot	• Eat at least thirty grams of protein every four hours • Almost always trade starch and sweets for protein and non-starchy vegetables • Almost always be too full for dessert • Eat unlimited low-quality food twice a month Which amounts to eating this daily: • 1 serving of starch or sweets • 5 thirty gram servings of protein • 9 servings of non-starchy vegetables • 4 servings of berries or citrus fruits • 1 quarter cup of milled flax seeds Exercise less—smarter.
How to Become a Fitness Model	• Eat at least thirty grams of protein every three hours • Always trade starch and sweets for protein and non-starchy vegetables • Almost always be too full for dessert • Eat unlimited low-quality food once a month Which amounts to eating this daily: • 0 servings of starch or sweets • 6 thirty gram servings of protein • 12 servings of non-starchy vegetables • 5 servings of berries or citrus fruits • 1.5 quarter cups of milled flax seeds Exercise less—smarter.

Before we turn to exercising less—smarter—here are some SANE food lists to help you achieve your specific fat loss goal as deliciously as possible.

Non-Starchy Vegetables (10+ servings per day)[18]

- Alfalfa Sprouts
- Artichoke
- Arugula
- Asparagus
- Avocado
- Bean Sprouts
- Beets
- Bell Peppers
- Bok Choy
- Broccoflower
- Broccoli
- Brussels Sprouts
- Cabbage
- Carrots
- Cauliflower
- Celery
- Chard
- Chives
- Collards
- Cucumber
- Dandelion Greens
- Eggplant
- Endive
- Escarole
- Garlic
- Green Beans
- Kale
- Leaf Amaranth
- Leeks
- Lemon Grass
- Mixed greens
- Mushrooms
- Mustard Greens
- Onion
- Parsley
- Peas
- Peppers
- Pumpkin
- Romaine Lettuce
- Sauerkraut
- Shallot
- Snow Peas
- Spinach
- Squash
- Sugar Snap Peas
- Tomatoes
- Turnip Greens
- Zucchini

Protein (5+ servings per day)[19]

- Bison
- Catfish
- Chicken
- Clams
- Cod
- Cornish Hen
- Crab
- Croaker
- Egg Whites
- Eggs
- Elk
- Extra Lean Beef
- Eye of Round
- Fat Free or Low Fat Cottage Cheese
- Fat-Free or Low-Fat Plain Greek Yogurt
- Flank Steak
- Flounder
- Haddock
- Halibut
- Ham
- Herring
- Lamb
- Lobster
- Mackerel
- Mahi Mahi
- Mussels
- Octopus
- Oysters
- Perch
- Pollock
- Pork
- Rabbit
- Rump Roast
- Salmon
- Sardines (& Anchovies)
- Scallops
- Sea Bass
- Shad
- Shrimp
- Sirloin Steak
- Sirloin Tip
- Snapper
- Sole
- Soy Protein Powder
- Soybeans
- Squid (Calamari)
- Swordfish
- Tenderloin
- Tilapia
- Tofu
- Top Loin
- Top Round
- Trout
- Tuna
- Turkey
- Venison
- Whey Protein Powder
- Whitefish

Fruits (4+ servings per day)

- Apricots
- Avocado
- Blackberries
- Blueberries
- Cantaloupe
- Cherries
- Grapefruit

- Guava
- Honeydew Melon
- Kiwifruit
- Mango
- Orange
- Papaya
- Peaches

- Pear
- Pineapple
- Plums
- Raspberries
- Strawberries
- Tangerine
- Watermelon[20]

Nuts and Seeds (4+ servings per day)

- Almonds
- Brazil Nuts
- Cashews
- Chestnuts
- Chia Seeds
- Hazelnuts

- Hemp Seeds
- Kola Nut
- Macadamia Nuts
- Milled Flax Seeds
- Peanuts
- Pecans

- Pistachios
- Pumpkin Seeds
- Sesame Seeds
- Squash Seeds
- Sunflower Seeds
- Walnuts[21]

• • •

That is how to make eating more—smarter—inexpensive and easy. If this part of the program sounds promising, just wait till part 7 when we review the research on exercising less—smarter.

While we already know that the key to long-term body-fat burning is unclogging, and that the key to unclogging is healing our hormones, what we are about to cover is that the most potent prescription to heal our hormones is high-quality exercise. A little high-quality exercise clears clogs more effectively than a lot of traditional exercise thanks to its extreme potency. Let's find out how to make it work for you.

What About Cultures Whose Diets Revolve Around Rice?

"Attempting to get at truth means rejecting stereotypes and clichés."
HAROLD EVANS, JOURNALIST

At some point you will be talking about the solution to our fat-loss struggles and someone will say: "What about cultures whose diets revolve around rice? If starch is fattening, why aren't these cultures the heaviest in the world?"

Here is what I say: "If a rice-centric diet is working for a culture, that is great. But a starch-centric diet is not working for us, so why not try a more SANE approach?"[4]

You could also use some statistics to spin their stereotype around. Specifically, the top rice- and grain-producing cultures in the world are China, the United States of America, and India. Rank those cultures by starch produced per person and you get:

Starch Centric Cultures

Thousands of Tons of Cereal Produced Divided by Millions of Residents

Now add in data from the Food and Agriculture Organization of the United Nations, and you'll find the amount of starch in the average Chinese or Indian diet is lower than the amount of starch in the average American diet.[22]

I would also mention how anecdotal cultural comparisons gloss over all sorts of factors. For example, the average person in America has six times the income of the average person in China and fourteen times the income of the average person in India. Hundreds of millions of people being too poor to afford anything other than a cup or two of rice a day may play a large role in these countries' lower obesity rates.[23]

Bottom line: Clichés confuse the issue. "Countries around Asia are starch-centric and slim" is a cliché. The countries American Samoa, Kiribati, and French Polynesia are the first, second, and third heaviest countries in the world.[24]

Encourage the uninformed to skip stereotypes and to stick with science.

4 And that is a big "if." About 200,000,000 people in China are overweight.

PART 7

Solution: Exercise Less–Smarter™

"About almost any subject, there are the facts 'everyone knows' and then there are the real ones."
ERNEST G. ROSS

CHAPTER 27

How to Exercise Less—Smarter

"We thought the findings [regarding exercising less—smarter] were star-tling because it suggests the overall volume of exercise people need to do is lower than what's recommended."
M. GIBALA, MCMASTER UNIVERSITY[1]

Traditional fat-loss programs require five to ten hours of exercise per week. This re-quirement alone accounts for much of their 95% failure rate. Who has that much spare time?

Fortunately, scientists have discovered a smarter alternative: a form of high-quality exer-cise that unclogs us in just ten to twenty minutes per week.

Let's quickly compare traditional exercise with this higher-quality alternative. Tradition-al exercise is rooted in the false *Calories In—Calories Out* theory of fat loss. It aims to burn calories and is done frequently, for a long time, and uses a little resistance. On the other hand, high-quality exercise is rooted in the science of the set-point. It aims to clear our hormonal clog and is done infrequently, for a short period of time, and uses a lot of resistance. This unique approach to exercise has been proven not only to heal our hor-mones, but also to give us all the benefits of traditional exercise—and then some—320% more efficiently.[2]

<table>
<tr><th>Traditional Exercise</th><th>High-Quality Exercise</th></tr>
</table>

☐ Done Frequently   ☐ Done Infrequently

☐ Done For A Long Period Of Time   ☐ Done For A Short Period Of Time

☐ Done With A Little Resistance   ☐ Done With A Lot Of Resistance

High-quality exercise is a smarter and more productive way to think about exercise. But before getting into the details, it is important to address a common fear: that using the amount of resistance required to increase the quality of exercise makes women look like men and men look like bulldogs. The best way to address the fear of using more resistance during exercise is to understand your body. Everyone has a gene called GDF-8, and it controls a substance called myostatin, which controls the amount of muscle we have and how much it develops naturally. The base levels of myostatin and muscle in basically all women and most men make it impossible for them to naturally build *bulky* muscles. It does not matter how much resistance we use. The majority of us—especially women—do not have the genes to build bulky muscles using any form of exercise.[3]

> "*Gradually, weight lifting [resistance training] changed the way I looked. The alteration was not dramatic, but I loved it. My back became broader, which makes my hips look smaller; my arms and legs are firmer and more shapely. I never grew big muscles, but they are defined; you can see their outlines. I feel different, too, more confident of my body's strength and of my ability to do almost any movement in daily life with little effort.*"
> GINA KOLATA, REPORTER FOR *THE NEW YORK TIMES*[4]

It is useful to think about muscle size as being much like muscle speed. Few people are fast because few people have "fast genes." No matter how much most people run, they will never get faster than their genes allow. However, if people do have the genes for speed, they will naturally be faster than most people without ever training. Similarly, few people can become bulky because few people—particularly women—have "bulky genes."

No matter how much most people resistance train, they will never develop more muscle than their genes allow them to.

When people say, "I do more repetitions with less weight because I do not want big muscles," they have a point...it is just the wrong point. Not only will doing all those low-quality repetitions prevent them from getting big muscles, it will prevent them from getting any substantial benefit from their exercise.

The point of exercise is to work the most muscle possible so that the most clog-clearing hormones get released (see chapter 28 and chapter 29). The less force an exercise requires, the less muscle it works. Combine this with the fact that it is impossible to naturally develop bulky muscles, unless you were born with bulky muscles, and you can see why doing a lot of reps with a little weight isn't optimal. In an effort to avoid something which will not happen anyway, high-reps, low-weight exercisers doom themselves to poor results.

> *"Women have been sold a myth of becoming big. They do not have the genetics."*
> **WILLIAM KRAEMER, EDITOR OF THE *JOURNAL OF STRENGTH AND CONDITIONING RESEARCH*[5]**

One last point to help us overcome any remaining fear of resistance training. Beyond being hard to develop, muscle tissue is small. This is why trainers will tell you, "Muscle weighs more than body fat." While muscle does not in fact weigh more than body fat, muscle does take up less space. This is why most female fitness models are about 5'6" and weigh 140 pounds. People look at them, and judging by their size, think they weigh 110 pounds. They do not. See those defined legs? That is quite a bit of muscle tissue taking up a little space, while clearing out quite a bit of clog.[6]

With our fears replaced with facts, let's move on to the specifics of high-quality exercise.

The Five Principles of High-Quality Exercise

In the same way we use SANE calories to increase the quality of our diet, we use deep, hormonal, infrequent, eccentric, and brief movements to increase the quality of our exercise.

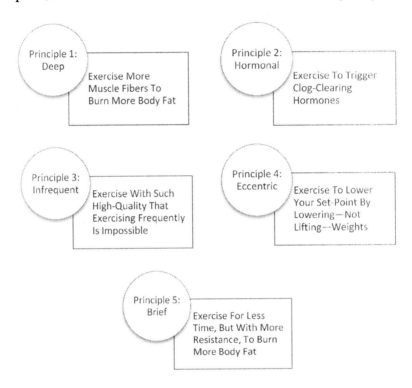

Principle 1: Deep — Exercise More Muscle Fibers To Burn More Body Fat

Principle 2: Hormonal — Exercise To Trigger Clog-Clearing Hormones

Principle 3: Infrequent — Exercise With Such High-Quality That Exercising Frequently Is Impossible

Principle 4: Eccentric — Exercise To Lower Your Set-Point By Lowering—Not Lifting—Weights

Principle 5: Brief — Exercise For Less Time, But With More Resistance, To Burn More Body Fat

Like all the advice in the book, this form of exercise is based on scientific findings. For example, Y. Izumiya of Boston University studied mice in a clinical setting and learned that development of the specific type of muscle fibers targeted by high-quality exercise "can regress obesity and resolve metabolic disorders in obese mice." The researcher then described how these muscle fibers cleared hormonal clogs by improving "insulin sensitivity and [causing] reductions in blood glucose, insulin, and leptin levels." Most encouraging, Dr. Izumiya noted: "These effects occurred despite a *reduction* in physical activity."[7]

High-quality exercise is the key to exercising less—*smarter*. Let's dig into the first principle.

CHAPTER 28

Deep—Exercise More Muscle Fibers to Burn More Body Fat

"These findings indicate that type II muscle [Deep muscle fiber] has a previously unappreciated role in regulating whole-body metabolism [un-clogging].... These data also suggest that strength training [resistance training]...may be of particular benefit to overweight individuals."
Y. IZUMIYA, BOSTON UNIVERSITY[1]

Why do people bike to burn body fat instead of drawing pictures of bikes to burn body fat? After all, both activities exercise muscles. They bike because of the *amount* of muscles it exercises. Riding bikes exercises a lot of muscle (the large leg muscles) while drawing bikes works a little muscle (the small hand muscles). The more muscle exercised, the better our results. Obvious, you say.

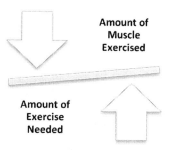

209

Here is what is not so obvious. Just as we get more results in less time by working more muscles within our body, we get even more results in even less time by working more of the muscle fibers which make up our muscles.

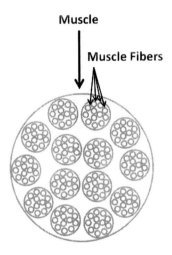

In addition to going broader—working more muscle—we can also go Deeper—working more muscle fibers.

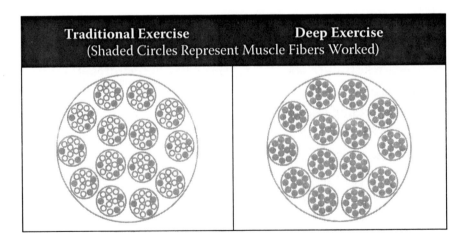

Just as working more muscle generates better results in less time, working more muscle fibers within more muscles generates even better results in even less time. That is why studies show that high-quality Deep exercise clears clogs and burns fat in only ten to twenty minutes per week. That's the kind of exercise regime that can fit into anybody's schedule.

Exercising More Muscle Fibers Burns More Body Fat Faster

The Deep principle is as simple as it gets. The physiology of our muscle fibers, and how exercising *less*—but Deeper—works more of them, is complicated, but the basic concept is easy once you understand three basic principles of how our muscles function:

1. We have different types of muscle fibers that do different things.
2. The Deeper the muscle fiber, the more force it generates and the less endurance it has.
3. Working our Deepest muscle fibers works all of our other muscle fibers.

Just as we have different muscles to do different things, we have different muscle fibers to do different things. Type 1 fibers on the surface of our muscles generate a little force for many hours. They keep us walking around all day. Type 2b fibers buried deep within our muscles generate a lot of force for a few seconds. They enable us to lift furniture briefly.

	Little Force for a Long Time
Shallow	Type 1 Fibers
	Type 2a Fibers
	Type 2x Fibers
Deep	Type 2b Fibers
	Lots of Force for Little Time

The great advantage of exercising Deeply is that when you and I work our Deepest muscle fibers, we automatically work the rest of them. Why does it work that way? If we ask our body to move something, our muscles first try to generate enough force with our shallow Type 1 fibers. If those do not generate enough force, our muscles dig Deeper and get our more forceful Type 2a fibers to help. Still not enough? Bring out the stronger Type 2x fibers. More? Here come our most powerful Type 2b fibers.

This *orderly recruitment* of muscle fibers means it is impossible for us to work our Deepest Type 2b fibers without working all of our muscle fibers. This aspect of our physiology

211

makes exercise simpler because now we know how to work more muscle fibers. We focus on activities that require enough force to exercise our Deepest—most forceful—fibers. It also happens to flip how we think about exercising to burn body fat on its head.[2]

The more force a muscle fiber generates, the more energy it uses. Similarly, the more muscle fibers exercised, the more energy used. Put these together and you can see why any exercise working our Deepest fibers—and therefore all of our muscle fibers—cannot be done for long. I am talking seconds. Not minutes. And definitely not hours. Activities such as jogging fire only a few of our least forceful fibers and therefore use so little energy that we can keep them up for hours. On the other hand, activities such as forceful resistance training fire all our fibers and use so much energy that we can only keep them up for seconds. The more muscle we use, the faster our energy runs out, and the less we can exercise.

How the Physiology of Our Muscle Fiber
Flips Exercising to Burn Body Fat on Its Head

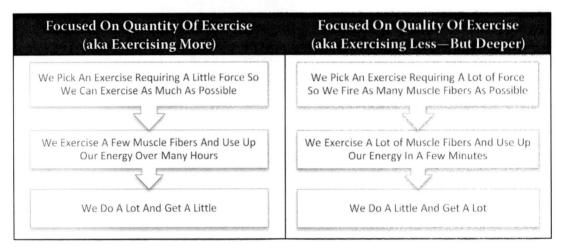

Once we understand how our muscles work, why exercise more? That requires exercising less forcefully, working less muscle, and getting worse results. Shouldn't we exercise less—but more forcefully—so we work more muscle and get better results?

Yes.

R.N. Carpinelli at Adelphi University says, "There is little scientific evidence, and no theoretical physiological basis, to suggest that a greater volume [quantity] of exercise elicits greater increases in strength or hypertrophy [results]."[3]

So why are we told to work less muscle fibers for a longer time? More exercise time means more profits. More exercise equipment, more personal training sessions, more aerobics classes, more gym memberships, more overeating after we exercise, more supplements to get us through the exercise, more medical care to take care of the injuries we get while exercising, and on and on. More exercise is better for the food, fitness, and pharmaceutical industries, but worse for us.

Enough with worrying about increasing the *quantity* of exercise we are getting, so that others increase the quantity of money they are making. Let's focus instead on increasing the *quality* of exercise we are getting by exercising less, but more forcefully. By exercising more muscle fibers. By exercising Deeper.[4]

> **Important Note:** Exercising Deeply and forcefully does not mean putting a lot of stress on our joints, ligaments, etc. The techniques you and I will use to exercise forcefully are "lower impact" than walking. Anyone can exercise forcefully if they have the right information.

CHAPTER 29

Hormonal—Exercise to Trigger Clog-Clearing Hormones

"We work out entirely too much. We waste time. A friend of mine runs marathons. He always talks about this 'runner's high,' but he has to go twenty-six miles for it. That is why I smoke and drink. I get the same feeling from a flight of stairs."
LARRY MILLER

Traditional exercise is all about "burning calories." Traditional exercise is all wrong. High-quality exercise ignores the quantity of calories burned by exercising. It focuses on triggering the release of the clog-clearing hormones that lower our set-point.[1]

All we need to harness these hormones is to apply the first exercise principle: Deep. By exercising more muscle—especially our deepest Type 2b fibers—we trigger more clog-clearing hormones. Here is the simplified version of how this works.[2]

One of the reasons our fat metabolism system slows down and burns muscle before it burns body fat is because burning body fat is hard. Until we get the right combination of hormones, we are not burning through anything meaningful other than muscle tissue.

The other reason is that our fat metabolism system does not want to burn body fat. It is unfortunate for fat loss, but it makes perfect survival sense. Our fat metabolism system stores body fat to protect us from starving. If it burns body fat, it cannot protect us. Therefore, it avoids burning body fat unless it has no other option.

"Hard to do" plus "do not want to do" generally equals "it's not happening." That is, unless our fat metabolism system has no other option. The way to achieve this is simple: require it to expend a huge amount of energy quickly. Exercise Deeply. Work all muscle fibers.

As we know, when our fat metabolism system needs a lot of energy it can do four things: Make us eat more. Slow down. Burn muscle. Burn body fat. However, when we exercise Deeply, we eliminate three of these options. Making us eat more will not work because digestion takes a long time. It is too late to slow us down because the energy demands have already been made. Burning muscle is out of the question since high-quality exercise stimulates muscle rather than destroying it. Left with no other option, our fat metabolism system is forced to produce hormones which free up energy stored as body fat.[3]

How Deep Hormonal Exercise Burns Body Fat Long Term

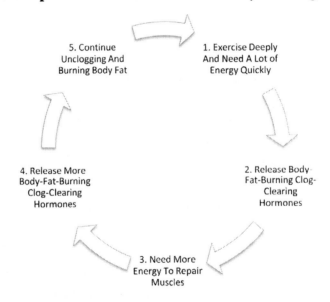

5. Continue Unclogging And Burning Body Fat

1. Exercise Deeply And Need A Lot of Energy Quickly

2. Release Body-Fat-Burning Clog-Clearing Hormones

3. Need More Energy To Repair Muscles

4. Release More Body-Fat-Burning Clog-Clearing Hormones

Forget calories. Focus on hormones. Clear your clog. Lower your set-point. Burn body fat forever.

CHAPTER 30

Infrequent–Exercise Less Often, but with Higher Quality

"This novel time-efficient training paradigm can be used as a strategy to reduce metabolic risk factors in young and middle-aged sedentary populations who otherwise would not adhere to time-consuming traditional aerobic exercise regimes."

J.A. Babraj, Heriot-Watt University, Edinburgh[1]

If we cut grass lower, we can mow our lawn less often. That is not some too-good-to-be-true gimmick. That is common sense. The more grass we cut off, the more time is needed to grow it back. Similarly, by exercising our muscles Deeply, we can exercise less often. The more muscle fibers we exercise, the more time we need to recover.[2]

How long your muscles take to recover is a great way to tell if you are exercising Deeply enough. If you are able to exercise on Monday and then do the same thing a day or two later, then you are not exercising Deeply. If Monday's workout is forceful enough to exercise all of your muscle fibers, they will not be ready to go again one, two, three, four, or even five days later. Deep Type 2b muscle fibers need at least six days to recover.[3]

So, if we are exercising often, we are either not exercising Deeply or not giving our clog-clearing hormones enough time to fix our fat metabolism system. Either way we are spending more time exercising and burning less body fat. Enough of that. Let's do a little high-quality exercise and then sit back while our unclogged fat metabolism system burns body fat for us.

CHAPTER 31

Eccentric–Exercise to Lower Your Set-Point By Lowering Weights

"Exercise with a maximal-eccentric [lowering] component can induce increases in muscle...with shorter durations of work than other modes [traditional resistance training]."

M. WERNBOM, GÖTEBORG UNIVERSITY[1]

High-quality resistance training does not require lifting weights. You are going to focus on lowering weights.

Every resistance training exercise has two parts: lifting the resistance and lowering the resistance. Lifting the resistance is called the *concentric* portion of the exercise. Concentric is when the muscle contracts. Lowering the resistance is called the *eccentric* portion of the exercise. Eccentric is when the muscle extends. Lifting weights—the concentric action—gets more attention from your buff friends, but lowering weights—the eccentric action—gets more results.[2]

While lifting weights helps boys feel like men, safely and slowly lowering weights works muscles up to 50% Deeper. That enables more muscle fibers to be worked and more clog-clearing hormones to be triggered. More clog-clearing hormones mean more results in less time. Mark Roig at the University of British Columbia ran tests and concluded: "Eccentric

219

training performed at high intensities [with high-quality] was shown to be more effective in promoting increases in muscle."[3]

Focusing on the eccentric—lowering—portion of resistance training works so well because it allows our muscles to generate more force. To test this principle, walk up a flight of stairs and then walk back down them. Notice how the trip down was easier? That is because you are doing eccentric—lowering—actions on the way down. Since our muscles can develop more force on the trip down—eccentric actions—it is easier than the trip up—concentric actions. Lowering your body down the stairs is easier than lifting it up the stairs because your muscles are literally stronger on the way down. Researcher N.D Reeves at Manchester Metropolitan University states: "Muscles are capable of developing much higher forces when they contract eccentrically compared with when they contract concentrically."[4]

Once we know that muscles generate more force when lowering resistance, and that the Depth of exercise is determined by the amount of force muscles are asked to generate, we can see that it is ineffective to focus on lifting resistance.

Forget lifting resistance. Lower it. Here's how.

How to Exercise Eccentrically
Exercising eccentrically is simple:

1. Get warmed up by walking briskly or riding a bike for a few minutes.
2. Pick a resistance you cannot lift with one arm or one leg—depending on the exercise—but can easily lift with both arms or both legs. Let's say 20 pounds.
3. Lift the resistance with both arms or both legs. Each arm or leg lifts half the weight—10 pounds in this example.
4. Lower the resistance with only one arm or one leg for ten seconds. Each arm or leg lowers all the weight—20 pounds in our example—slowly.
5. Repeat until it is impossible to lower the resistance with only one arm or one leg for ten seconds. If this takes more than six repetitions, gradually add resistance until it only takes six repetitions.

With this technique you can exercise Eccentrically in the comfort of your own home and bend most resistance training machines at your local gym to your every Eccentric whim. But before we go get Eccentric, there are two important rules to keep in mind.

First, if we choose to exercise Eccentrically on resistance training machines at our local gym, then we should only use machines that work both of our arms or both of our legs *together*. This is the only way to have less resistance on the way up and more on the way down. If we pick machines that work our arms and legs independently, we will lift and lower the same amount of resistance. That defeats the whole purpose. Think about it this way. Say you grab a gallon of milk in each hand, lift them above your head, and then drop the one in your right hand to increase the resistance for your left hand. That does not work because lifting milk jugs works your arms independently. However, if you lifted one milk jug with each arm, but then lowered both jugs with only your left arm, you would lower more resistance with your left arm than you lifted with your left arm. Resistance training machines which work both of our arms or both of our legs together do the same thing.

Second, exercise Eccentrically only when *little, if any, balance is needed*. Just as you would not pick up a giant flat-screen TV with two hands and then let go with one, you should only exercise Eccentrically when minimal balance is needed.

Let's put the two rules together: We could do a push-up with our knees on the floor (to reduce the resistance), and then lift our knees and lower ourselves (to increase the resistance). Our arms *work together* to lift a shared source of resistance (our body), and *little, if any, balance is needed*.

We will cover complete "at home" and "at the gym" Eccentric exercise programs in chapters 34 and 35, but for now, Deep, Hormonal, and Infrequent Eccentric exercise is as simple as one, two, three:

1. Lift resistance with both arms or both legs. Lower resistance slowly with one arm or one leg.
2. Pick exercises which work both arms or both legs together.
3. Pick exercises which require minimal balance.

CHAPTER 32

Brief—Exercise for Less Time, but with More Resistance

"Vigorous exercise favors negative energy and lipid [fat] balance to a greater extent than exercise of low to moderate intensity. Moreover, the metabolic adaptations taking place in the skeletal muscle in response to the HIIT [high-quality Brief exercise] program appear to favor the process of lipid oxidation [fat burning]."
A. Tremblay, Laval University[1]

To recap: the first principle—Deep—revealed how we get more results by exercising more muscle, less, instead of less muscle, more. The second principle—Hormonal—showed that exercise is most effective when it triggers hormones that burn body fat automatically, long term. The third principle—Infrequent—demonstrated that exercising enough muscle fibers to trigger a Hormonal response is extremely taxing and therefore cannot be done often.

Then along came the fourth principle—Eccentric. It covered the technique used to make resistance training Deep, Hormonal, and Infrequent. Now it is time for the fifth principle—Brief. It covers the technique used to make cardiovascular exercises Deep, Hormonal, and Infrequent. Conrad Earnest at the Pennington Biomedical Research Center reports: "Interval [Brief] training will provide a more powerful stimulus for improving insulin sensitivity [unclogging] than low-quality-high-quantity cardiovascular exercise." But for the technique to make sense, we need to update the way we think about cardiovascular exercises.[2]

Contrary to popular belief, cardiovascular exercises and resistance training exercises are not completely different. Traditional cardiovascular exercises are resistance-training exercises that require little force and work only our weakest muscle fibers.

Say we get on a leg press resistance training machine, add no resistance, and move our legs up and down for thirty minutes. Did we do resistance training or cardiovascular exercise? Who cares? Our muscles did not have to generate much force, so we did not exercise Deeply or Hormonally, and that is all that matters. Or say we get on a stair stepper cardiovascular exercise machine, add no resistance, and move our legs up and down for thirty minutes. Did we do resistance training or cardiovascular exercise? Who cares?

Now let's say we get on a stationary bike, increase the resistance so much that the only way we can generate enough force to move the pedals is to lift our butt off the seat. Let's say we then pedal as hard as we can for thirty seconds, at which point we have to stop because we cannot move the pedals anymore. Did we do:

1. Resistance training?
2. Cardiovascular exercise?
3. Neither?
4. Both?
5. It does not matter—our muscles had to generate a lot of force and therefore were exercised Deeply and Hormonally?

Answer: 5. Our fat metabolism system does not respond in terms of resistance training exercises or cardiovascular exercises. It responds in terms of how many muscle fibers an exercise works. So the question of the day is: "How do we make cardiovascular exercises work more muscle fibers?"

Easy. Make them require more force. Perform high-quality Brief cardiovascular exercise.

High-Quality Brief Cardiovascular Exercise—How and Why

High-quality Brief cardiovascular exercise is simple:[3]

1. Hop on an upright stationary bike—the ones that look like regular bikes, not the ones that look like recliners.
2. Pedal at a moderate pace, with moderate resistance, to get warmed up.
3. Increase the bike's resistance so you can pedal only by standing up on the pedals and pushing down on them as hard as you can.
4. Pedal like that for thirty seconds. If you can pedal for longer than thirty seconds, increase the resistance until you cannot.
5. Rest for two minutes.
6. Repeat the steps 4 and 5 three times.
7. Smile, because that took ten minutes and you are done with cardiovascular exercise for the week.

Sounds too good to be true? Let's look at the studies.

University of Virginia researcher B.A. Irving took two groups of women and had them do traditional low-quality cardiovascular exercise or high-quality Brief cardiovascular exercise. The two groups burned the same number of calories exercising, but the high-quality Brief cardiovascular exercise group spent significantly less time exercising, while losing significantly more belly fat.[4]

McMaster University researcher M. Gibala separated people into high-quality Brief cardiovascular exercise and traditional cardiovascular exercise groups. Over the course of the two-week study, the Brief cardiovascular group exercised for two-and-a-half hours while the traditional cardiovascular exercise group exercised for ten-and-a-half hours. At the end of the study both groups got the same results even though the high-quality Brief cardiovascular exercise group spent 320% less time exercising than the traditional cardiovascular exercise group. The researcher put it like this: "We thought there would be benefits, but we did not expect them to be this obvious. It shows how effective short intense [high-quality Brief] exercise can be."[5]

Many more studies show the same encouraging results and further prove that hours of exercising per week are not needed to help our weight and health. Consider this small sample:[6]

- "Vigorous [high-quality Brief] activities are associated with a reduced risk of coronary heart disease, whereas moderate or light [low-quality] activities have no clear association with the risk of coronary heart disease," says H.D. Sesso at Harvard University[7]
- "The intensity [quality] of effort was more important than the quantity of energy output in deterring hypertension and preventing premature mortality," found R.S. Paffenbarger Jr. of Stanford University[8]
- "There is an inverse association between relative intensity [quality] of physical activity and risk of coronary heart disease," states I.M. Lee, also at Harvard University.[9]
- "Vigorous-intensity [high-quality Brief] activities may have greater benefit for reducing cardiovascular disease and premature mortality than moderate-intensity physical activities [traditional exercise]," noted the American Heart Association[10]
- "Exercise training reduces the impact of the metabolic syndrome [the clog] and that the magnitude of the effect depends on exercise intensity [quality]," discovered P.M. Haram of the Norwegian University of Science and Technology[11]

Even day-to-day cardiovascular benefits, like not being out of breath after walking up a few flights of stairs, are achieved faster with high-quality exercise. Edward Coyle's research at the University of Texas found: "Interval [high-quality Brief] training in untrained people can markedly increase aerobic endurance...This serves as a dramatic reminder of the potency of exercise intensity [quality]...Interval [high-quality Brief] training is very time efficient with much 'bang for the buck.'" Old Dominion University researcher D.P. Swain adds: "Vigorous intensity [high-quality Brief] exercise has been shown to increase aerobic fitness more effectively than moderate intensity [traditional] exercise, suggesting that the former may confer greater cardioprotective [health] benefits."[12]

> **Time Saving Tip:** Since high-quality Brief cardiovascular exercise only takes ten minutes per week, going to a gym to do it may not make a lot of sense. To save yourself time and money, consider investing in your own upright stationary bike. Simple upright stationary bikes cost less than $150.

High-quality cardiovascular exercise has clearly emerged as the right way to help lose weight faster. You can trade quantity for quality and get more for less by increasing the force of your exercise. You can also grab back all that time spent pounding the pavement with those six o'clock jogs. The new way to wellness is Brief.[13]

Traditional Cardiovascular Exercise Is a Terrible Way to Burn Body Fat

"For Americans to begin losing weight through [traditional cardiovascular] exercise, the current USDA exercise guideline would have to be increased by almost 200%.... Americans would need to start exercising at least two hours a day, six days a week."
ERIC J. OLIVER, UNIVERSITY OF CHICAGO[14]

Traditional cardiovascular exercise helps people to be more active, but it is not a useful way to unclog. Traditional cardiovascular exercise does not touch the clog. At best, it increases our need to eat more, slow down, and then burn something. It is not even good at that job. Thirty minutes of jogging only consumes 170 more calories than we would have burned spending thirty minutes of quality time with our family and friends.

Putting 170 calories into perspective, our livers burn over three times that amount per day. In other words, you and I would have to do 90 minutes of traditional cardiovascular exercise every single day to burn as many calories as our liver does every day. Three-quarters of the calories we burn every day have nothing to do with moving, let alone traditional cardiovascular exercise.[15]

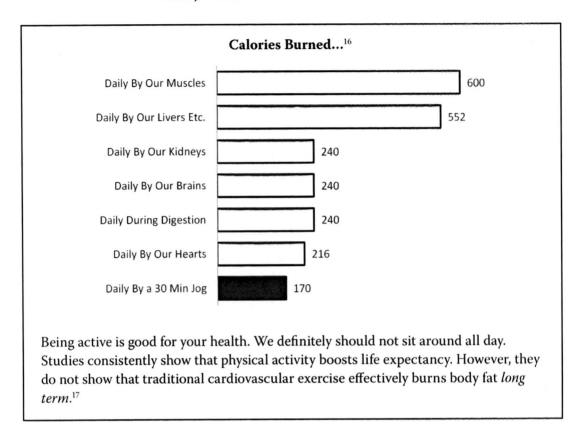

Calories Burned...[16]

Daily By Our Muscles	600
Daily By Our Livers Etc.	552
Daily By Our Kidneys	240
Daily By Our Brains	240
Daily During Digestion	240
Daily By Our Hearts	216
Daily By a 30 Min Jog	170

Being active is good for your health. We definitely should not sit around all day. Studies consistently show that physical activity boosts life expectancy. However, they do not show that traditional cardiovascular exercise effectively burns body fat *long term*.[17]

CHAPTER 33

The High Quality Exercise Program: More for Less

"Muscular strengthening activities...promote the development and maintenance of metabolically active lean muscle mass, which is particularly important for enhancing glucose metabolism [unclogging]."
AMERICAN HEART ASSOCIATION[1]

Inspired by author Michael Pollan, here is the high-quality exercise program summed up in seven words: *Exercise Forcefully. Not Too Often. Mostly Eccentric.*

The high-quality exercise program takes at most twenty minutes per week, so it cannot be complex. Sure, there are all sorts of ways to exercise forcefully, not too often, mostly Eccentric. Plenty of people at your local gym are happy to take your money to complicate things. However, if you want a simple, proven plan, then use four Eccentric exercises, for ten minutes once per week, along with ten minutes of high-quality Brief cardiovascular exercise once per week (this can be done at home or at a gym).

Here is the program. It is simple because staying healthy and fit is simple once we know the science. The next few sections cover the details.

- Day 1: 10 minutes of high-quality Eccentric resistance training
- Day 2: Relax and recover

- Day 3: Relax and recover
- Day 4: 10 minutes of high-quality Brief cardiovascular exercise
- Day 5: Relax and recover
- Day 6: Relax and recover
- Day 7: Relax and recover

After the discussion about needing a week to recover from high-quality exercise, you may be wondering why you would do both high-quality Eccentric resistance training and high-quality Brief cardiovascular exercise each week. Great catch. Two high-quality workouts per week make sense only for people new to high-quality exercise.

It is important to put safety first and ease your way into high-quality exercise. So it will take a while before you work your muscles Deeply. Since your Deepest muscle fibers will not be getting exercised right from the start, two high-quality workouts per week are fine. Once you are comfortable exercising as Deeply as possible, you can skip the high-quality Brief cardiovascular exercise.

Here is how you can tell when to cut back to one high-quality workout per week:

1. Do high-quality Eccentric resistance training and write down the amount of resistance used. For example: "Did six Eccentric shoulder presses with 20 pounds."
2. Rest for two days.
3. Do high-quality Brief cardiovascular exercise.
4. Rest for three days.
5. Do high-quality Eccentric resistance training with the same resistance used last time.

If steps three and five are possible, you are not exercising Deeply yet and should stick with two high-quality workouts per week. If you were exercising Deeply, your high-quality Brief cardiovascular exercise would have gone badly. Your exhausted Type 2 muscle fibers would not have worked well. If you somehow dragged your exhausted muscles through the high-quality Brief cardiovascular exercise, they would be unable to meet the demands of high-quality Eccentric resistance training three days later.

As you are getting used to high-quality low-quantity exercise, two ten-minute workouts per week are fine. When you are comfortable exercising as Deeply as possible during Eccentric resistance training, you will only need one ten-minute workout per week. For women there is an extra bonus. "There is a special sense of empowerment with strength [resistance] training. You do not feel as intimidated by being in a room full of men, or by many of the tasks that face us in our daily lives. Carrying groceries, carrying a child, opening heavy doors—these are things that for some women are really burdens. With strength [resistance] training, a relatively small woman can see a big difference," reports Jan Todd at the University of Texas at Austin.[2]

This does not mean you have to give up all other forms of exercise. You can still do whatever additional exercises you like, but only after high-quality exercise, and only if it does not compromise your ability to do high-quality exercise. Or you can skip traditional exercise all together. The point is not that traditional exercise is bad and should be avoided. It's just not needed once we know how to exercise less—smarter.

Ten Minutes of High-Quality Eccentric Resistance Training

If you are familiar with resistance training, you are familiar with sets and reps. If you are not familiar, you are better off because sets and reps are irrelevant. Muscle fibers do not care how many sets or reps we do. Ralph Carpinelli at Adelphi University says: "There are fifty-seven studies…that show no statistically significant difference in the magnitude of strength gains or muscular hypertrophy [results] as a result of performing a greater number of sets."[3]

All our muscle fibers care about is how much force they need to generate. So let's focus on making as many muscle fibers as possible generate as much force as possible, doing whichever set of the following exercises we would like, *once* per week.

Home Exercises   Gym Exercises

<table>
<tr><td>█████████████</td><td>█████████████</td></tr>
</table>

☐ Assisted Eccentric Squats   ☐ Eccentric Leg Presses

☐ Assisted Eccentric Pull-Ups   ☐ Eccentric Rows

☐ Assisted Eccentric Push-Ups   ☐ Eccentric Chest Presses

☐ Assisted Eccentric Shoulder Press   ☐ Eccentric Shoulder Presses

More exercises provide little if any value. Think about doing more exercises to make your set-point lower as being like heating boiling water more to make it hotter. In both cases we would just be wasting energy.[4]

For each exercise, raise the resistance at a controlled speed with two legs or arms, and then lower it with one leg or arm for ten seconds. Repeat that six times per leg or arm. If you can do it a seventh time, increase the resistance. Each exercise takes about two and a half minutes—a little over a minute per arm or leg. After each exercise, move immediately to the next one. Ten minutes later, get on with your day.[5]

Specific instructions on how to do these Eccentric exercises are coming up in the next two chapters, but if you have ever sat down, opened a door, pushed something, or lifted anything above your head, you are most of the way to being an Eccentric exercise expert.

Keep in mind that while the Smarter workout is simple, it is not easy. We are trading quantity for quality, and that is hard. For example, go back to the staircase, walk up it normally, and note how you feel. Now wait a few minutes and walk up the same staircase two steps at a time. Notice how that is more tiring? In both cases you did the same quantity of exercise, but taking two steps at a time requires more force and works more muscle fibers.

Ten minutes of high-quality Eccentric resistance training should be like walking up a dozen stairs at a time. You will generate more force and work more muscle fibers than you ever have before. At the end of each exercise you will be exhausted. It will not be fun, but the results are incredible. Plus, it is encouraging to know that you only have to do it once per week for ten minutes.

You do not need to do arm- and ab-specific exercises. Our goal is to work as many muscle fibers as possible, and arm- and ab-specific exercises work few muscle fibers. Besides, our four Eccentric exercises work our arms and abs along with a bunch of other muscles, and the Hormonal impact of these "big" exercises benefits our arms and abs more than bicep curls or crunches ever could.

In my favorite study of all time, researchers at the University of Southern Denmark divided people into two groups. The first group only trained one of their arms. The second group trained only one arm exactly the same way as the first group, but also trained both legs. With this creative setup, researchers could see what impacted people's arm muscles more: direct arm training or the hormones triggered by all the muscle fibers worked using leg exercises. They could answer the following questions. How much stronger does an arm get if people:[6]

- do not train it?   [untrained arm + untrained legs]
- train only it?   [trained arm + untrained legs]
- do not train it, but do train their legs? [untrained arm + trained legs]
- train it and train their legs?   [trained arm + trained legs]

Here are the results:

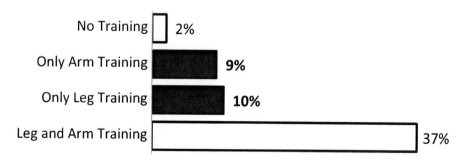

% Increase in *Arm* Strength

No Training	2%
Only Arm Training	9%
Only Leg Training	10%
Leg and Arm Training	37%

Clearly training legs along with arms is our best bet, but the fun part is the middle two bars. Resistance training only the legs increased *arm* strength more than resistance training only the arms. Why? Leg training worked more muscle and therefore triggered more whole-body-transforming Hormones than arm training. All those whole-body-transforming Hormones benefit seemingly unrelated muscles more than exercising those muscles directly. That is why we will work our biggest muscle groups (legs, back, chest, and shoulders) directly and our small muscle groups (arms, abs, etc.) indirectly. By focusing on the big things directly and the little things indirectly, we will take care of the little things better than we could any other way.

But seriously, what about our abdominal muscles? Don't we want a flat, toned tummy? Absolutely. But doing abdominal-only exercises before we lower our body fat percentage to the mid-teens is like worrying about how shiny a ring looks while wearing a boxing glove over it. The fastest way to "get abs" has nothing to do with exercising our abdominal muscles. You have to uncover your abdominal muscles—that is, unclog and drop your set-point.

CHAPTER 34

How to Do the Four Clog-Clearing Exercises at Home

"An increase in fast/glycolytic muscle mass [Deeper muscle fibers] can result in the regression of obesity and metabolic improvement [unclogging]."
Y. IZUMIYA, BOSTON UNIVERSITY[1]

Here is how to get a Deep workout without buying a gym membership. Combine the specific steps covered in this chapter with the general Eccentric guidelines covered in chapter 31, and you will be exercising Deeply, Hormonally, Infrequently, and safely, within minutes. The next chapter covers how to exercise Eccentrically on resistance training machines.

You need to keep in mind two points while exercising Eccentrically. First and foremost, nothing is more important than safety. The quickest way to compromise clog-clearing is to get hurt. Eccentric resistance training is designed specifically to minimize injury—it is slow and controlled, requires minimal balance, and you can spot yourself—but you still need to ease into it and to keep perfect form.

Second, once you have the hang of safely executing the four clog-clearing exercises, you have to push yourself as hard as you safely can. You are trading quantity for quality, so it is particularly important that you maximize the quality of these exercises. If you do not, you will have thrown quantity *and* quality out the window. That is not exercising less—smarter. That is just exercising less.

You have to push yourself as hard as you safely can and then continue to push yourself more and more by gradually adding resistance at least every couple of workouts. As you improve the quality of your health and fitness, you must improve the quality of your exercise to keep progressing.[2]

You will only exercise for ten to twenty minutes a week, so be sure to make it count.

Assisted Eccentric Squats

Muscle groups worked: legs and butt.

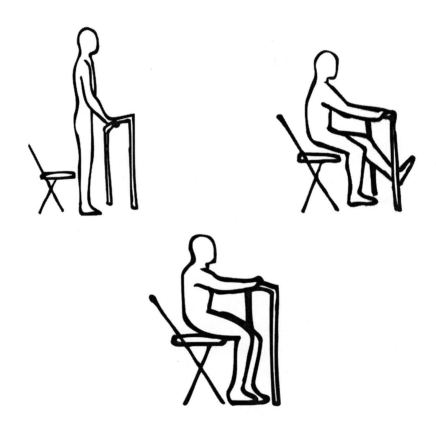

1. Stand with your feet shoulder-width apart in front of something sturdy that you can hold on to with both hands. I use a railing or a doorknob. Put a chair behind you.

2. Grab the sturdy thing in front of you and lean back until your arms are fully extended. Stand with all of your weight on one of your heels. Make sure to keep your head and shoulders back while sticking your chest and butt out.

3. Keeping all of your weight on one of your heels, and keeping yourself balanced by holding onto that sturdy thing in front of you, sit down using only the one leg you put all of your weight on. Use your non-weight-bearing leg to keep your balance and to ensure that you can lower yourself slowly and safely for ten seconds. If you can lower yourself for longer than ten seconds, then you are using your other leg too much. If you cannot lower yourself for ten seconds, then you are not using your other leg enough.

4. Make sure that your knees never stick out farther than your toes while you are lowering yourself.

5. Stop lowering yourself with one leg once your butt touches the chair. Keep holding on to the sturdy thing in front of you. Stand back up using both legs.

6. Repeat this five more times and then do the same thing with your other leg.

7. As you get stronger, remove the chair and try to squat down as far as you comfortably can without your heel lifting off the ground or your knees sticking out farther than your toes.

Assisted Eccentric Pull-Ups

Muscle groups worked: back and arms.

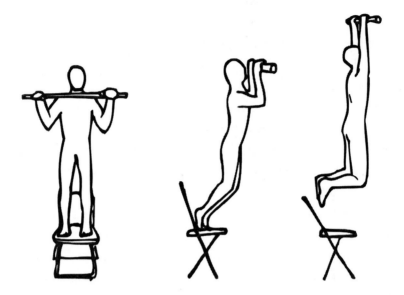

1. Find something sturdy to hang from. It should be no lower than your chin if you are standing on the ground, and no higher than your chin if you are standing on a chair. Common options include: jungle gyms/swing-sets, construction scaffolding, tree branches, or I-beams in your basement or attic.
2. Stand on the ground or on a chair so that your chin is slightly above the thing you are going to hang from.
3. With your arms slightly wider than shoulder-width apart, put your hands on top of the thing you are going to hang from. Grip it as tightly as you can. Stick your chest out and squeeze your shoulder blades together.
4. With a firm grip, start to bend your legs so that you begin to hang from whatever it is you are holding on to. The more you bend your legs, the more challenging it will be to hang on.
5. Bend your legs enough that you cannot hang on for longer than ten seconds. If you can hang on for longer than ten seconds, bend your legs more. If you cannot hang on for ten seconds, bend your legs less. Depending on your strength level, you may not need to use your legs at all.

6. While you are hanging on, your back and arms will get tired and you will slowly lower down until your arms are fully extended. If your arms fully extend in less than ten seconds, you are using your legs too little. If your arms fully extend in more than ten seconds, you are using your legs too much.

7. While your arms are extending and you are lowering down, keep your shoulders back, chest out, look up, and keep your arms as even with your torso as possible—that is, do not let your arms creep out in front of you.

8. After your arms have fully extended, keep hanging on and stand up to get your chin back above the bar.

9. Repeat five more times without resting.

Assisted Eccentric Push-Ups

Muscle groups worked: chest, shoulders, and arms.

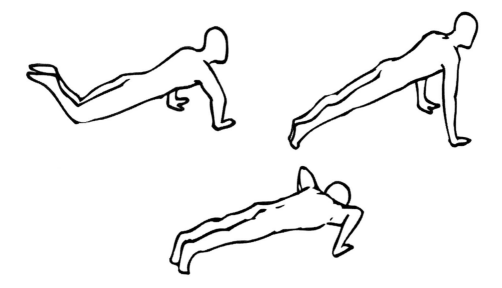

1. Lie face down on a clean floor and put your arms out to your sides so that your hands are even with your upper chest and slightly wider than shoulder-width apart.

2. Keeping your knees on the floor, push yourself up through the palms of your hands until just before your elbows lock. You will now have only your knees and your hands touching the floor.

3. Lift your knees off the floor and shift your weight to your toes. You will now have only your toes and hands touching the floor.

4. With your shoulders back and your chest out, slowly lower yourself until just before any other part of your body touches the ground. Hold that position for ten seconds. Make sure you keep your body in a straight line throughout the movement. Do not let your chest or hips bow down.

5. After ten seconds, put your knees back on the floor and push yourself back up like you did originally. Once you have lowered yourself six times—for ten seconds each time without resting in between —you are done.

6. If you cannot lower yourself six times—for ten seconds each time—put your knees back on the floor until you can.

7. If you can lower yourself more than six times—for ten seconds each time—do not ever let your knees touch the floor. Always have just your hands and toes touching the floor. If that is still too easy, put your toes on something six to twelve inches off the ground. If that is still too easy, put your toes on something six to twelve inches off the ground and put something heavy on your back.

Assisted Eccentric Shoulder Press

Muscle groups worked: shoulders and arms.

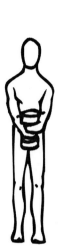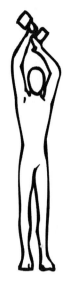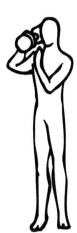

1. Find something that you can safely lift above your head using both arms. You should also be able to safely hold it above your head with one arm. This means it should be small. Ideally you would use a dumbbell. Hold it in both hands.

2. Lift it above your head using both hands. You should now be standing with your shoulders back and your chest out, holding something above your head with both arms extended as much as they can without locking at the elbows.

3. Very carefully release one hand but keep it close to whatever you are holding above your head to help lower it if needed.

4. Keep the arm supporting the resistance to your side—that is, do not let it creep in front of you—and slowly lower the resistance for ten seconds, always keeping your other hand close by.

5. If you can lower the resistance for more than ten seconds, you need something heavier. If you cannot lower the resistance for ten seconds, you need something lighter.

6. Repeat this five more times—without resting—and then do the same thing with your other arm.

CHAPTER 35

How to Do the Four Clog-Clearing Exercises at a Gym

"My gym has two-pound weights. If you are using two-pound weights, how did you even open the door to the gym? What's your dream? To pump up and open your mail?"
DAVE ATTELL

Before you get Eccentric at your local gym, keep in mind that every brand of exercise machine is slightly different. Read the instructions on the machines you will be using to learn specifically how to lower the resistance, raise the resistance, position the seat, and position the handles. Also, remember to inhale deeply before lowering resistance and to exhale when lifting resistance. Finally, all of the general Eccentric guidelines from before still apply. Get warmed up. Pick resistance you cannot lift with one arm or one leg, but can easily lift with both arms or both legs. Lift the resistance with both arms or both legs. Lower the resistance with only one arm or one leg for ten seconds. Repeat until it is impossible to lower the resistance with only one arm or one leg for ten seconds. If this takes more than six repetitions, gradually add resistance until it only takes six repetitions. Push yourself as hard as you can while staying safe.

Eccentric Leg Presses

Muscle groups worked: legs and butt.

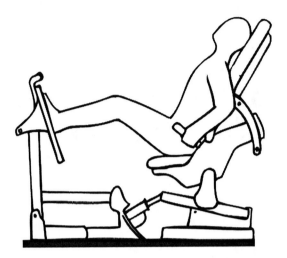

1. Sit on the leg press machine with your back against the pad. Make sure to keep your head and shoulders back, while sticking your chest out. Think about how military personnel stand at attention. Do that with your head, shoulders, and back while sitting on the machine. This protects your back from injury. Never, ever, round your back forward during any exercise.

2. Put your feet on the platform. Space your feet slightly wider than shoulder-width apart—whatever is most comfortable for you. Make sure your feet are high enough on the platform that your toes stay higher than your knees when you lower the resistance.

3. When you lower and raise the resistance, make sure your knees stay lined-up with your feet. Do not bow your legs in or out. Make sure your knees never stick out farther than your toes.

4. Always push on the platform through your heels, while keeping your abs tight and your back against the pad, with your shoulders back, and your chest out.

5. Lower the resistance for ten seconds with one leg, as low as you comfortably can without your back coming off the pad or your heels lifting off the platform.

6. When you lift the resistance—with both legs—avoid locking your knees at the top of the movement. Right before you begin to lock your knees, start lowering the resistance with one leg again.

7. Repeat this five more times—without resting—and then do the same thing with your other leg.

Eccentric Rows

Muscle groups worked: back and arms.

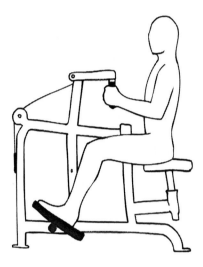

1. Sit on the row machine and put your chest against the pad, if there is one. Either way, make sure to keep your back perpendicular with the floor with your head and shoulders back, while sticking your chest out. Imagine trying to pinch a playing card between your shoulder blades. Do that with your back and shoulders while you lift and lower the resistance.
2. Put your feet flat on the floor or flat on the machine's platform. Keep them there.
3. When you lift and lower the resistance, keep your torso still. Use only your back and arm muscles to lift the resistance. Do not move your torso to generate momentum to help your back and arms.
4. Lift with both arms, then lower the resistance for ten seconds with one arm until your arm extends as far as it can, without causing you to round your back or to lock your elbow. Repeat "shoulders back, chest out" in your mind during this and all other exercises.
5. Just before your elbow begins to lock, use both arms to lift the resistance again.
6. Repeat this five more times—without resting—and then do the same thing with your other arm.

Eccentric Chest Press

Muscle groups worked: chest, shoulders, and arms.

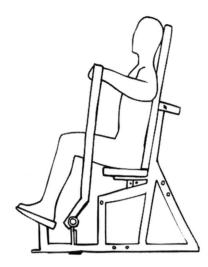

1. Sit on the chest press machine with your back against the pad, like you did with the leg press machine. Make sure to keep your head and shoulders back, while sticking your chest out.
2. Put your feet flat on the floor or flat on the machine's platform. Keep them there.
3. When you lower and lift the resistance, make sure you keep your shoulders and head back, abs tight, and chest out. Do not lift your lower back off the pad.
4. When you lift the resistance with both arms, extend your arms as far as they will go without locking your elbows or moving your shoulders forward. Just before your elbows begin to lock, start slowly lowering the resistance.
5. Lower the resistance for ten seconds with one arm until your hand is about even with your rib cage.
6. Repeat this five more times—without resting—and then do the same thing with your other arm.

Eccentric Shoulder Press

Muscle groups worked: shoulders and arms.

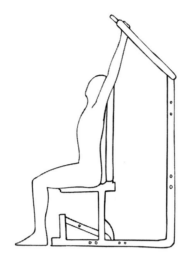

1. Sit on the shoulder press machine with your back against the pad like you did with the chest press machine. Make sure to keep your head and shoulders back, while sticking your chest out.
2. Put your feet flat on the floor or flat on the machine's platform. Keep them there.
3. When you lower and lift the resistance, make sure you keep your shoulders and head back, abs tight, and chest out. Do not lift your lower back off the pad.
4. When you lift the resistance with both arms, extend your arms as far as they will go without locking your elbows or moving your shoulders up. Just before your elbows begin to lock, start slowly lowering the resistance.
5. Lower the resistance for ten seconds with one arm until your hand is about even with your shoulders.
6. Repeat this five more times—without resting—and then do the same thing with your other arm.

CHAPTER 36

Ten Minutes of High-Quality Brief Cardiovascular Exercise

"The efficacy of a high intensity [high-quality Brief cardiovascular] exercise protocol, involving only ~250 kcal [calories] of work each week, to substantially improve insulin action [unclog] in young sedentary subjects is remarkable."

J.A. Babraj, Heriot-Watt University, Edinburgh[1]

Since you already know how to pedal on an upright stationary bike and since we already covered how to use an upright stationary bike Briefly but more forcefully, you are ready to go do high-quality Brief cardiovascular exercise:

1. Hop on an upright stationary bike.
2. Get warmed up by pedaling at a moderate pace with moderate resistance to get warmed up.
3. Increase the bike's resistance so that you can only pedal by standing up on the pedals and pushing down on them as hard as you can.
4. Pedal like that for thirty seconds. If you can pedal for longer than thirty seconds, increase the resistance until you cannot.
5. Rest for two minutes.
6. Repeat the steps 4 and 5 three times.

The key thing to keep in mind when doing high-quality Brief cardiovascular exercise is that we are not doing *high-quality* Brief cardiovascular exercise if we get on an upright stationary bike and flail around uncontrollably for thirty seconds. Sounds silly, but that is exactly what will happen if you do not bump the resistance way up on the bike. Assuming you are not a highly trained athlete—moving your body very quickly will eventually lead to an injury. However, after you add resistance, you can move at a normal, controllable, and safe rate, while working as forcefully as you possibly can.

As a general rule of thumb, *high-quality* Brief cardiovascular exercise is not about moving faster. It's about trying to move more resistance.

Smarter Success

Before we wrap things up, please download your free companion ebook *Smarter Success*. This quick read sets you up for long-term success as you put *The Smarter Science of Slim* into practice.

http://TheSmarterScienceOfSlim.com/Smarter-Success

Inside you will find:

- Details on when you can expect results and how to measure them.
- A five-step plan to get you started eating SANEly and exercising eccentrically.
- Access to reader-only resources such as recipes, meal plans, serving size guides, how-to videos, workout logs, grocery lists, and more.

Fighting Body Fat With Biological Facts

"True scientists put the solution to a medical problem first and not the preservation of their own hypothesis, no matter how clever the hypothesis may seem or how proud of themselves they may be for creating it."
UFFE RAVNSKOV, M.D., PH.D.[1]

If two billion people can be selective about what they eat, so can you. Take the dietary restrictions of the Islamic, Hindu, and Jewish religions, add diabetics and vegetarians, assume a third of these people skip the restrictions, and we end up with about two billion people worldwide who eat in a way that is much tougher than eating more—smarter. Also, most people spend an average of over twenty-four minutes per day driving to and from work. Everyone has ten to twenty minutes per *week* to spend driving hormonal clogs from their body. We have all done more difficult and less beneficial things than eating more and exercising less—smarter. Now, armed with the right information, you have the ability to burn body fat forever.[2]

As you start becoming slim, people will ask questions that mask their envy. "Don't you like food?" is a common remark. Eating more—smarter—is the opposite of disliking food. You are eating more food. Your disapproving peers are the ones trying to eat less of it. Sure, you are selective about what you eat, but to say that means you dislike food is like saying that being selective about what you listen to means you dislike music. Dr. Seuss put it best when he noted that "those who mind do not matter and those who matter do not mind."

Beyond specific food-related jabs, the envious will generally try to bring you back to "normal." The best way to deal with the constant coaxing is to keep some simple logic in mind: If you do not want what everyone else has, you should not do what everyone else does. Put differently: If you do not want typical results, you should not do what is typically done.

As we have seen throughout this book, eating more and exercising less—smarter—is based on scientific findings, not on opinion. It is not an opinion that our fat metabolism system regulates our weight automatically. Calories do have different qualities. Hormones are as important as calories. Starches are more harmful than helpful. Added sweeteners cause metabolic chaos. A balanced intake of natural carbohydrate, protein, and fat is healthy. And it is not an opinion that we get better results by exercising more muscle.

Speaking of science, here is the summary of the smarter science of slim:

- Gaining or losing body fat is controlled by our fat metabolism system. It automatically regulates our body fat levels around a set-point. Gaining body fat is the result of a hormonal clog in our fat metabolism system that raises our set-point.

- Long-term fat loss comes from clearing this hormonal clog and lowering our set-point. Long-term fat loss comes from making our fat metabolism system work like the fat metabolism systems of people who eat whatever they want and do not get fat. Long-term fat loss comes from improving our basic biological functions. We improve them by increasing the quality of calories we eat and the quality of exercises we do.

- Temporary fat loss comes from ignoring our clog while fiddling with the *quantity* of calories we eat and exercise off. Temporary fat loss comes from making our fat metabolism system think it is starving. This approach causes us to slow down, hold on to body fat, burn muscle, and gain back more body fat than we lost.

- Studies show that *Calories In—Calories Out, A Calorie Is a Calorie, Calories Are All That Matter* and the rest of the manually-balance calories mythology fails because it ignores the set-point, calorie quality, and our hormonal clog. Traditional fat loss theories ignore all of the factors controlling fat loss. That is why studies show they fail 95% of the time.

- By focusing on calorie quality, we eat as much SANE—high-Satiety, low-Aggression, high-Nutrition, and low-Efficiency—food as possible, and sit back while our body takes care of itself. Our hormones get healed, our clog clears, our set-point drops, and we burn body fat all day, automatically.

- Eating SANE food is simple. We eat natural foods packed with water, fiber, and protein. We eat the way our ancestors ate for 99.8% of our evolutionary history. We eat the way people ate before obesity and all its related diseases became a problem. We eat normally instead of typically. We eat pragmatically for our good instead of profitably for corporate greed.

- Sadly, our government promotes disproven, imbalanced, and unnatural *Dietary Guidelines* that encourage the inSANE eating that in turn causes the obesity, diabetes, heart disease, and cardiovascular disease epidemics.

- Big food, fitness, and pharmaceutical corporations pile on the inSANE "food" and spread misinformation because the worse we do, the better they do.

- We do not burn more body fat by exercising more. We burn more body fat by unclogging. We unclog by working more muscle fibers and triggering clog-clearing hormones. This type of deep and hormonal exercise is performed by moving eccentrically, briefly, and infrequently. Exercise helps us burn body fat forever when we do less of it—smarter.

- Eating less and exercising more lead to what we didn't want—weight gain. Eating more and exercising less—smarter—leads to what we want—weight loss.

- Eating more—smarter—provides the unique combination of more nutrients, more satisfaction, and more clog clearing, while preventing us from overeating. Add in exercising less—smarter—and we stimulate our clog-clearing hormones. More nutrients plus less overeating and less clog quickly convince our fat metabolism system to lower our set-point and burn body fat for us automatically. Since we are eating *more* while exercising less than ever, we easily can keep this up long-term.

The Smarter Science of Slim

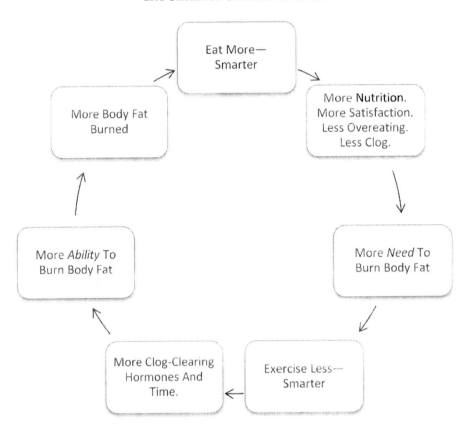

The science is simple. The lifestyle is easy. The results are amazing.

Here's to a lifetime of fighting fat with facts instead of getting frustrated by fat-loss fiction.

AFTERWORD

Spread the Word

"We cannot solve problems by using the same kind of thinking we used when we created them."
ALBERT EINSTEIN

In the past, the "truth" was determined by profitability. This does not have to be the case anymore. The truth can be determined by science. You and I simply need to get the word out.

Please help spread this scientific news using every outlet available to you. Let me know how I can help (TheSmarterScienceofSlim.com/contact). And please make sure you credit the researchers who spent years of their lives discovering this data.

If every one of us spends a few seconds sharing this scientific news, we can create a healthier and happier world.

P.S. If you'd like more guidance during your first five weeks of eating more and exercising less—smarter, check-out *The Smarter Science of Slim Workbook*. In addition to providing a specific five-week program which will lower your set-point weight, it also provides simple tools which can help you overcome subconscious roadblocks which could derail your fat loss efforts regardless of how much science you know.

You can find additional information on this book's companion websites: TheSmarterScienceofSlim.com and JonathanBailor.com.

Finally, as eating more and exercising less—smarter—makes you healthier, hotter, and happier, I would love to hear about it. Please share your good news with me at www.TheSmarterScienceofSlim.com/contact.

Appendices

APPENDIX 1

Food Groups' SANEity Scores

The quality of a calorie is calculated by averaging how Satiating, unAggressive, Nutritious, and inEfficient it is. Here are the scores from each of the four calorie quality factors, averaged and stacked ranked.

Type Of Food	Satiety Rating	unAggressive Rating	Nutrition Rating	inEfficiency Rating	SANEity Rating
Non-Starchy Vegetables	5	5	5	4	★★★★★
Seafood/Lean Meat/ Egg Whites/Whey Protein/Select Dairy	5	5	4	5	★★★★★
Nuts, Flax Seeds	3	5	3	2.5	★★★⌐
Fruits	3.5	3	4	2	★★★
Legumes	4	3	3	3	★★★
Most Dairy	2.5	2	2	2.5	★★⌐
Oils	2	5	0	0	★★⌐
Whole Grain Starch	2.5	0.5	1	1	★⌐
Processed Starch	1	0	0	0.5	⌐
Sweeteners	0	0	0	0	

APPENDIX 2

Products That Make Long-Term Fat Loss Easier

Note that I am not receiving any compensation from anyone for these recommendations. None of them are required for you to lose fat in the long-term. They simply save you time and money in the long-term.

Whey Protein Powder

Many supplement companies advertise that their whey protein is best. Do not believe the hype. Just make sure your protein powder does not contain a bunch of extra ingredients. Any product with more than two grams of sugar per twenty-five grams of protein is low-quality and should be avoided.

When choosing flavors, think about how you are going to eat the protein. If you plan to blend it with fruits and vegetables, then I recommend vanilla, strawberry, or some other fruit flavor. Other flavors are risky with fruits and vegetables. If you plan on mixing the whey protein with only water, ice, and milled flax seeds, get whatever flavor sounds appealing to you.

Membership at a Bulk Wholesale Store

With the cash-back my wife and I get thanks to our "executive" membership, Costco ends up paying us a few dollars per year for our membership.

High-Quality Blender

If you want to make smoothies, a good blender costs between $300 and $400. If you blend frequently, cheap blenders cost you more over the long run because they have to be replaced every year.

You will also find that high-quality blenders are significantly better at making tasty smoothies. Cheap blenders break food into small chunks, and it is no fun drinking grainy, chunky smoothies. High-quality blenders create smooth and delightful smoothies.

For example, if you put spinach into a $100 blender, you will get bits of spinach. However, if you put spinach in a $400 blender, you will get smooth spinach juice. Or consider whole flax seeds. Cheap blenders mix them up and leave you with whole flax seeds. High-quality blenders liquefy them. If you had a grainy, chunky, and overall bad experience with blending in the past, blame the blender and give smoothies another shot with a better blender.

I use a Vitamix blender, which costs about $400. There are other great ones out there. I chose the Vitamix because it has an impressive seven-year warranty and comes with a large jar—to blend a lot at once—and a handy plunger—to push food down in the blender without splattering all over the place. If your time is scarce, I think a $400 blender is worth the investment. If it lasts you seven years—which it will if it has a seven-year warranty—that is $57 a year.

Natural Peanut Butter

Try to buy your peanut butter from a store with a peanut butter machine—a machine that pulverizes peanuts into perfect natural peanut butter right before your eyes. This way the oil doesn't separate out, and you don't have to remix your peanut butter before you eat it.

Buying *natural* peanut butter is critical. The ingredients should read: peanuts. Traditional peanut butter contains added sugar and hydrogenated fats. Added sugar is bad news and hydrogenated fats are as bad for us as high-fructose corn syrup.

Bulk Unsweetened Cocoa

If you like chocolate, buying unsweetened cocoa in bulk is a great cost saver. Amazon.com's Subscribe and Save service is the way to go here. Unlike chocolate, pure cocoa is one of the most SANE foods in the world. I mix chocolate protein powder, natural peanut butter, cocoa, cinnamon, flax seed oil, and Splenda to make chocolate-peanut-butter fudge that takes care of my sweet tooth while keeping me SANE. It can also be baked into SANE brownies.

Stevia or Splenda

If you would like to sweeten certain foods, use Stevia (natural sweetener) or Splenda (artificial sweetener). Both are much healthier than sugar, high-fructose corn syrup, or any other traditional sweetener.

Indoor Grill

A must-have for easy meat and seafood preparation. George Foreman's is the most common. There are other great ones. My only recommendation is to get one where you can detach the grilling "plates" for easy washing.

Stand-alone Freezer

If many people in your house are going SANE, a stand-alone freezer is helpful. All this freezer space allows you to buy non-starchy vegetables, meat, seafood, and fruit in bulk, and saves you money and time.

APPENDIX 3

A Higher-Quality Diet with the Least Effort Possible

If you want to try going SANE with even less effort, you can follow these three steps.

- Step 1: Buy whey protein powder, wheat grass powder or something like it, and milled flax seeds.
- Step 2: Mix a heaping scoop of the whey protein, a heaping tablespoon of the milled flax seeds, and two heaping tablespoons of the wheat grass with as much water as you like, and drink it before breakfast, lunch, and dinner.
- Step 3: Eat as SANEly as possible at breakfast, lunch, and dinner.

With as little time and effort as possible, this will dramatically increase the SANEity of your diet.

APPENDIX 4

How to Eat Before and After Workouts

"Studies show that carbohydrates combined with...protein creates a better muscle refueling and building response."
NANCY CLARK, AMERICAN COLLEGE OF SPORTS MEDICINE[1]

We can enhance the results of deep, hormonal, infrequent, eccentric, and brief exercise by making two simple additions to our SANE diet. First, consume about thirty grams of whey protein powder immediately before all workouts. Second, consume about thirty grams of whey protein powder, and eat two servings of fruit, immediately after all workouts. And I mean immediately afterwards. Not a half hour later. Take the food with you and eat it the second you finish your workout.[2]

> **Important Note:** If you would like to splurge on starch or sweets, do it immediately after high-quality exercise to minimize clogging. [3]

A Summary of the Five Benefits of Eating More–Smarter

"U.S. dietary guidelines advocate a low-fat, high-complex-carbohydrate, lower-protein diet although several recent studies have reported that replacing a portion of carbohydrate intake with dietary protein and/or fat may be as, if not more, effective in promoting weight loss and reducing disease risk."

P.J. ARCIERO, SKIDMORE COLLEGE[4]

Giving our fat metabolism system more of the fuel it is designed for makes all sorts of good things happen. In a study of over 105,000 people, the American Cancer Society found: "The dietary pattern represented by the AHEI [a more SANE way of eating] predicted lower incidence of major chronic disease in men and women."[5]

I discovered thousands of pages worth of research that confirm the health benefits of eating more—smarter. Consider just the additional fiber from SANE food. David Ludwig, at Children's Hospital Boston, found "[Fiber intake is] inversely associated with insulin levels [and] weight gain." Tulane University researcher Lydia Bazzano adds: "A higher intake of dietary fiber, particularly water-soluble fiber, reduces the risk of coronary heart disease."[6]

Here is a quick summary of the top five benefits of boosting our biology by eating more—smarter.

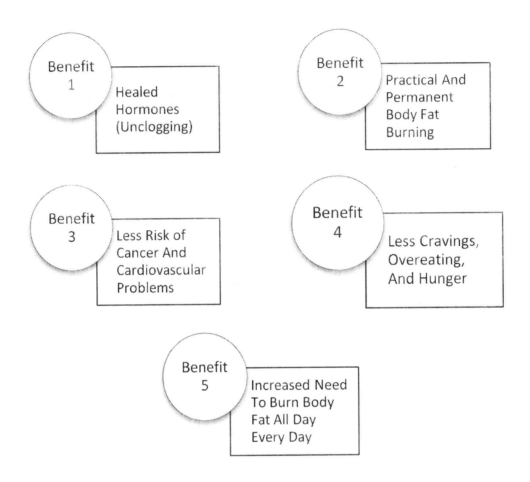

Benefit 1—Healed Hormones (Unclogging)

"A weight loss diet with moderate carbohydrate, moderate protein results in more favorable changes in body composition...[and] insulinemic response [unclogging] compared to a high carbohydrate, low protein diet suggesting an additional benefit beyond weight management to include augmented risk reduction for metabolic disease."

D.A. LASKER, UNIVERSITY OF ILLINOIS[7]

"Even short-term consumption of a paleolithic type [SANE] diet improves blood pressure and glucose tolerance, decreases insulin secretion, increases insulin sensitivity and improves lipid profiles [clears clogs]."
L.A. FRASSETTO, UNIVERSITY OF CALIFORNIA, SAN FRANCISCO[8]

A higher quantity of high-quality food causes the fat metabolism system to produce less body-fat-storing hormones and more body-fat-burning hormones. This helps us to clear our hormonal clog, lower our set-point, and burn body fat automatically, like naturally thin people. University of Illinois researcher D.K. Layman tells us: "Evidence is convincing that reduction in total dietary carbohydrates to less than 40% of total energy is the most effective way to improve glycemic regulations [to unclog]." With about a third of our calories coming from non-starchy vegetables and fruit, a third coming from natural fats, and the other third coming from lean protein, we will heal our hormones and clear our clog quickly and easily.[9]

Benefit 2—Practical and Permanent Body Fat Burning

"A balanced carbohydrate/protein [SANE] diet results in greater improvement in body composition...than a program comprised of a traditional diet... regimen commonly recommended for weight loss."
P.J. ARCIERO, SKIDMORE COLLEGE[10]

"Additional protein consumption results in a significantly lower body weight regain after weight loss."
M.S. WESTERTERP-PLANTENGA, MAASTRICHT UNIVERSITY[11]

If anyone ever says they have a program, pill, or product that enables you to burn more body fat faster and longer, ignore them unless they have third-party studies to prove it. Here is a sampling of studies that prove you will burn body fat more practically and permanently than ever before by eating more—smarter.[12]

Study 1

The Journal of Nutrition published a 2003 study where women were put into two groups: let's call them inSANE and SANE. The inSANE people followed the government's guidelines. The SANE group ate a more balanced ratio of protein, carbohydrate, and fat from more natural foods. Both groups ate the same quantity of calories per day. The only difference between the groups was the quality of their diets.

After ten weeks, the SANE group lost 75% more body fat than the inSANE group.[13]

Study 2

The International Journal of Obesity published a study in 2004 in which people were put into two groups, eating as many calories as they wanted to. The only thing that varied between the groups was the SANEity of their diets. The study lasted one year. Keep in mind that everyone in the study ate an unlimited quantity of food. The only thing that varied was the quality of their calories.

After six months, the more SANE group lost nearly 80% more fat. After twelve months, the more SANE group had lost 50% more body fat and shrunk their bellies 367% more. Beyond being visually appealing, a 367% greater decrease in belly size is important since abdominal fat and waist circumference—rather than total body fat—are what most accurately predict weight-related health issues.[14]

Study 3

In 2009, the journal *Cardiovascular Diabetology* reported that researchers found a SANE diet burned body fat 35% more effectively than exactly the same number of calories from less SANE sources. Researchers also noted that the SANE diet was "more beneficial with respect to cardiovascular risk factors." The researchers concluded: "Since mean energy intake and energy expenditure did not differ between the two groups, the differences in [weight reduction, belly fat lost, and blood pressure] are most likely due to differences in macronutrient relations [calorie quality]."[15]

Study 4

In 2007, the journal *Applied Physiology, Nutrition, and Metabolism* reported a study in which researchers divided people into four groups. All of the groups ate the same number of calories but varied how SANE their diets were and how much they exercised.

- **SANE + Exercise:** This group ate a SANE diet and exercised three times per week.
- **Almost SANE + No Exercise:** This group ate an almost SANE diet and did not exercise.
- **InSANE + Exercise:** This group ate a mostly inSANE diet and exercised three times per week.
- **InSANE + No Exercise:** This group ate an inSANE diet and did not exercise.

Here are the results:

Pounds Lost in Twelve Weeks

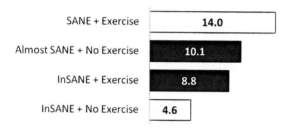

Look at the middle two bars. The *quality* of calories, not the *quantity* of exercise, played the biggest role in burning body fat. Put differently, adding exercise to an inSANE diet led to less body fat being burned than skipping exercise altogether, while eating a more SANE diet. The researchers noted that a SANE diet "was superior to a low-fat, high-carbohydrate diet [the government's diet] either alone or *when combined with an aerobic/resistance-training program* in promoting weight loss."[16]

Study 5

Last but not least and more related to the permanent fat loss side of things, in 2006 the journal *Nutrition & Metabolism* researchers followed up with people a year and a half after a weight-loss study. The people in the more SANE group still weighed 15 pounds less, even though they had stopped eating the SANE diet from the study.[17]

Benefit 3—Less Risk of Cancer and Cardiovascular Problems

"One of the more surprising findings from nutrition research over the past decade is that people who regularly eat nuts are less likely to have heart attacks or die from heart disease than those who rarely eat them."
W.C. WILLETT, HARVARD UNIVERSITY[18]

"These prospective data suggest that consumption of seafood at least once per week may reduce the risk of sudden cardiac death in men."
C.M. ALBERT, HARVARD UNIVERSITY[19]

Let's get straight to the point. Eating more non-starchy vegetables has been associated with drops in the risk of nearly all diseases. Eating more fruit and nuts contributes to a reduced risk of cardiovascular disease. Eating more seafood and chicken drops our risk of heart disease and cancer. The list goes on. As you would expect, eating high-quality food leads to high-quality health.[20]

Benefit 4—Less Cravings, Overeating, and Hunger

"The difference in intake was striking with the lower protein group consuming 621 more calories."
T.L. HALTON, HARVARD UNIVERSITY[21]

We covered this in detail when we discussed Satiety, but here are a few other interesting findings. Studies at Temple University show high-quality calories causing a "spontaneous reduction in energy intake" to an appropriate level for healthy and sustained fat loss. Other research reveals getting a natural balanced amount of protein—about a third of calories—causes people to effortlessly avoid hundreds of excess calories per day. By eating more good food, it is easy to avoid bad food while keeping the fat metabolism system from thinking that it is starving.[22]

Benefit 5—Increased Need to Burn Body Fat All Day, Every Day

> *"Higher protein diets increase loss of body weight and body fat and attenuate [slow] loss of lean tissue when compared with commonly recommended high carbohydrate low fat low protein diets."*
> **D.K. LAYMAN, UNIVERSITY OF ILLINOIS**[23]

While eating less of the same old inSANE diet drops our need to burn body fat, eating more of a SANE diet increases it. Consider an American University of Beirut study. There was a SANE diet group and a group that adhered to governmental dietary guidelines. After a month, the SANE group lost six pounds more than the inSANE group and still needed 250 more calories per day than the relatively heavier inSANE group. In other words, they lost weight without losing their need to burn body fat.[24]

Glossary

Ability to Burn Body Fat: When our body is capable of efficiently burning body fat for energy.
Example—An unclogged fat metabolism system has the *ability to burn body fat*.

Added Sweeteners: Substances that contain calories and are infused into foods to "enhance" taste. The most inSANE and clog-causing substance in the world.
Example—Sugar, high-fructose corn syrup, and evaporated cane juice are common *added sweeteners*.

Aggression: A measure of how likely calories are to be stored as body fat.
Example—Starches and sweets are basically pure glucose and therefore provide an abundance of *Aggressive* calories.

Amino Acids: What our bodies initially convert protein into.
Example—Excess *amino acids* must be converted into glucose and then converted into fatty acids before they can be stored as body fat.

Balance Scale Analogy: The myth that people can practically regulate the calories they take in and burn off with enough precision to impact their weight in the long term.
Example—The second chapter of the USDA's *2010 Dietary Guidelines for Americans* promotes the *balance scale analogy*. The chapter is titled: *Balancing Calories to Mange Weight.*

Balanced Diet: Eating about the same amount of calories from protein, carbohydrate, and fat.
Example—The government's guidelines and graphics tell people to get about 65% of their calories from carbohydrate, 20% from fat, and 15% from protein. That is not a *balanced diet*.

Body-Fat-Burning Hormones: Substances such as epinephrine, adrenaline, noradrenaline, growth hormone, ACTH, glucagon, thyroid hormone, and lipase that enable the fat metabolism system to burn body fat.

Example—High-quality eating and exercise trigger *body-fat-burning hormones*.

Body-Fat-Storing Hormones: Substances such as insulin that enable the fat metabolism system to store body fat.

Example—Low-quality eating triggers *body-fat-storing hormones*.

Brief Exercise: A key characteristic of high-quality cardiovascular exercise.

Example—By doing forceful *Brief exercise* on a low-impact cardiovascular exercise machine for ten minutes per week, Jane felt and looked better than when she did five hours of traditional cardiovascular exercise per week.

Caloric Sweeteners: The type of sweeteners proven to cause clogs in the fat metabolism system and to destroy our health. Also see *Added Sweeteners*.

Example—Non-caloric sweeteners such as Splenda and Equal are not great for us, but they are not nearly as bad for us as *caloric sweeteners*.

Calorie Quality Factors: The four measurements which determine if a calorie is high- or low-quality: Satiety, Aggression, Nutrition, Efficiency.

Example—*A Calorie Is A Calorie* cannot be true given the *calorie quality factors*.

Calorie Quality: What determines if a calorie will clog or clear the fat metabolism system. What determines if a calorie will trigger body-fat-burning or body-fat-storing hormones.

Example—Low *calorie quality* is the cause of long-term body fat gain.

Calorie Quantity Theory of Fat Loss: A myth that gaining body fat is *caused* by eating too many calories and exercising away too few calories, and that burning body fat is *caused* by eating less calories and exercising away more calories.

Example—According to the *calorie quantity theory of fat loss,* Jane will gain about 1,000 pounds over the next ten years if she eats about 1,000 too many calories per day.

Cholesterol: A substance produced by the liver or intestines or acquired from food that is required for the production of new cells and hormones.

Example—"In [a famous cardiovascular disease study] the more saturated fat one ate, the more *cholesterol* one ate, the more calories one ate, the lower people's serum [total] *cholesterol*."—W.P. Castelli, Framingham Cardiovascular Institute[1]

Clog: An analogy that explains the fat metabolism system's inability to respond to hormonal signals that cause it to burn—rather than store—excess calories.

Example—The cause of weight gain is a *clog* in the fat metabolism system.

Clogged Fat Metabolism System: When the hormonal signals that otherwise automatically regulate body weight around a set-point do not function properly.

Example—Studies show that even when obese people eat nothing, their *clogged fat metabolism system* prevents them from burning body fat effectively.

Deep Exercise: An activity that requires so much force and works so many muscle fibers that it can only be done for a matter of seconds, once per week.

Example—A great *deep exercise* you can do at home is to increase the resistance on a stationary bike so that you have to push on the pedals as hard as you can in order to move them.

Deep Muscle Fibers: The parts of muscles that trigger the most clog-clearing hormones and that can only be exercised by making the muscle generate as much force as possible.

Example—Slowly lowering as much resistance as possible for ten seconds works your *deep muscle fibers*.

Dietary Guidelines: A government document that was first released in 1980—and has been rereleased every five years since—that recommends a high-carbohydrate-low-fat-low-protein diet which is only practical if you eat unnatural amounts of starches and sweeteners.

Example—Combine the governments' *Dietary Guidelines* with the profitability of highly-processed high-carbohydrate-low-fat-low-protein starch and sweetener based foods, and we get the weight and health problems we have today.

Diseases of Civilization: Obesity, diabetes, heart disease, cardiovascular disease, and other diet related diseases which were not a problem before starches and sweeteners became the cornerstone of our diet.

Example—The remaining hunter-gather populations stay free of the *diseases of civilization* well into old age.

Eccentric Exercise: A technique that enables us to safely increase the quality of resistance training by allowing us to use more resistance when muscles are stronger and less resistance when our muscles are weaker.

Example— Because it is so safe, *eccentric exercise* enables everyone to make their muscles generate more force.

Efficiency: A measure of how many calories from a given food could ever be stored as body fat.

Example—Only about a third of calories from protein can ever be stored as body fat, thanks to their low *Efficiency*.

Exercise Quality: Determined by the amount of clog-clearing hormones triggered by an activity.

Example—Focusing on *exercise quality* rather than exercise quantity is one of the keys to long-term health and long-term body fat loss.

Fat Metabolism System: An analogy that explains how a series of hormonal and neural signals regulate food intake, energy expenditure, and body fat.

Example—When our *fat metabolism system* becomes clogged, we are prone to store body fat regardless of how many calories we eat.

Fat Super Accumulation: The primary long-term side effect of eating less.

Example—After eating less, rats gained body fat twenty times faster than normal. They experienced *fat super accumulation*.

Glucose: The primary source of fuel for our bodies. What carbohydrate is immediately converted into during digestion.

Example—We gain body fat from eating low-quality foods that trigger the creation of more *glucose* than our body needs at any point in time.

Glycemic Index: A measure of a food's Aggression.

Example—Foods with a high *glycemic index* are more likely to be stored as body fat since they are converted into glucose faster than foods with a low *glycemic index.*

Glycemic Load: A measures of a food's Aggression combined with the calories in a portion of it.

Example—One of the reasons starches and sweets are so fattening is because of their high *glycemic load.*

Government Guidelines and Graphics: A set of disproven dietary principles and pictures which encourage a diet made up of 65% carbohydrate—much of which comes from starch—20% fat, and 15% protein.

Example—While they have become prettier over time, the *government's guidelines and graphics* still recommend the same harmful and fattening diet.

High-Fructose Corn Syrup: An especially clog-causing caloric sweetener.

Example—Starches, sweets, and most dairy products are common sources of *high-fructose corn syrup.*

High-Protein Diet: Getting more than about a third of your calories from protein.

Example—If someone who needs 2,400 calories per day consistently eats eleven chicken breasts per day, they would get 55% of their calories from protein and would be eating a *high-protein diet.*

High-Quality Brief Cardiovascular Exercise: Accomplished by increasing the resistance on cardiovascular exercise machines so much that the exercise can only be done for a few thirty-second bursts per week.

Example—Adding resistance to an upright stationary bike until you can only move the pedals by standing up and pushing as hard as you can is the first step to *high-quality Brief cardiovascular exercise.*

High-Quality Eccentric Resistance Training: Accomplished by lowering as much resistance as possible for ten seconds.

Example—Using exercises that require no balance and use a shared source of resistance, you can do *high-quality Eccentric resistance training* by using both limbs to lift the resistance and one limb to lower it.

High-Quality Exercise: An activity that is done infrequently, for a short period of time, using a lot of resistance, and provides all the benefits of traditional cardiovascular exercise, but much more efficiently, and unclogs the fat metabolism system.
  Example—The key to long-term body fat loss is not a lot of low-quality exercise. The key to long-term body fat loss is a little *high-quality exercise*.

High-Quality Foods: See *SANE Foods*.

Hormonal Exercise: An activity that unclogs the fat metabolism system.
  Example—Eccentric leg press is a very *hormonal exercise*.

Hormones: The substances that control our set-point, fat metabolism system, and many other bodily systems. The substances significantly influenced by the quality of the food that we eat.
  Example—Calorie quality significantly influences *hormones. Hormones* control our fat metabolism system and set-point. Therefore, we can significantly influence our fat metabolism system and set-point by controlling the quality of our calories.

Imbalanced Diet: Getting more than about a third of calories from carbohydrate, protein, or fat.
  Example—The diet recommended by the government's guidelines and graphics is a grossly *imbalanced diet*.

inSANE Foods: Water-, fiber-, and protein-poor foods that have low Satiety, high Aggression, low Nutrition, and high Efficiency.
  Example—Starches and sweets are *inSANE foods*.

Insulin: A hormone that enables body fat to be stored while preventing body fat from being burned.
  Example—When we eat inSANE starches and sweets, we produce too much *insulin* and lose the ability to burn body fat effectively regardless of how much we starve ourselves.

Insulin Resistance: When the body must produce excess insulin to get energy into our cells.

Example—When we are *insulin resistant,* we are clogged-up with excess insulin and cannot burn body fat effectively.

Internal Starvation: When the fat metabolism system is so broken down that it encourages us to overeat to compensate for all the calories it is leaking into our fat cells.

Example—When insulin can only effectively get energy into fat cells while removing our ability to burn stored energy for fuel, we experience *internal starvation.*

Lean Meat: Meat that has at least 80% of its calories coming from protein.

Example—White-meat skinless turkey and white-meat skinless chicken are the most common sources of *lean meat.*

Low-Carbohydrate Diet: Getting less than about a third of your calories from carbohydrate.

Example—*The Atkins Diet* is the most famous *low-carbohydrate diet.*

Lowered Set-Point: The result of eating more and exercising less—smarter. What happens when the hormonal clog is cleared. The key to practical and permanent fat loss.

Example—A *lowered set-point* will do automatically what is completely impractical to do manually: burn body fat all day, every day.

Low-Fat Diet: Getting less than about a third of your calories from fat.

Example—The government's *Dietary Guidelines* and graphics promote a *low-fat diet.*

Low-Quality Exercise: An activity that is done frequently, for a long period of time, using little resistance, and improves health, but does not unclog the fat metabolism system.

Example—Jogging and walking are *low-quality exercises.*

Low-Quality Foods: See inSANE Foods.

Macronutrients: The three primary sources of calories.

Example—The three *macronutrients* are carbohydrate, fat, and protein.

Manually Balance Calories Theory of Fat Loss: The myth that people can effectively burn body fat long-term by consciously regulating the amount of calories they take in and exercise off.

Example—Anyone who thinks eating less and exercising more is an effective long-term approach to burning body fat believes the *manually balance calories theory of fat loss.*

Milled Flax Seeds: An extremely SANE food that provides an incredible amount of nutrients—such as omega-3 fatty acids—which are otherwise hard to get.

Example—An easy way to incorporate *milled flax seeds* into your diet is to add a tablespoon or two to smoothies.

Monounsaturated Fats: The second most healthy type of fat.

Example—Meat, fish, select dairy, nuts, avocados, olive oil, and canola oil are good sources of *monounsaturated fats.*

Natural Balanced Diet: Eating about an equal amount of carbohydrate, fat, and protein from foods that can be hunted or gathered.

Example—The easiest way to clear your clog and lower your set-point is to eat a *natural balanced diet.*

Natural Food: The foods that humans ate for 99.8% of their evolution. The foods that humans ate prior to agriculture and civilization. The foods that help us to avoid the diseases of civilization.

Example—Non-starchy vegetables, seafood, meat, fruit, eggs, flax seeds, and nuts are *natural foods.* Organic bread, organic cereal, and organic pasta are not *natural foods.*

Need to Burn Body Fat: When the fat metabolism system has insufficient calories from food, but sufficient nutrition to avoid slowing down or burning muscle.

Example—It is easy to create the *need to burn body fat* instead of the need to slow down and burn muscle when we eat more SANE foods. SANE foods provide an abundance of Satiety and Nutrition in relatively few unAggressive and inEfficient calories.

Non-Caloric Sweeteners: Any substance that is sweet and does not contain calories. The healthier alternative to caloric sweeteners.

Example—The most common *non-caloric sweeteners* are acesulfame potassium (Sunett, Sweet One), aspartame (Equal, NutraSweet), neotame, saccharin (Sweet 'N Low), sucralose (Splenda), stevia (Sweet Leaf, Honey Leaf), and tagatose (Naturlose).

Non-Starchy Vegetables: The most SANE vegetables. Essentially, anything other than corn, potatoes, turnips, yams, parsnips, radishes, and most other root vegetables.

Example—Common *non-starchy vegetables* include: Broccoli, carrots, cauliflower, celery, cucumber, eggplant, lettuce, mushrooms, onions, peas, peppers, spinach, squash, and zucchini. Generally speaking, vegetables that grow above ground—except corn...which is a starch—are non-starchy vegetables.

Nutrients: The substances in foods that our bodies need to function optimally.

Example—Protein, vitamins, minerals, and essential fatty acids (aka omega-3 and 6 fatty acids) are key *nutrients.*

Nutrition: A measure of how many nutrients are provided per calorie of a given food. Primarily determined by the amount of water, fiber, and protein in a food.

Example—Water-, fiber-, and protein-packed non-starchy vegetables contain more *Nutrition* than any other type of food.

Omega-3 Fatty Acids: An exceptionally healthy type of polyunsaturated fat that is very difficult to eat enough of, unless you eat milled flax seeds.

Example—You can easily ensure that you get enough *omega-3 fatty acids* by adding a tablespoon of milled flax seeds to everything you can. They have very little taste, so adding them to food does nothing but make you healthier and slimmer.

Polyunsaturated Fats: The healthiest type of fat.[2]

Example—Milled flax seeds, salmon, herring, sardines, mackerel, halibut, tuna, swordfish, and walnuts are good sources of *polyunsaturated* fats.

Raised Set-Point: Abnormal levels of hormones that make the fat metabolism system think abnormal levels of body fat are normal. When the hormonal systems that normally keep us thin get clogged-up by inSANE low-quality foods and then malfunction.

Example—Once we are hormonally clogged, we have a *raised set-point* and will stay heavy, in the long term, 95% of the time, no matter how many calories we cut or exercise away.

SANE Foods: Water-, fiber-, and protein-packed foods that have high Satiety, low Aggression, high Nutrition, and low Efficiency.

Example—The easiest way to eat the most *SANE foods* possible is to eat as much as you want, whenever you want, from foods you could hunt or gather.

Satiety: A measure of how likely calories are to prevent us from overeating.

Example—Non-starchy vegetables and seafood have higher *Satiety* than any other foods.

Saturated Fats: The third healthiest fat. Note: The only unhealthy fat is unnatural trans-fat (an artificial form of fat added to starches and sweets).

Example—Healthy amounts of *saturated fats* are found in SANE foods such as seafood, lean meat, select dairy, nuts, and seeds.

Select Dairy: Dairy products that have more than 60% of their calories coming from protein and do not contain any added sweeteners.

Example—The most common examples of *select dairy* are fat-free or low-fat cottage cheese and fat-free or low-fat *plain Greek* yogurt.

Set-Point: The weight our fat metabolism system automatically works to keep us at, regardless of the quantity of calories we take in or exercise off.

Example—Eating less and exercising more fail 95% of the time because they fight against our *set-point*.

Smarter Eating: Eating so much more SANE high-quality foods that you are too full for inSANE low-quality foods.

Example—Thanks to *smarter eating*, Jane cleared her clog, dropped her set-point, and automatically stayed slim for the rest of her life, much like a naturally thin person.

Smarter Exercise: See *High-Quality Exercise*.

Smarter Science of Slim: Eating so much high-quality food and doing so little—but such high-quality—exercise that you are able to clear your clog and lower your set-point practically and permanently.

Example—The *smarter science of slim* is a proven and practical way to burn body fat long term.

Starch: A food that is basically pure glucose.

Example—Sugar is unhealthy and fattening because it is nothing more than glucose. So is *starch*. Whole grain *starch* sprinkles a little fiber, vitamins, and minerals on glucose. Whole grain *starch* is like adding a sliver of a vitamin and dash of a fiber supplement to soda.

Starchy Vegetables: A food that is basically pure glucose. The type of vegetables we should avoid.

Example—*Starchy vegetables* include any form of corn and potato, as well as turnips, yams, parsnips, radishes, and most other root vegetables. Avoid corn and non-sweet potatoes completely. Everything else can be enjoyed in moderation.

Sweeteners: See *Added Sweeteners.*

Traditional Cardiovascular Exercise: Activities that can be done for a long time, require little force, exercise only a small fraction of our muscle fibers, release little if any clog-clearing hormones, and must be done for hours to impact our health and weight.

Example—The most common forms of *traditional cardiovascular exercise* are walking, biking, and jogging.

Traditional Exercise: See *Low-Quality Exercise.*

Traditional Weight Loss Approach: Eat less food and spend more time exercising. Became mainstream in the 1970's. Ignores the three things that control long-term weight: the set-point, calorie quality, and a hormonal clog in the fat metabolism system.

Example—Studies show that the *traditional weight loss approach* fails long-term 95% of the time.

Unclogged Fat Metabolism System: A bodily system that balances calories with 99.83% accuracy.[3]

Example—An *unclogged fat metabolism system* does automatically what we could never do manually, long term.

Unnatural Diet: Eating foods other than those eaten for 99.8% of human evolution.

Example—Eating starches and sweets is eating an *unnatural diet*.

Weight Lifting: See *High-Quality Eccentric Resistance Training*.

Whey Protein Powder: A high-quality, inexpensive, SANE, tasty, and convenient source of protein that is derived from milk.

Example—Drinking thirty grams of whey protein powder mixed with a tablespoon of milled flax seeds, two tablespoons of finely ground wheat grass, and water before breakfast, lunch, and dinner is the easiest way to eat a more SANE diet.

Online Resources, Extras, and Bonuses

For more science, please visit TheSmarterScienceofSlim.com and JonathanBailor.com. They both have all sorts of free tools, recipes, videos, articles, etc.

Index

To easily find specific topics in this book, visit the searchable digital version at http://books.google.com. Simply search for *The Smarter Science of Slim* and then search within it for the given topic.

Bibliography

Introduction

1   Friedman JM. Modern science versus the stigma of obesity. Nat Med. 2004 Jun;10(6):563-9. Review. PubMed PMID: 15170194.
2   A sampling of supporting research:
  • "To avoid overweight, consume only as much energy as is expended; if overweight, decrease energy intake and increase energy expenditure." Senate Select Committee on Nutrition and Human Needs (U.S.). Dietary goals for the United States. 2nd ed. Washington: Government Printing office; 1977.
  • http://www.cdc.gov/brfss/. Data from the Behavioral Risk Factor Surveillance System reveal that nearly half of women and a third of men are dieting and about fifty million Americans pay for gym memberships.
  • Petersen CB, Thygesen LC, Helge JW, Grønbaek M, Tolstrup JS. Time trends in physical activity in leisure time in the Danish population from 1987 to 2005. Scand J Public Health. 2010 Mar;38(2):121-8. Epub 2010 Jan 11. PubMed PMID: 20064919.
  • http://www.time.com/time/health/article/0,8599,1914857,00.html#ixzz0Wz0PTtHj
  • http://apps.who.int/bmi/index.jsp
  • Oliver, J. Eric. Fat Politics: The Real Story behind America's Obesity Epidemic. New Ed ed. New York: Oxford University Press, USA, 2006. Print.
  • Nestle M, Jacobson MF. Halting the obesity epidemic: a public health policy approach. Public Health Rep. 2000 Jan-Feb;115(1):12-24. PubMed PMID: 10968581; PubMed Central PMCID: PMC1308552.
  • Petersen CB, Thygesen LC, Helge JW, Grønbaek M, Tolstrup JS. Time trends in physical activity in leisure time in the Danish population from 1987 to 2005. Scand J Public Health. 2010 Mar;38(2):121-8. Epub 2010 Jan 11. PubMed PMID: 20064919.
  • Roberts, Seth. The Shangri-La Diet: The No Hunger Eat Anything Weight-Loss Plan. Chicago: Perigee Trade, 2007. Print.
3   http://www.cdc.gov/brfss/
4   Wooley SC, Garner DM. Dietary treatments for obesity are ineffective. BMJ. 1994 Sep 10;309(6955):655-6. PubMed PMID: 8086992; PubMed Central PMCID: PMC2541482.
5   Stunkard, A., and M. McClaren-Hume. 1959. "The Results of Treatment for Obesity: A Review of the Literature and a Report of a Series." Archives of Internal Medicine. Jan.;103(I):79-85.
6   P.J. Skerrett, and W.C. Willett. Eat, Drink, and Be Healthy: The Harvard Medical School Guide to Healthy Eating. Free Press Trade Pbk. New York City: Free Press, 2005. & Weinberg SL. The diet-heart hypothesis: a critique. J Am Coll Cardiol. 2004 Mar 3;43(5):731-3. Review. PubMed PMID: 14998608.
7   A sampling of supporting research:
  • Roberts, Paul. The End of Food. New York: Mariner Books, 2009. Print.
  • In 1990 the following report estimated that United States consumers spend more than $33 billion yearly on weight loss products and services.The U.S. Congress H. Deception and Fraud in the Diet Industry, Part 1. 101st Congress, 2nd Session. 1990. Committee on Small Business, Subcommittee on

Regulation, Business Opportunities, and Energy. Nearly twenty years later this number is estimated to have grown to $50 billion. See: Freedhoff Y, Sharma AM. "Lose 40 pounds in 4 weeks": regulating commercial weight-loss programs. CMAJ. 2009 Feb 17;180(4):367-8. English, French. PubMed PMID: 19221340; PubMed Central PMCID: PMC2638047. the European diet market is estimated at 100B Euros. See: Cannon, Geoffrey. Dieting Makes You Fat: The Scientifically Proven Way to be Slim without Lowering Your Food Intake. Revised edition ed. None: Virgin Books, 2008. Print.

- Cassels, Alan, and Ray Moynihan. Selling Sickness: How the World's Biggest Pharmaceutical Companies Are Turning Us All Into Patients. 1 ed. New York City, New York: Nation Books, 2006. Print
- "Economics of the Food and Fiber System." USDA Economic Research Service—Home Page. N.p., n.d. Web. 13 June 2010. <http://www.ers.usda.gov/amberwaves/February04/DataFeature/>.
- http://www.kraftfoodscompany.com/assets/pdf/kraft_foods_fact_sheet.pdf
- "Investor Relations." Nestle Global—Homepage template. N.p., n.d. Web. 13 June 2010. <http://www.nestle.com/InvestorRelations/>.
- Cassels, Alan, and Ray Moynihan. Selling Sickness: How the World's Biggest Pharmaceutical Companies Are Turning Us All Into Patients. 1 ed. New York City, New York: Nation Books, 2006. Print.
- Brownell, Kelly, and Katherine Battle Horgen. Food Fight. 1 ed. New York: McGraw-Hill, 2004. Print.

8 A sampling of supporting research:
- Crawford D, Jeffery RW, French SA. Can anyone successfully control their weight? Findings of a three year community-based study of men and women. Int J Obes Relat Metab Disord. 2000 Sep;24(9):1107-10. PubMed PMID: 11033978.
- Summerbell CD, Cameron C, Glasziou PP. WITHDRAWN: Advice on low-fat diets for obesity. Cochrane Database Syst Rev. 2008 Jul 16;(3):CD003640. Review. PubMed PMID: 18646093.
- Pirozzo S, Summerbell C, Cameron C, Glasziou P. Should we recommend low-fat diets for obesity? Obes Rev. 2003 May;4(2):83-90. Review. Erratum in: Obes Rev. 2003 Aug;4(3):185. PubMed PMID: 12760443.
- " A word about quitting success rates ." American Cancer Society :: Information and Resources for Cancer: Breast, Colon, Prostate, Lung and Other Forms. N.p., n.d. Web. 11 Jan. 2011. <http://www.cancer.org/Healthy/StayAwayfromTobacco/GuidetoQuittingSmoking/guide-to-quitting-smoking-success-rates>.

9 Johnson D., Drenick E. J. (1977) therapeutic fasting in morbid obesity: long-term fellow-up. Arch. Intern. Med. 137:1381–1382.

10 A sampling of supporting research:
- Farnsworth E, Luscombe ND, Noakes M, Wittert G, Argyiou E, Clifton PM. Effect of a high-protein, energy-restricted diet on body composition, glycemic control, and lipid concentrations in overweight and obese hyperinsulinemic men and women.Am J Clin Nutr. 2003 Jul;78(1):31-9.
- Arora SK, McFarlane SI. The case for low carbohydrate diets in diabetes management. Nutr Metab (Lond). 2005 Jul 14;2:16. PubMed PMID: 16018812; PubMed Central PMCID: PMC1188071.
- Augustin LS, Franceschi S, Jenkins DJ, Kendall CW, La Vecchia C. Glycemic index in chronic disease: a review. Eur J Clin Nutr. 2002 Nov;56(11):1049-71.Review. PubMed PMID: 12428171.
- Baba NH, Sawaya S, Torbay N, Habbal Z, Azar S, Hashim SA: High protein vs high carbohydrate hypoenergetic diet for the treatment of obese hyperinsulinemic subjects. Int J Obes23 :1202–1206, 1999.
- Børsheim E, Bui Q-UT, Tissier S, Kobayashi H, Ferrando AA, Wolfe RR. Effect of amino acid supplementation in insulin sensitivity in elderly. Fed Proc (in press).
- Brand-Miller J. Diets with a low glycemic index: From theory to practice. Nutrition Today. 1999;34:64–72.
- Brehm BJ, Seeley RJ, Daniels SR, D'Alessio DA: A randomized trial comparing a very low carbohydrate diet and a calorie restricted low fat diet on body weight and cardiovascular risk factors in healthy women. J Clin Endocrinol Metab88 :1617 –1623,2003
- Despres JP, Moorjani S, Lupien PJ, Tremblay A, Nadeau A, Bouchard C. Regional distribution of body

fat, plasmalipoproteins, and cardiovascular disease. rteriosclerosis 1990;10: 497–511.

- Despres JP. Dyslipidaemia and obesity. Baillieres Clin Endocrinol Metab 1994; 8: 629–660.
- Due A, Toubro S, Skov AR, Astrup A. Effect of normal-fat diets, either medium or high in protein, on body weight in overweight subjects: a randomised 1-year trial. Int J Obes Relat Metab Disord. 2004 Oct;28(10):1283-90. PubMed PMID:15303109.
- Foster GD, Wyatt HR, Hill JO, McGuckin BG, Brill C, Mohammed S: A randomized trial of a low-carbohydrate diet. N Eng J Med348 :2082 –2090,2003
- Frisch S, Zittermann A, Berthold HK, Götting C, Kuhn J, Kleesiek K, Stehle P, Körtke H. A random-ized controlled trial on the efficacy of carbohydrate-reduced or fat-reduced diets in patients attend-ing a telemedically guided weight loss program. Cardiovasc Diabetol. 2009 Jul 18;8:36. PubMed PMID: 19615091; PubMed Central PMCID: PMC2722581.
- Frost G, Keogh B, Smith D, Akinsanya K, Leeds A. (1996). The effect of low-glycemic carbohydrate on insulin and glucose response in vivo and in vitro in patients with coronary heart disease. Metabo-lism, 45: 669-672.
- Gannon MC, Nuttall FQ, Saeed A, Jordan K, Hoover H. An increase in dietary protein improves the blood glucose response in persons with type 2 diabetes. Am J Clin Nutr. 2003 Oct;78(4):734-41. PubMed PMID: 14522731.
- Harrison BC, Leinwand LA. Fighting fat with muscle: bulking up to slim down.Cell Metab. 2008 Feb;7(2):97-8. Review. PubMed PMID: 18249167.
- Izumiya Y, Hopkins T, Morris C, Sato K, Zeng L, Viereck J, Hamilton JA, Ouchi N, LeBrasseur NK, Walsh K. Fast/Glycolytic muscle fiber growth reduces fat mass and improves metabolic parameters in obese mice. Cell Metab. 2008 Feb;7(2):159-72. PubMed PMID: 18249175.
- Kissebah AH, Krakower GR. Regional adiposity and morbidity. Physiol Rev 1994; 74: 761–811.
- Lasker DA, Evans EM, Layman DK. Moderate carbohydrate, moderate protein weight loss diet re-duces cardiovascular disease risk compared to high carbohydrate, low protein diet in obese adults: A randomized clinical trial. Nutr Metab (Lond). 2008 Nov 7;5:30. PubMed PMID: 18990242; PubMed Central PMCID: PMC2585565.
- Layman DK, Boileau RA, Erickson DJ, Painter JE, Shiue H, Sather C, Christou DD. A reduced ratio of dietary carbohydrate to protein improves body composition and blood lipid profiles during weight loss in adult women. J Nutr. 2003 Feb;133(2):411-7. PubMed PMID: 12566476.
- Lejeune MP, Kovacs EM, Westerterp-Plantenga MS. Additional protein intake limits weight regain after weight loss in humans. Br J Nutr. 2005 Feb;93(2):281-9. PubMed PMID: 15788122.
- Low-carbohydrate diet in type 2 diabetes. Stable improvement of bodyweight and glycemic control during 22 months follow-up Jørgen Vesti Nielsen and Eva Joensson Nutr Metab (Lond). 2006; 3: 22. Published online 2006 June 14. doi: 10.1186/1743-7075-3-22. PMCID: PMC1526736
- McAuley KA, Hopkins CM, Smith KJ, McLay RT, Williams SM, Taylor RW, Mann JI. Comparison of high-fat and high-protein diets with a high-carbohydrate diet in insulin-resistant obese women. Diabetologia. 2005 Jan;48(1):8-16.
- McAuley KA, Smith KJ, Taylor RW, McLay RT, Williams SM, Mann JI. Long-term effects of popu-lar dietary approaches on weight loss and features of insulin resistance. Int J Obes (Lond). 2006 Feb;30(2):342-9.
- Meckling KA, Sherfey R. A randomized trial of a hypocaloric high-protein diet, with and without exercise, on weight loss, fitness, and markers of the Metabolic Syndrome in overweight and obese women. Appl Physiol Nutr Metab. 2007 Aug;32(4):743-52. PubMed PMID: 17622289.
- Noakes M, Keogh JB, Foster PR, Clifton PM. Effect of an energy-restricted, high-protein, low-fat diet relative to a conventional high-carbohydrate, low-fat diet on weight loss, body composition, nutritional status, and markers of cardiovascular health in obese women. Am J Clin Nutr. 2005 Jun;81(6):1298-306.

- Nuttall FQ, Gannon MC. Metabolic response of people with type 2 diabetes to a high protein diet. Nutr Metab (Lond). 2004 Sep 13;1(1):652.
- Nuttall FQ, Gannon MC. The metabolic response to a high-protein, low-carbohydrate diet in men with type 2 diabetes mellitus. Metabolism. 2006 Feb;55(2):243-51.
- Parker, B., Noakes, M., Luscombe, N. & Clifton, P. (2002) Effect of a high-protein, monounsaturated fat weight loss diet on glycemic control and lipid levels in type 2 diabetes. Diabetes Care 25:425-430.
- Piatti PM, Monti F, Fermo I, Baruffaldi L, Nasser R, Santambrogio G, Librenti MC, Galli-Kienle M, Pontiroli AE, Pozza G. Hypocaloric high-protein diet improves glucose oxidation and spares lean body mass: comparison to hypocaloric high-carbohydrate diet. Metabolism. 1994 Dec;43(12):1481-7. PubMed PMID: 7990700.
- Samaha FF, Iqbal N, Seshadri P, Chicano KL, Daily D, Mcgrory J: A low carbohydrate as compared with a low fat diet in severe obesity. N Eng J Med348 :2074 –2081,2003 .
- Skov AR, Toubro S, Rønn B, Holm L, Astrup A. Randomized trial on protein vs carbohydrate in ad libitum fat reduced diet for the treatment of obesity. Int J Obes Relat Metab Disord. 1999 May;23(5):528-36. PubMed PMID: 10375057.
- Skov, A. R., Toubro, S., Ronn, B., Holm, L. & Astrup, A. (1999) Randomized trial on protein vs carbohydrate in ad libitum fat reduced diet for the treatment of obesity. Int. J. Obes. 23:528-536.
- Weigle DS, Breen PA, Matthys CC, Callahan HS, Meeuws KE, Burden VR, Purnell JQ. A high-protein diet induces sustained reductions in appetite, ad libitum caloric intake, and body weight despite compensatory changes in diurnal plasma leptin and ghrelin concentrations. Am J Clin Nutr. 2005 Jul;82(1):41-8
- Westerterp-Plantenga MS, Lejeune MP, Nijs I, van Ooijen M, Kovacs EM. High protein intake sustains weight maintenance after body weight loss in humans. Int J Obes Relat Metab Disord. 2004 Jan;28(1):57-64.
- Wolfe RR. The underappreciated role of muscle in health and disease. Am J Clin Nutr. 2006 Sep;84(3):475-82. Review. PubMed PMID: 16960159.
- Worthington BS, Taylor LE: Balanced low calorie vs high protein, low carbohydrate reducing diets. J Am Diet Assoc64 :47 –51,1974 .
- Yancy Jr WS, Olsen MK, Guyton JR, Bakst RP, Westman EC: A low-carbohydrate, ketogenic diet versus a low-fat diet to treat obesity and hyperlipidemia. Ann Intern Med140 :769 –777,2004

11 Arciero PJ, Gentile CL, Martin-Pressman R, Ormsbee MJ, Everett M, Zwicky L, Steele CA. Increased dietary protein and combined high intensity aerobic and resistance training improves body fat distribution and cardiovascular risk factors. Int J Sport Nutr Exerc Metab. 2006 Aug;16(4):373-92. PubMed PMID: 17136940.

Chapter 1

1 Jensen AR How much can we boost IQ and scholastic achievement? Harvard Educ Rev 1969;39:1–123.
2 Wooley SC, Wooley OW, Dyrenforth S. The case against radical interventions. Am J Clin Nutr. 1980 Feb;33(2 Suppl):465-71. PubMed PMID: 7355820.
3 Havel PJ. Dietary fructose: implications for dysregulation of energy homeostasis and lipid/carbohydrate metabolism. Nutr Rev. 2005 May;63(5):133-57. Review. PubMed PMID: 15971409.
4 Sampling of supporting research:
   - Stetten, D. J. Biol. Chem. 147: 327, 1943
   - Bessard T, Schutz Y, Jéquier E. Energy expenditure and postprandial thermogenesis in obese women before and after weight loss. Am J Clin Nutr. 1983 Nov;38(5):680-93. PubMed PMID: 6637860.
   - Eckel RH. Adipose Tissue Lipoprotein Lipase. In: Borensztajn J, edl Lipoprotein Lipase. Chicago: Evener, 1987: 79-132.
   - Arner P, Eckel R. Adipose Tissue as a Storage Organ In: Bray GA, Couchard d, James WP, eds. Hand-

book of Obesity. New York: Marcel Dekker, 1997: 379-396.

- Jequier E. Thermogenic responses induced by nutrients in man: Their importance in energy balance regulation. Experientia Suppl. 1983;44:26-44. Review. PubMed PMID: 6357848.
- Schutz Y, Bessard T, Jéquier E. Diet-induced thermogenesis measured over a whole day in obese and nonobese women. Am J Clin Nutr. 1984 Sep;40(3):542-52. PubMed PMID: 6540980.

5 Kelesidis T, Kelesidis I, Chou S, Mantzoros CS. Narrative review: The role of leptin in human physiology: emerging clinical applications. Ann Intern Med. 2010 Jan 19;152(2):93-100. Review. PubMed PMID: 20083828; PubMed Central PMCID:PMC2829242.

6 Rolland-Cachera MF, Bellisle F. No correlation between adiposity and food intake: why are working class children fatter? Am J Clin Nutr. 1986 Dec;44(6):779-87. PubMed PMID: 3788830. & Keen H, Thomas BJ, Jarrett RJ, Fuller JH. Nutrient intake, adiposity, and diabetes. Br Med J. 1979 Mar 10;1(6164):655-8. PubMed PMID: 435710

7 Howard BV, Manson JE, Stefanick ML, Beresford SA, Frank G, Jones B, Rodabough RJ, Snetselaar L, Thomson C, Tinker L, Vitolins M, Prentice R. Low-fat dietary pattern and weight change over 7 years: The Women's Health Initiative Dietary Modification Trial. JAMA. 2006 Jan 4;295(1):39-49. PubMed PMID: 16391215.

8 Keesey RE, Powley TL. The regulation of body weight. Annu Rev Psychol. 1986;37:109-33. PubMed PMID: 3963779. & Benedict, Francis Gano. Human Vitality and Efficiency under Prolonged Restricted Diet,. Washington: Carnegie Institution of Washington, 1919. Print.

9 A sampling of supporting research:
- Keesey RE, Powley TL. The regulation of body weight. Annu Rev Psychol. 1986;37:109-33. PubMed PMID: 3963779.
- http://www.mayoclinic.com/health/insulin-and-weight-gain/DA00139
- Flatt JP. Conversion of carbohydrate to fat in adipose tissue: an energy-yielding and, therefore, self-limiting process. J Lipid Res. 1970 Mar;11(2):131-43. PubMed PMID: 4392141.
- Acheson KJ, Schutz Y, Bessard T, Anantharaman K, Flatt JP, Jéquier E. Glycogen storage capacity and de novo lipogenesis during massive carbohydrate overfeeding in man. Am J Clin Nutr. 1988 Aug;48(2):240-7. PubMed PMID: 3165600.
- Keys, Ancel. The biology of human starvation. New York: Oxford U.P, 1950. Print.

10 Friedman JM. Modern science versus the stigma of obesity. Nat Med. 2004 Jun;10(6):563-9. Review. PubMed PMID: 15170194.

11 Jeevanandam M, Young DH, Schiller WR. Obesity and the metabolic response to severe multiple trauma in man. J Clin Invest. 1991 Jan;87(1):262-9. PubMed PMID: 1985100; PubMed Central PMCID: PMC295040.

12 A sampling of supporting research:
- Goldberg M, Gordon E. Energy Metabolism In Human Obesity. Plasma Free Fatty Acid, Glucose, And Glycerol Response To Epinephrine. JAMA. 1964 Aug 24;189:616-23. PubMed PMID: 14162576.
- E.A. Newsholme and C. Start. Regulation of Metabolism. 173 ISBN: 0471635308
- Frayn, K. N. Metabolic Regulation: a Human Perspective. London: Portland, 1996. Print.

13 A sampling of supporting research:
- Layman DK. Dietary Guidelines should reflect new understandings about adult protein needs. Nutr Metab (Lond). 2009 Mar 13;6:12. PubMed PMID: 19284668; PubMed Central PMCID: PMC2666737.
- Harvey RF. Gut peptides and the control of food intake. Br Med J (Clin Res Ed). 1983 Nov 26;287(6405):1572-4. PubMed PMID: 6416508; PubMed Central PMCID:PMC1549802.
- Comparison of the Action of Macronutrients on the Expression of Appetite in Lean and Obese Human Subjects ANDREW J. HILL, JOHN E. BLUNDELL Annals of the New York Academy of Sciences Volume 575 , Issue, Pages 529 — 531 1989 the New York Academy of Sciences
- Weigle DS, Breen PA, Matthys CC, Callahan HS, Meeuws KE, Burden VR, Purnell JQ. A high-protein diet induces sustained reductions in appetite, ad libitum caloric intake, and body weight despite

compensatory changes in diurnal plasma leptin and ghrelin concentrations. Am J Clin Nutr. 2005 Jul;82(1):41-8. PubMed PMID: 16002798.

- Hill AJ, Blundell JE: Macronutrients and satiety; the effects of a high protein or high carbohydrate meal on subjective motivation to eat and food preferences. Nutr Behav3 :133 –144,1986 .
- Barkeling B, Rössner S, Björvell H. Effects of a high-protein meal (meat) and a high-carbohydrate meal (vegetarian) on satiety measured by automated computerized monitoring of subsequent food intake, motivation to eat and food preferences. Int J Obes. 1990 Sep;14(9):743-51. PubMed PMID: 2228407.
- Booth DA, Chase A, Campbell AT. Relative effectiveness of protein in the late stages of appetite suppression in man. Physiol Behav. 1970 Nov;5(11):1299-302.PubMed PMID: 5524514.
- 1998: Poehlman E T; Mepoundy C Resistance training and energy balance. International journal of sport nutrition 1998;8(2):143-59.
- Weigle DS, Sande KJ, Iverius PH, Monsen ER, Brunzell JD. Weight loss leads to a marked decrease in nonresting energy expenditure in ambulatory human subjects. Metabolism. 1988 Oct;37(10):930-6. PubMed PMID: 3173112.
- King, J., Panton, L., Broeder, C., Browder, K., Quindry, J., & Rhea, L. (2001). A comparison of high intensity vs. low intensity exercise on body composition in overweight women. Medicine and Science in Sports & Exercise, 33, A2421
- Gibala MJ, McGee SL. Metabolic adaptations to short-term high-intensity interval training: a little pain for a lot of gain? Exerc Sport Sci Rev. 2008 Apr;36(2):58-63. Review. PubMed PMID: 18362686.
- Larosa JC, Fry AG, Muesing R, Rosing DR: Effects of high-protein, low-carbohydrate dieting on plasma lipoproteins and body weight. J Am Diet Assoc 1980, 77(3):264-270.
- Miller BV, Bertino J, Reed TG, Burrington C, Davidson LK, Green A, Gartung A, Nafziger A: An Evaluation of the Atkins' Diet. Metabolic Syndrome and Related Disorders 2003, 1:299-309.
- Koopmans, Henry S. Experimental studies on the control of food intake.. In: Bray GA, Couchard d, James WP, eds. Handbook of Obesity. New York: Marcel Dekker, 1997: 273-311.
- Eaton SB, Cordain L, Sparling PB. Evolution, body composition, insulin receptor competition, and insulin resistance. Prev Med. 2009 Oct;49(4):283-5. Epub 2009 Aug 15. PubMed PMID: 19686772.
- Craig BW, Everhart J, Brown R. The influence of high-resistance training on glucose tolerance in young and elderly subjects. Mech Ageing Dev. 1989 Aug;49(2):147-57. Review. PubMed PMID: 2677535.
- Miller WJ, Sherman WM, Ivy JL. Effect of strength training on glucose tolerance and post-glucose insulin response. Med Sci Sports Exerc. 1984 Dec;16(6):539-43. PubMed PMID: 6392812.
- Muscle logic : escalating density training changes the rules for maximum-impact strength training / Charles Staley.
- Poehlman ET, Mepoundy C. Resistance training and energy balance. Int J Sport Nutr. 1998 Jun;8(2):143-59. Review. PubMed PMID: 9637193.
- Hunter GR, Wetzstein CJ, Fields DA, Brown A, Bamman MM. Resistance training increases total energy expenditure and free-living physical activity in older adults. J Appl Physiol. 2000 Sep;89(3):977-84. PubMed PMID: 10956341.
- Boden G, Sargrad K, Homko C, Mozzoli M, Stein TP: Effect of a low-carbohydrate diet on appetite, blood glucose levels, and insulin resistance in obese patients with type 2 diabetes. Ann Intern Med 2005, 142(6):403-411.
- Volek JS, Feinman RD. Carbohydrate restriction improves the features of Metabolic Syndrome. Metabolic Syndrome may be defined by the response to carbohydrate restriction. Nutr Metab (Lond). 2005 Nov 16;2:31. PubMed PMID:16288655; PubMed Central PMCID: PMC1323303.

14 Miller WC, Lindeman AK, Wallace J, Niederpruem M. Diet composition, energy intake, and exercise in relation to body fat in men and women. Am J Clin Nutr. 1990 Sep;52(3):426-30. PubMed PMID: 2393005.

15 A sampling of supporting research:
   - Koopmans, Henry S. Experimental studies on the control of food intake. In: Bray GA, Couchard d, James WP, eds. Handbook of Obesity. New York: Marcel Dekker, 1997: 273-311
   - Friedman JM. A war on obesity, not the obese. Science. 2003 Feb7;299(5608):856-8. PubMed PMID: 12574619.
   - Friedman JM. Modern science versus the stigma of obesity. Nat Med. 2004 Jun;10(6):563-9. Review. PubMed PMID: 15170194.
16 Haskell WL, Lee IM, Pate RR, Powell KE, Blair SN, Franklin BA, Macera CA, Heath GW, Thompson PD, Bauman A; American College of Sports Medicine; American Heart Association. Physical activity and public health: updated recommendation for adults from the American College of Sports Medicine and the American Heart Association. Circulation. 2007 Aug 28;116(9):1081-93. Epub 2007 Aug 1. PubMed PMID: 17671237. & American Heart Association complete guide to women's heart health: The Go Red for Women way to well-being & vitality. New York: Clarkson Potter, 2009. Print.

Chapter 2

1 Weigle DS. Human obesity. Exploding the myths. West J Med. 1990 Oct;153(4):421-8. Review. PubMed PMID: 2244378; PubMed Central PMCID: PMC1002573.
2 A sampling of supporting research:
   - Weigle DS. Human obesity. Exploding the myths. West J Med. 1990 Oct;153(4):421-8. Review. PubMed PMID: 2244378; PubMed Central PMCID: PMC1002573.
   - Hirsch J, Hudgins LC, Leibel RL, Rosenbaum M. Diet composition and energy balance in humans. Am J Clin Nutr. 1998 Mar;67(3 Suppl):551S-555S. Review. PubMed PMID: 9497169.
   - Hirsch J. The regulation of food intake. Discussion. Adv Psychosom Med. 1972;7:229-42. PubMed PMID: 4485878.
   - James W. Reeds P. Nutrient Partitioning In: Bray GA, Couchard d, James WP, eds. Handbook of Obesity. New York: Marcel Dekker, 1997: 555-571.
   - Keesey RE, Hirvonen MD. Body weight set-points: determination and adjustment. J Nutr. 1997 Sep;127(9):1875S-1883S. Review. PubMed PMID: 9278574.
   - Keesey RE. The body-weight set point. What can you tell your patients? Postgrad Med. 1988 May 1;83(6):114-8, 121-2, 127. Review. PubMed PMID: 3283713.
3 A sampling of supporting research:
   - Lönnqvist F, Arner P, Nordfors L, Schalling M. Overexpression of the obese (ob) gene in adipose tissue of human obese subjects. Nat Med. 1995 Sep;1(9):950-3. PubMed PMID: 7585223.Frayn, K. N. Metabolic Regulation: a Human Perspective. London: Portland, 1996. Print.
   - Havel PJ. Dietary fructose: implications for dysregulation of energy homeostasis and lipid/carbohydrate metabolism. Nutr Rev. 2005 May;63(5):133-57.Review. PubMed PMID: 15971409.
   - Garner, David, and Paul Garfinkel. Handbook of Treatment for Eating Disorders: 2nd Edition. 2 Sub ed. New York: The Guilford Press, 1997. Print.
   - Friedman JM. A war on obesity, not the obese. Science. 2003 Feb 7;299(5608):856-8. PubMed PMID: 12574619.
4 Woods SC, Porte D Jr, Bobbioni E, Ionescu E, Sauter JF, Rohner-Jeanrenaud F, Jeanrenaud B. Insulin: its relationship to the central nervous system and to the control of food intake and body weight. Am J Clin Nutr. 1985 Nov;42(5 Suppl):1063-71. Review. PubMed PMID: 3904396. & Weigle DS. Appetite and the regulation of body composition. FASEB J. 1994 Mar 1;8(3):302-10. Review. PubMed PMID: 8143936.
5 A sampling of supporting research:
   - Hirsch J, Hudgins LC, Leibel RL, Rosenbaum M. Diet composition and energy balance in humans. Am J Clin Nutr. 1998 Mar;67(3 Suppl):551S-555S. Review. PubMed PMID: 9497169.
   - Hirsch J. The regulation of food intake. Discussion. Adv Psychosom Med. 1972;7:229-42. PubMed

PMID: 4485878.
- Sims EAH and Horton ES: Endocrine and metabolic adaptations to obesity and starvation. Am J Clin Nutr 21: 1455, 1968
- Trans Assoc Am Physicians. 1968;81:153-70. Experimental obesity in man. Sims EA, Goldman RF, Gluck CM, Horton ES, Kelleher PC, Rowe DW.
- Obesity and leanness. Basic aspects. Stock, M., Rothwell, N., Author Affiliation: Dep. Physiology, St. George's Hospital Medical School, London Univ., London, UK.

6   A sampling of supporting research:
- Sims EAH and Horton ES: Endocrine and metabolic adaptations to obesity and starvation. Am J Clin Nutr 21: 1455, 1968
- Trans Assoc Am Physicians. 1968;81:153-70. Experimental obesity in man. Sims EA, Goldman RF, Gluck CM, Horton ES, Kelleher PC, Rowe DW.
- Obesity and leanness. Basic aspects. Stock, M., Rothwell, N., Author Affiliation: Dep. Physiology, St. George's Hospital Medical School, London Univ., London, UK.

7   A sampling of supporting research:
- Stunkard AJ, Foch TT, Hrubec Z. A twin study of human obesity. JAMA. 1986 Jul 4;256(1):51-4. PubMed PMID: 3712713.
- Weigle DS. Human obesity. Exploding the myths. West J Med. 1990 Oct;153(4):421-8. Review. PubMed PMID: 2244378; PubMed Central PMCID: PMC1002573.
- Stunkard AJ, Sorensen TI, Hanis C, Teasdale TW, Chakraborty R, Schull WJ, Schulsinger F: An adoption study of human obesity. N Engl J Med314 : 193–198,1986
- Allison DB, Kaprio J, Korkeila M, Koskenvuo M, Neale MC, Hayakawa K. The heritability of body mass index among an international sample of monozygotic twins reared apart. Int J Obes Relat Metab Disord. 1996 Jun;20(6):501-6. PubMed PMID: 8782724.
- Stunkard AJ, Harris JR, Pedersen NL, McClearn GE. The body-mass index of twins who have been reared apart. N Engl J Med. 1990 May 24;322(21):1483-7. PubMed PMID: 2336075.
- From Research to Practice/The Art and Science of Obesity Management: Betsy B. Dokken andTsu-Shuen Tsao the Physiology of Body Weight Regulation: Are We Too Efficient for Our Own Good? Diabetes Spectrum July 2007 20:166-170; doi:10.2337/diaspect.20.3.166
- Friedman JM. A war on obesity, not the obese. Science. 2003 Feb 7;299(5608):856-8. PubMed PMID: 12574619.
- Hainer V, Stunkard A, Kunesova M, Parizkova J, Stich V, Allison DB: A twin study of weight loss and metabolic efficiency. Int J Obes Relat Metab Disord 25:533 –537, 2001
- Bouchard C, Tremblay A, Despres JP, Nadeau A, Lupien PJ, theriault G, Dussault J, Moorjani S, Pinault S, Fournier G: The response to long-term overfeeding in identical twins. N Engl J Med 322:1477 –1482, 1990
- Levine JA, Eberhardt NL, Jensen MD. Role of nonexercise activity thermogenesis in resistance to fat gain in humans. Science. 1999 Jan 8;283(5399):212-4. PubMed PMID: 9880251.

8   Friedman JM. Modern science versus the stigma of obesity. Nat Med. 2004 Jun;10(6):563-9. Review. PubMed PMID: 15170194. & Havel PJ. Dietary fructose: implications for dysregulation of energy homeostasis and lipid/carbohydrate metabolism. Nutr Rev. 2005 May;63(5):133-57. Review. PubMed PMID: 15971409.

9   A sampling of supporting research:
- Koopmans, Henry S. Experimental studies on the control of food intake.. In: Bray GA, Couchard d, James WP, eds. Handbook of Obesity. New York: Marcel Dekker, 1997: 273-311.
- Trans Assoc Am Physicians. 1968;81:153-70. Experimental obesity in man. Sims EA, Goldman RF, Gluck CM, Horton ES, Kelleher PC, Rowe DW.
- Rosenbaum M, Vandenborne K, Goldsmith R, Simoneau JA, Heymsfield S, Joanisse DR, Hirsch J, Murphy E, Matthews D, Segal KR, Leibel RL. Effects of experimental weight perturbation on

skeletal muscle work efficiency in human subjects. Am J Physiol Regul Integr Comp Physiol. 2003 Jul;285(1):R183-92. Epub 2003 Feb 27. PubMed PMID: 12609816.

- Havel PJ. Dietary fructose: implications for dysregulation of energy homeostasis and lipid/carbohydrate metabolism. Nutr Rev. 2005 May;63(5):133-57. Review. PubMed PMID: 15971409.
- Havel PJ. Update on adipocyte hormones: regulation of energy balance and carbohydrate/lipid metabolism. Diabetes. 2004 Feb;53 Suppl 1:S143-51. Review. PubMed PMID: 14749280.

10 A sampling of supporting research:

- Jéquier E. Leptin signaling, adiposity, and energy balance. Ann N Y Acad Sci. 2002 Jun;967:379-88. Review. PubMed PMID: 12079865.
- Kelesidis T, Kelesidis I, Chou S, Mantzoros CS. Narrative review: The role of leptin in human physiology: emerging clinical applications. Ann Intern Med. 2010 Jan 19;152(2):93-100. Review. PubMed PMID: 20083828.
- Havel PJ. Update on adipocyte hormones: regulation of energy balance and carbohydrate/lipid metabolism. Diabetes. 2004 Feb;53 Suppl 1:S143-51. Review. PubMed PMID: 14749280.
- Friedman JM. Modern science versus the stigma of obesity. Nat Med. 2004Jun;10(6):563-9. Review. PubMed PMID: 15170194.
- Flier JS. The adipocyte: storage depot or node on the energy information superhighway? Cell. 1995 Jan 13;80(1):15-8. Review. PubMed PMID: 7813011.
- Fried S, Russell C. Diverse Roles of Adipose Tissue in the Regulation of Systemic Metabolism and Energy Balance In: Bray GA, Couchard d, James WP, eds. Handbook of Obesity. New York: Marcel Dekker, 1997: 379-396.
- ANAND BK, DUA S, SHOENBERG K. Hypothalamic control of food intake in cats and monkeys. J Physiol. 1955 Jan 28;127(1):143-52. English, Finnish. PubMed PMID: 14354634; PubMed Central PMCID: PMC1365844.
- Hoebel BG, Teitepoundaum P. Weight regulation in normal and hypothalamic hyperphagic rats. J Comp Physiol Psychol. 1966 Apr;61(2):189-93. PubMed PMID: 5909295.
- Porte D Jr, Woods SC. Regulation of food intake and body weight in insulin.Diabetologia. 1981 Mar;20 Suppl:274-80. PubMed PMID: 7014326.
- Woods SC, Decke E, Vasselli JR. Metabolic hormones and regulation of body weight. Psychol Rev. 1974 Jan;81(1):26-43. PubMed PMID: 4812879.
- Bernardis LL, Goldman JK. Origin of endocrine-metabolic changes in the weanling rat ventromedial syndrome. J Neurosci Res. 1976;2(2):91-116. PubMed PMID: 950680.
- Goralski KB, Sinal CJ. Type 2 diabetes and cardiovascular disease: getting to the fat of the matter. Can J Physiol Pharmacol. 2007 Jan;85(1):113-32. Review. PubMed PMID: 17487251.
- Cherhab FF, Mounzih K, Lu R, Lim ME: Early onset of reproductive function in normal female mice treated with leptin. Science 275:88, 1997.
- Clement K, Vaisse C, Lahlou N, et al: A mutation in the human leptin receptor gene causes obesity and pituitary dysfunction. Nature 392:398, 1998.
- Considine RV, Sinha MK, Heiman ML etc: Serum immunoreactive-leptin concentrations in normal-weight and obese humans. New Eng J Med 334:292, 1996.
- Friedman JM, Halaas JL: Leptin and the regulation of body weight in mammals. Nature 395:763, 1998.
- Halaas JL, Gajiwala KS, Maffel M, etc: Weight-reducing effects of the plasma protein encoded by the obese gene. Science 269:543, 1995.
- Montague CT, Faroozi IS, Whitehead JP, etc: Congenital leptin deficiency is associated with severe early-onset obesity in humans. Nature 387:903, 1997.
- Pelleymounter MA, Cullen MJ, Baker MB, etc: Effects of the obese gene product on body weight regulation in ob/ob mice. Science 269:540, 1995.
- Zhang Y, Proenca R, Maffei M, etc: Positional cloning of the mouse obese gene and its human homo-

logue. Nature 372:425, 1994.

- Bowen, R.. "Pathophysiology of the Endocrine System." arbl.cvmbs.colostate.edu. N.p., n.d. Web. 24 May 2010. <http://www.vivo.colostate.edu/hbooks/pathphys/endocrine/index.html>.

- Meier U, Gressner AM. Endocrine regulation of energy metabolism: review of pathobiochemical and clinical chemical aspects of leptin, ghrelin, adiponectin,and resistin. Clin Chem. 2004 Sep;50(9):1511-25. Epub 2004 Jul 20. Review. PubMed PMID: 15265818.

11 A sampling of supporting research:

- Kelesidis T, Kelesidis I, Chou S, Mantzoros CS. Narrative review: The role of leptin in human physiology: emerging clinical applications. Ann Intern Med. 2010 Jan 19;152(2):93-100. Review. PubMed PMID: 20083828; PubMed Central PMCID:PMC2829242.

- Weigle DS. Appetite and the regulation of body composition. FASEB J. 1994 Mar 1;8(3):302-10. Review. PubMed PMID: 8143936.

- Keesey RE, Powley TL. The regulation of body weight. Annu Rev Psychol. 1986;37:109-33. PubMed PMID: 3963779.

- Havel PJ. Peripheral signals conveying metabolic information to the brain: short-term and long-term regulation of food intake and energy homeostasis. Exp Biol Med (Maywood). 2001 Dec;226(11):963-77. Review. PubMed PMID: 11743131.

- Schwartz MW, Figlewicz DP, Baskin DG, Woods SC, Porte D Jr. Insulin in the brain: a hormonal regulator of energy balance. Endocrinol Rev 13:387–414, 1992.

- Woods SC, Chavez M, Park CR, Riedy C, Kaiyala K, Richardson RD, Figlewicz DP, Schwartz MW, Porte D Jr., Seeley RJ. The evaluation of insulin as a metabolic signal influencing behavior via the brain. Neurosci Biobehav Rev 20:139–144, 1996.

- Teff KL, Grudziak J, Townsend RR, Dunn TN, Grant RW, Adams SH, Keim NL, Cummings BP, Stanhope KL, Havel PJ. Endocrine and metabolic effects of consuming fructose- and glucose-sweetened beverages with meals in obese men and women: influence of insulin resistance on plasma triglyceride responses. J Clin

- Endocrinol Metab. 2009 May;94(5):1562-9. Epub 2009 Feb 10. PubMed PMID: 19208729; PubMed Central PMCID: PMC2684484.

- Chan JL, Mantzoros CS. Role of leptin in energy-deprivation states: normal human physiology and clinical implications for hypothalamic amenorrhoea and anorexia nervosa. Lancet. 2005 Jul 2-8;366(9479):74-85. Review. PubMed PMID: 15993236.

- Goralski KB, Sinal CJ. Type 2 diabetes and cardiovascular disease: getting to the fat of the matter. Can J Physiol Pharmacol. 2007 Jan;85(1):113-32. Review. PubMed PMID: 17487251.

- Porte D Jr, Woods SC. Regulation of food intake and body weight in insulin.Diabetologia. 1981 Mar;20 Suppl:274-80. PubMed PMID: 7014326.

- Considine RV, Sinha MK, Heiman ML, Kriauciunas A, Stephens TW, Nyce MR, Ohannesian JP, Marco CC, McKee LJ, Bauer TL, et al. Serum immunoreactive-leptin concentrations in normal-weight and obese humans. N Engl J Med. 1996 Feb 1;334(5):292-5. PubMed PMID: 8532024.

- Funahashi T, Shimomura I, Hiraoka H, Arai T, Takahashi M, Nakamura T, Nozaki S, Yamashita S, Takemura K, Tokunaga K, et al. Enhanced expression of rat obese (ob) gene in adipose tissues of ventromedial hypothalamus (VMH)-lesioned rats. Biochem Biophys Res Commun. 1995 Jun 15;211(2):469-75. PubMed PMID: 7794258.

- Maffei M, Fei H, Lee GH, Dani C, Leroy P, Zhang Y, Proenca R, Negrel R, Ailhaud G, Friedman JM. Increased expression in adipocytes of ob RNA in mice with lesions of the hypothalamus and with mutations at the db locus. Proc Natl Acad Sci U S A. 1995 Jul 18;92(15):6957-60. PubMed PMID: 7624352; PubMed Central PMCID: PMC41450.

- Considine RV, Considine EL, Williams CJ, Nyce MR, Magosin SA, Bauer TL, Rosato EL, Copounderg J, Caro JF. Evidence against either a premature stop codon or the absence of obese gene mRNA in human obesity. J Clin Invest. 1995 Jun;95(6):2986-8. PubMed PMID: 7769141; PubMed Central

PMCID: PMC295988.

- Hamilton BS, Paglia D, Kwan AY, Deitel M. Increased obese mRNA expression in omental fat cells from massively obese humans. Nat Med. 1995 Sep;1(9):953-6. PubMed PMID: 7585224.
- Lönnqvist F, Arner P, Nordfors L, Schalling M. Overexpression of the obese (ob) gene in adipose tissue of human obese subjects. Nat Med. 1995 Sep;1(9):950-3. PubMed PMID: 7585223.
- Frederich RC, Löllmann B, Hamann A, Napolitano-Rosen A, Kahn BB, Lowell BB, Flier JS. Expression of ob mRNA and its encoded protein in rodents. Impact of nutrition and obesity. J Clin Invest. 1995 Sep;96(3):1658-63. PubMed PMID: 7657836; PubMed Central PMCID: PMC185793.
- Myers MG, Cowley MA, Münzberg H. Mechanisms of leptin action and leptin resistance. Annu Rev Physiol. 2008;70:537-56. Review. PubMed PMID: 17937601.
- Heymsfield SB, Greenberg AS, Fujioka K, Dixon RM, Kushner R, Hunt T, Lubina JA, Patane J, Self B, Hunt P, McCamish M. Recombinant leptin for weight loss in obese and lean adults: a randomized, controlled, dose-escalation trial. JAMA. 1999 Oct 27;282(16):1568-75. PubMed PMID: 10546697.
- Roth JD, Roland BL, Cole RL, Trevaskis JL, Weyer C, Koda JE, Anderson CM, Parkes DG, Baron AD. Leptin responsiveness restored by amylin agonism in diet-induced obesity: evidence from nonclinical and clinical studies. Proc Natl Acad Sci U S A. 2008 May 20;105(20):7257-62. Epub 2008 May 5. PubMed PMID: 18458326; PubMed Central PMCID: PMC2438237.
- Friedman JM. Modern science versus the stigma of obesity. Nat Med. 2004 Jun;10(6):563-9. Review. PubMed PMID: 15170194.

12 Keesey RE, Hirvonen MD. Body weight set-points: determination and adjustment. J Nutr. 1997 Sep;127(9):1875S-1883S. Review. PubMed PMID: 9278574.

13 Woods SC, Porte D Jr, Bobbioni E, Ionescu E, Sauter JF, Rohner-Jeanrenaud F, Jeanrenaud B. Insulin: its relationship to the central nervous system and to the control of food intake and body weight. Am J Clin Nutr. 1985 Nov;42(5 Suppl):1063-71. Review. PubMed PMID: 3904396.

Chapter 3

1 Keesey RE, Powley TL. The regulation of body weight. Annu Rev Psychol. 1986;37:109-33. PubMed PMID: 3963779.

2 Rolls BJ, Rowe EA, Turner RC. Persistent obesity in rats following a period of consumption of a mixed, high energy diet. J Physiol. 1980 Jan;298:415-27. PubMed PMID: 6987379; PubMed Central PMCID: PMC1279126.

3 Peck JW. Rats defend different body weights depending on palatability and accessibility of their food. J Comp Physiol Psychol. 1978 Jun;92(3):555-70. PubMed PMID: 98538.

4 Rothwell NJ, Stock MJ. Energy expenditure of 'cafeteria'-fed rats determined from measurements of energy balance and indirect calorimetry. J Physiol. 1982 Jul;328:371-7. PubMed PMID: 7131317; PubMed Central PMCID: PMC1225664.)

5 A sampling of supporting research:

- Obesity and leanness. Basic aspects. Stock, M., Rothwell, N., Author Affiliation: Dep. Physiology, St. George's Hospital Medical School, London Univ., London, UK.
- Rothwell NJ, Stock MJ. Regulation of energy balance in two models of reversible obesity in the rat. J Comp Physiol Psychol. 1979 Dec;93(6):1024-34. PubMed PMID: 521518.
- Rothwell NJ, Stock MJ. Energy expenditure of 'cafeteria'-fed rats determined from measurements of energy balance and indirect calorimetry. J Physiol. 1982 Jul;328:371-7. PubMed PMID: 7131317; PubMed Central PMCID: PMC1225664.
- Tordoff MG. Obesity by choice: The powerful influence of nutrient availability on nutrient intake. Am J Physiol Regul Integr Comp Physiol. 2002 May;282(5):R1536-9. PubMed PMID: 11959698.
- Peckham SC, Entenman C. The influence of a hypercaloric diet on gross body and adipose tissue composition in the rat. Res Dev Tech Rep. 1962 Feb 5:23. PubMed PMID: 14484833.

- Sclafani A, Springer D. Dietary obesity in adult rats: similarities to hypothalamic and human obesity syndromes. Physiol Behav. 1976 Sep;17(3):461-71. PubMed PMID: 1013192.
- Haines H, Hackel Db, Schmidt-Nielsen K. Experimental Diabetes Mellitus Induced By Diet In the Sand Rat. Am J Physiol. 1965 Feb;208:297-300. Pubmed Pmid: 14259964.

Chapter 4

1   Bray, George and Claude Bouchard. Handbook of Obesity. Oxford Oxfordshire: Oxford University Press, 1998.
2   Sampling of research showing that eating less drops the fat metabolism system's need to burn fat:
- Leibel RL, Rosenbaum M, Hirsch J. Changes in energy expenditure resulting from altered body weight. N Engl J Med. 1995 Mar 9;332(10):621-8. Erratum in: N Engl J Med 1995 Aug 10;333(6):399. PubMed PMID: 7632212.
- Keys, Ancel. The Biology of Human Starvation: Volume I. Minneapolis: University of Minnesota Press, 1950. Print.
- Leibel RL, Hirsch J: Diminished energy requirements in reduced-obese patients. Metabolism 1984; 33:164-170
- Geissler CA, Miller DS, Shah M: The daily metabolic rate of the postobese and the lean. Am J Clin Nutr 1987; 45:914-920
- Bray GA: Effect of caloric restriction on energy expenditure in obese patients. Lancet 1969; 2:397-398
- Ravussin E, Burnand B, Schutz Y, et al: Energy expenditure before and during energy restriction in obese patients. Am J Clin Nutr 1985; 41:753-759
- Shah M, Miller DS, Geissler CA. Lower metabolic rates of post-obese versus lean women: Thermogenesis, basal metabolic rate and genetics. Eur J Clin Nutr. 1988 Sep;42(9):741-52. PubMed PMID: 3181107.
- Weigle DS, Sande KJ, Iverius PH, Monsen ER, Brunzell JD. Weight loss leads to a marked decrease in nonresting energy expenditure in ambulatory human subjects. Metabolism. 1988 Oct;37(10):930-6. PubMed PMID: 3173112.
- Jéquier E. Leptin signaling, adiposity, and energy balance. Ann N Y Acad Sci. 2002 Jun;967:379-88. Review. PubMed PMID: 12079865.
- Sampling of research showing that eating less drops the fat metabolism system's ability to burn fat:
- Rosenbaum M, Murphy EM, Heymsfield SB, Matthews DE, Leibel RL. Low dose leptin administration reverses effects of sustained weight-reduction on energy expenditure and circulating concentrations of thyroid hormones. J Clin Endocrinol Metab. 2002 May;87(5):2391-4. PubMed PMID: 11994393.
- Friedman JM, Halaas JL. Leptin and the regulation of body weight in mammals. Nature. 1998 Oct 22;395(6704):763-70. Review. PubMed PMID: 9796811.
- Jéquier E. Leptin signaling, adiposity, and energy balance. Ann N Y Acad Sci. 2002 Jun;967:379-88. Review. PubMed PMID: 12079865.
- Walks D, Lavau M, Presta E, Yang MU, Björntorp P. Refeeding after fasting in the rat: effects of dietary-induced obesity on energy balance regulation. Am J
- Clin Nutr. 1983 Mar;37(3):387-95. PubMed PMID: 6338694.
- Dulloo AG, Girardier L. Adaptive changes in energy expenditure during refeeding following low-calorie intake: evidence for a specific metabolic component favoring fat storage. Am J Clin Nutr. 1990 Sep;52(3):415-20. PubMed PMID: 2393003.
- Björntorp P, Yang MU. Refeeding after fasting in the rat: effects on body composition and food efficiency. Am J Clin Nutr. 1982 Sep;36(3):444-9. PubMed PMID: 7113950.
- Dulloo AG, Jacquet J, Girardier L. Autoregulation of body composition during weight recovery in human: The Minnesota Experiment revisited. Int J Obes Relat Metab Disord. 1996 May;20(5):393-405.

PubMed PMID: 8696417.

3   A sampling of supporting research:
- Kelesidis T, Kelesidis I, Chou S, Mantzoros CS. Narrative review: The role of leptin in human physiology: emerging clinical applications. Ann Intern Med. 2010 Jan 19;152(2):93-100. Review. PubMed PMID: 20083828; PubMed Central PMCID:PMC2829242.
- Jéquier E. Energy metabolism in human obesity. Soz Praventivmed.1989;34(2):58-62. PubMed PMID: 2750332.
- Jéquier E. Energy expenditure in obesity. Clin Endocrinol Metab. 1984 Nov;13(3):563-80. Review. PubMed PMID: 6391755.
- Rosenbaum M, Hirsch J, Gallagher DA, Leibel RL. Long-term persistence of adaptive thermogenesis in subjects who have maintained a reduced body weight. Am J Clin Nutr. 2008 Oct;88(4):906-12. PubMed PMID: 18842775.
- Poehlman ET, Mepoundy C. Resistance training and energy balance. Int J Sport Nutr. 1998 Jun;8(2):143-59. Review. PubMed PMID: 9637193.
- Hunter GR, Wetzstein CJ, Fields DA, Brown A, Bamman MM. Resistance training increases total energy expenditure and free-living physical activity in older adults. J Appl Physiol. 2000 Sep;89(3):977-84. PubMed PMID: 10956341.
- Muscle logic : escalating density training changes the rules for maximum-impact strength training / Charles Staley.
- Ballor DL, Katch VL, Becque MD, Marks CR. Resistance strength training during caloric restriction enhances lean body weight maintenance. Am J Clin Nutr. 1988 Jan;47(1):19-25. PubMed PMID: 3337037.
- Poehlman ET, Mepoundy CL, Goran MI. The impact of exercise and diet restriction on daily energy expenditure. Sports Med. 1991 Feb;11(2):78-101. Review.
- A.C. Guyton: 'Textbook of medical physiology' 3rd edn. Philadelphia: Saunders, 1966
- Weigle DS, Sande KJ, Iverius PH, Monsen ER, Brunzell JD. Weight loss leads to a marked decrease in nonresting energy expenditure in ambulatory human subjects. Metabolism. 1988 Oct;37(10):930-6. PubMed PMID: 3173112.
- Jen KL, Lu H, Savona L, Watkins A, Shaw M. Long-term weight cycling reduces body weight and fat free mass, but not fat mass in female Wistar rats. Int J Obes Relat Metab Disord. 1995 Oct;19(10):699-708. PubMed PMID: 8589763.

4   Thorpe GL. Treating overweight patients. J Am Med Assoc. 1957 Nov 16;165(11):1361-5. PubMed PMID: 13475044. & Dulloo AG, Girardier L. Adaptive changes in energy expenditure during refeeding following low-calorie intake: evidence for a specific metabolic component favoring fat storage. Am J Clin Nutr. 1990 Sep;52(3):415-20. PubMed PMID: 2393003.

5   Weigle DS. Human obesity. Exploding the myths. West J Med. 1990 Oct;153(4):421-8. Review. PubMed PMID: 2244378; PubMed Central PMCID: PMC1002573.

6   MacLean PS, Higgins JA, Johnson GC, Fleming-Elder BK, Donahoo WT, Melanson EL, Hill JO. Enhanced metabolic efficiency contributes to weight regain after weight loss in obesity-prone rats. Am J Physiol Regul Integr Comp Physiol. 2004 Dec;287(6):R1306-15. Epub 2004 Aug 26. PubMed PMID: 15331386. & Dulloo AG, Girardier L. Adaptive changes in energy expenditure during refeeding following low-calorie intake: evidence for a specific metabolic component favoring fat storage. Am J Clin Nutr. 1990 Sep;52(3):415-20. PubMed PMID: 2393003.

7   Sampling of supporting research:
- French SA Jeffery RW (1994) Consequences of dieting to lose weight: effects on physical and mental health Health Psychol 13 195—212
- McGuire MT Wing RR Hill JO Klem ML Lang W (1999) What predicts weight gain in a group of successful weight losers? J Consult Clin Psychol 67 177—185
- Korkeila M Rissanen A Kaprio J Sorensen TIA Koskenvuo M (1999) Weight-loss attempts and risk of

major weight gain: a prospective study in Finnish adults Am J Clin Nutr 70 965—975

- Juhaeri Stevens J Chambless LE Tyroler HA Harp J Jones D Arnett D (2001) Weight change among self-reported dieters and non-dieters in white and African American men and women Eur J Epidemiol 17 917 –

- Drapeau V Provencher V Lemieux S Despres J-P Bouchard C Tremblay A (2003) Do 6-y changes in eating behaviours predict changes in body weight? Results from the Quebec Family Study Int J Obes 27 808—814

- Klesges RC Klem ML Bene CR (1989) Effects of dietary restraint, obesity and gender on holiday eating behaviour and weight gain J Abnorm Psychol 98 499—503

- Klesges RC Isbell TR Klesges LM (1992) Relationship between dietary restraint, energy intake, physical activity, and body weight: a prospective analysis J Abnorm Psychol 101 668—674

- Stice E Cameron RP Killen JD Hayward C Barr Taylor C (1999) Naturalistic weight-reduction efforts prospectively predict growth in relative weight and onset of obesity among female adolescents J Consult Clin Psychol 67 967—974

- Young EA, Harris MM, Cantu TL, Ghidoni JJ, Crawley R. Hepatic response to a very-low-energy diet and refeeding in rats. Am J Clin Nutr. 1993 Jun;57(6):857-62. PubMed PMID: 8503353.

8   A sampling of supporting research:
- Dulloo AG, Jacquet J. Adaptive reduction in basal metabolic rate in response to food deprivation in humans: a role for feedback signals from fat stores. Am J Clin Nutr. 1998 Sep;68(3):599-606. PubMed PMID: 9734736. & Flier JS, Maratos-Flier E. What fuels fat. Sci Am. 2007 Sep;297(3):72-81. PubMed PMID: 17784627.

- Walks D, Lavau M, Presta E, Yang MU, Björntorp P. Refeeding after fasting in the rat: effects of dietary-induced obesity on energy balance regulation. Am J

- Clin Nutr. 1983 Mar;37(3):387-95. PubMed PMID: 6338694.

- A sampling of supporting research:

- Dulloo AG, Girardier L. 24 hour energy expenditure several months after weight loss in the underfed rat: evidence for a chronic increase in whole-body metabolic efficiency. Int J Obes Relat Metab Disord. 1993 Feb;17(2):115-23. PubMed PMID: 8384165.

- Dulloo AG, Calokatisa R. Adaptation to low calorie intake in obese mice: contribution of a metabolic component to diminished energy expenditures during and after weight loss. Int J Obes. 1991 Jan;15(1):7-16. PubMed PMID: 2010261.

- Shah M, Miller DS, Geissler CA. Lower metabolic rates of post-obese versus lean women: Thermogenesis, basal metabolic rate and genetics. Eur J Clin Nutr. 1988 Sep;42(9):741-52. PubMed PMID: 3181107.

- Weigle DS, Sande KJ, Iverius PH, Monsen ER, Brunzell JD. Weight loss leads to a marked decrease in nonresting energy expenditure in ambulatory human subjects. Metabolism. 1988 Oct;37(10):930-6. PubMed PMID: 3173112.

9   Leibel RL, Hirsch J. Diminished energy requirements in reduced-obese patients. Metabolism. 1984 Feb;33(2):164-70. PubMed PMID: 6694559. & Keesey RE, Powley TL. The regulation of body weight. Annu Rev Psychol. 1986;37:109-33. PubMed PMID: 3963779.

10 Garrow JS. The safety of dieting. Proc Nutr Soc. 1991 Aug;50(2):493-9. Review. PubMed PMID: 1749815.

11 Keys, Ancel. The biology of human starvation. New York: Oxford U.P, 1950. Print.

12 Brownell KD, Greenwood MR, Stellar E, Shrager EE. The effects of repeated cycles of weight loss and regain in rats. Physiol Behav. 1986 Oct;38(4):459-64. PubMed PMID: 3823159. & Blackburn GL, Wilson GT, Kanders BS, Stein LJ, Lavin PT, Adler J, Brownell KD. Weight cycling: The experience of human dieters. Am J Clin Nutr. 1989 May;49(5 Suppl):1105-9. PubMed PMID: 2718940.

13 Garner DM, Wooley SC. Confronting the failure of behavioral and dietary treatments for obesity. Clin Psychol Rev. 1991;11:729–780. doi: 10.1016/0272-7358(91)90128-H.

14 McCullough ML, Feskanich D, Stampfer MJ, Rosner BA, Hu FB, Hunter DJ, Variyam JN, Colditz GA,

Willett WC. Adherence to the Dietary Guidelines for Americans and risk of major chronic disease in women. Am J Clin Nutr. 2000 Nov;72(5):1214-22. PubMed PMID: 11063452.

15 Mann T, Tomiyama AJ, Westling E, Lew AM, Samuels B, Chatman J. Medicare's search for effective obesity treatments: diets are not the answer. Am Psychol. 2007 Apr;62(3):220-33. Review. PubMed PMID: 17469900.

16 A sampling of supporting research:

- Weigle DS. Human obesity. Exploding the myths. West J Med. 1990 Oct;153(4):421-8. Review. PubMed PMID: 2244378; PubMed Central PMCID: PMC1002573.

- Hill AJ. Does dieting make you fat? Br J Nutr. 2004 Aug;92 Suppl 1:S15-8. Review. PubMed PMID: 15384316.

- Green MW, Rogers PJ. Impaired cognitive functioning during spontaneous dieting. Psychol Med. 1995 Sep;25(5):1003-10. PubMed PMID: 8587997.

- Brownell KD, Rodin J. Medical, metabolic, and psychological effects of weight cycling. Arch Intern Med. 1994 Jun 27;154(12):1325-30. Review. PubMed PMID: 8002684.

- Mann T, Tomiyama AJ, Westling E, Lew AM, Samuels B, Chatman J. Medicare's search for effective obesity treatments: diets are not the answer. Am Psychol. 2007 Apr;62(3):220-33. Review. PubMed PMID: 17469900.

- Blackburn GL, Wilson GT, Kanders BS, Stein LJ, Lavin PT, Adler J, Brownell KD. Weight cycling: The experience of human dieters. Am J Clin Nutr. 1989 May;49(5 Suppl):1105-9. PubMed PMID: 2718940.

- Hamm P, Shekelle RB, Stamler J. Large fluctuations in body weight during young adulthood and twenty-five-year risk of coronary death in men. Am J Epidemiol. 1989 Feb;129(2):312-8. PubMed PMID: 2912043.

- Higgins M, D'Agostino R, Kannel W, Cobb J, Pinsky J. Benefits and adverse effects of weight loss. Observations from the Framingham Study. Ann Intern Med. 1993 Oct 1;119(7 Pt 2):758-63. Erratum in: Ann Intern Med 1993 Nov 15;119(10):1055. PubMed PMID: 8363211.

- Blair SN, Shaten J, Brownell K, Collins G, Lissner L. Body weight change, all-cause mortality, and cause-specific mortality in the Multiple Risk Factor Intervention Trial. Ann Intern Med. 1993 Oct 1;119(7 Pt 2):749-57. PubMed PMID: 8363210.

- Lissner L, Odell PM, D'Agostino RB, Stokes J 3rd, Kreger BE, Belanger AJ,Brownell KD. Variability of body weight and health outcomes in the Framingham population. N Engl J Med. 1991 Jun 27;324(26):1839-44. PubMed PMID: 2041550.

- Phinney SD. Weight cycling and cardiovascular risk in obese men and women. Am J Clin Nutr. 1992 Oct;56(4):781-2. PubMed PMID: 1414977.

17 Boyle PC, Storlien LH, Keesey RE. Increased efficiency of food utilization following weight loss. Physiol Behav. 1978 Aug;21(2):261-4. PubMed PMID: 693652.

Chapter 5

1 Layman DK. Dietary Guidelines should reflect new understandings about adult protein needs. Nutr Metab (Lond). 2009 Mar 13;6:12. PubMed PMID: 19284668; PubMed Central PMCID: PMC2666737. & Ross R, Janssen I. Physical activity, total and regional obesity: dose-response considerations. Med Sci Sports Exerc. 2001 Jun;33(6 Suppl):S521-7; discussion S528-9. Review. PubMed PMID: 11427779.

2 Rony, Hugo R.. Obesity and Leanness. London, Great Britian : Lea & Febiger, 1940. Print. & Friedman JM. Modern science versus the stigma of obesity. Nat Med. 2004 Jun;10(6):563-9. Review. PubMed PMID: 15170194.

3 A sampling of supporting research:

- Donnelly JE, Smith BK. Is exercise effective for weight loss with ad libitum diet? Energy balance, compensation, and gender differences. Exerc Sport Sci Rev. 2005 Oct;33(4):169-74. Review. PubMed

PMID: 16239833.

- Koopmans HS. Internal signals cause large changes in food intake in one-way crossed intestines rats. Brain Res Bull. 1985 Jun;14(6):595-603. PubMed PMID: 3875383.
  - http://www.time.com/time/health/article/0,8599,1914857,00.html#ixzz0Wz0PTtHj
  - http://www.foxnews.com/story/0,2933,403803,00.html
  - Cordain, Loren, and Joe Friel. The Paleo Diet for Athletes: A Nutritional Formula for Peak Athletic Performance. Emmaus, Pa.: Rodale Books, 2005. Print.

4   Church TS, Martin CK, Thompson AM, Earnest CP, Mikus CR, Blair SN. Changes in weight, waist circumference and compensatory responses with different doses of exercise among sedentary, overweight postmenopausal women. PLoS One. 2009;4(2):e4515. Epub 2009 Feb 18. PubMed PMID: 19223984; PubMed Central PMCID:PMC2639700.

5   Marion Nestle, quoted in : J.M. Hirsch, "Food Industry a Targe in Obesity Fight," March 19, 2006. www.forbes.com/feeds/ap/2006/03/18/ap2605096.html. & Simon, Michele. Appetite for Profit: How the food industry undermines our health and how to fight back. New York City, New York: Nation Books, 2006. Print.

6   National Soft Drink Association. Soft Drinks: Balance, Variety, Moderation.

7   Yudkin, John. Sweet and Dangerous. Washington D.C.: Natl Health Federation, 1978. Print.

Chapter 6

1   Haskell WL, Lee IM, Pate RR, Powell KE, Blair SN, Franklin BA, Macera CA, Heath GW, Thompson PD, Bauman A; American College of Sports Medicine; American Heart Association. Physical activity and public health: updated recommendation for adults from the American College of Sports Medicine and the American Heart Association. Circulation. 2007 Aug 28;116(9):1081-93. Epub 2007 Aug 1. PubMed PMID: 17671237.

2   Whitehead, Saffron A.; Nussey, Stephen (2001). Endocrinology: an integrated approach. Oxford: BIOS. pp. 122. ISBN 1-85996-252-1.

3   Petersen L, Torensen, TIA. Is physical inactivity the cause or the consequence of obesity? In: Bouchard, Claude, Alfredo Halpern, and Geraldo Medeiros-Neto. Progress in Obesity Research: 9. manhattan: Food & Nutrition Pr, 2003. Print. & Petersen L, Schnohr P, Sørensen TI. Longitudinal study of the long-term relation between physical activity and obesity in adults. Int J Obes Relat Metab Disord. 2004 Jan;28(1):105-12. PubMed PMID: 14647181.

4   Dr. Pauline, Entin. "History of Exercise Science." www2.nau.edu. Northern Arizona University, n.d. Web. 10 Feb. 2011. <http://jan.ucc.nau.edu/pe/exs190web/exs190history.htm>. & http://apps.who.int/bmi/index.jsp

5   Oliver, J. Eric. Fat Politics: The Real Story behind America's Obesity Epidemic. New Ed ed. New York: Oxford University Press, USA, 2006. Print.

6   Nestle M, Jacobson MF. Halting the obesity epidemic: a public health policy approach. Public Health Rep. 2000 Jan-Feb;115(1):12-24. PubMed PMID: 10968581; PubMed Central PMCID: PMC1308552.

7   A sampling of supporting research:
  - Schoenborn CA, Adams PF, Barnes PM. Body weight status of adults: United States, 1997–98. Adv Data 2002;330:1–15.
  - Phillip B. Goldblatt; Mary E. Moore; Apoundert J. Stunkard Social Factors in Obesity JAMA. 1965;192(12):1039-1044.
  - Fredericks, Carrie. Obesity (Compact Research Series). San Diego: Referencepoint Press, 2008. Print.
  - McCrady SK, Levine JA. Sedentariness at work: how much do we really sit? Obesity (Silver Spring). 2009 Nov;17(11):2103-5. Epub 2009 Apr 23. PubMed PMID: 19390526; PubMed Central PMCID: PMC2783690.
  - Drewnowski A, Specter SE. Poverty and obesity: The role of energy density and energy costs. Am J

Clin Nutr. 2004 Jan;79(1):6-16. Review. PubMed PMID: 14684391.

8   Blundell John E., Stubbs R. James. Diet Composition and the Control of Food Intake in Humans In: Bray GA, Couchard d, James WP, eds. Handbook of Obesity. New York: Marcel Dekker, 1997: 243-272. & Prentice AM, Black AE, Coward WA, Cole TJ. Energy expenditure in overweight and obese adults in affluent societies: an analysis of 319 doubly-labelled water measurements. Eur J Clin Nutr. 1996 Feb;50(2):93-7. PubMed PMID: 8641251.

Chapter 7

1   Keen H, Thomas BJ, Jarrett RJ, Fuller JH. Nutrient intake, adiposity, and diabetes. Br Med J. 1979 Mar 10;1(6164):655-8. PubMed PMID: 435710; PubMed Central PMCID: PMC1598272.

2   Volek J, Sharman M, Gómez A, Judelson D, Rubin M, Watson G, Sokmen B, Silvestre R, French D, Kraemer W. Comparison of energy-restricted very low-carbohydrate and low-fat diets on weight loss and body composition in overweight men and women. Nutr Metab (Lond). 2004 Nov 8;1(1):13. PubMed PMID:15533250; PubMed Central PMCID: PMC538279.

3   Samaha FF, Iqbal N, Seshadri P, Chicano KL, Daily DA, McGrory J, Williams T, Williams M, Gracely EJ, Stern L. A low-carbohydrate as compared with a low-fat diet in severe obesity. N Engl J Med. 2003 May 22;348(21):2074-81. PubMed PMID: 12761364.

4   Greene P, Willett W, et al. Pilot 12-week feeding weight loss comparison: low-fat vs. low-carbohydrate (ketogenic) diets [abstract]. Obes Res. 2003;11:A23.

5   Sondike, S., et al. "The Ketogenic Diet Increases Weight Loss But Not Cardiovascular Risk: A Random- ized Controlled Trial." Journal of Adolescent Health 26: 91, 2000

6   D. M. Lyon , And D. M. Dunlop, the Treatment of Obesity: A Comparison of the Effects of Diet And of Thyroid Extract, QJM 1: 331-352.

7   Levine JA, Eberhardt NL, Jensen MD. Role of nonexercise activity thermogenesis in resistance to fat gain in humans. Science. 1999 Jan 8;283(5399):212-4. PubMed PMID: 9880251.

8   A sampling of supporting research:

   • Leibel RL, Rosenbaum M, Hirsch J. Changes in energy expenditure resulting from altered body weight. N Engl J Med. 1995 Mar 9;332(10):621-8. Erratum in: N Engl J Med 1995 Aug 10;333(6):399. PubMed PMID: 7632212.

   • Gulick A: A study of weight regulation in the adult human body during overnutrition. Am J Physiol 1922; 60:371-395

   • Miller DS, Mumford P, Stock MJ: Gluttony-2. Thermogenesis in overeating man. Am J Clin Nutr 1967; 20:1223-1229

   • Apfepoundaum M Bostsarron J, Lacatis D: Effect of caloric restriction and excessive caloric intake on energy expenditure. Am J Clin Nutr 1971; 24:1405-1409

   • Whipp BJ, Bray G, Koyal SN: Exercise energetics in normal man following acute weight gain. Am J Clin Nutr 1973; 26:1284-1286

   • Friedman JM, Halaas JL. Leptin and the regulation of body weight in mammals. Nature. 1998 Oct 22;395(6704):763-70. Review. PubMed PMID: 9796811.

   • Jéquier E. Leptin signaling, adiposity, and energy balance. Ann N Y Acad Sci. 2002 Jun;967:379-88. Review. PubMed PMID: 12079865.

   • Riestra JL, Skowsky WR, Martinez I, Swan L. Passive transfer of an appetite suppressant factor. Proc Soc Exp Biol Med. 1977 Nov;156(2):236-40. PubMed PMID: 337318.

   • Fam BC, Morris MJ, Hansen MJ, Kebede M, Andrikopoulos S, Proietto J, Thorburn AW. Modulation of central leptin sensitivity and energy balance in a rat model of diet-induced obesity. Diabetes Obes Metab. 2007 Nov;9(6):840-52. PubMed PMID: 17924866.

   • Flier JS. The adipocyte: storage depot or node on the energy information superhighway? Cell. 1995 Jan 13;80(1):15-8. Review. PubMed PMID: 7813011.

- Bray GA. Obesity--a state of reduced sympathetic activity and normal or high adrenal activity (the autonomic and adrenal hypothesis revisited). Int J Obes. 1990;14 Suppl 3:77-91; discussion 91-2. Review. PubMed PMID: 2086518.
- Sopko G, Jacobs DR Jr, Taylor HL. Dietary measures of physical activity. Am J Epidemiol. 1984 Dec;120(6):900-11. PubMed PMID: 6507429.
- Levine JA. Non-exercise activity thermogenesis (NEAT). Best Pract Res Clin Endocrinol Metab. 2002 Dec;16(4):679-702. Review. PubMed PMID: 12468415.

9   http://www.cnpp.usda.gov/Publications/DietaryGuidelines/2010/PolicyDoc/Chapter2.pdf & http://www.health.gov/DietaryGuidelines/dga2005/document/html/chapter3.htm

10 Friedman JM. A war on obesity, not the obese. Science. 2003 Feb7;299(5608):856-8. PubMed PMID: 12574619.

11 http://www.cnpp.usda.gov/Publications/DietaryGuidelines/2010/PolicyDoc/Chapter2.pdf & McCullough ML, Feskanich D, Rimm EB, Giovannucci EL, Ascherio A, Variyam JN, Spiegelman D, Stampfer MJ, Willett WC. Adherence to the Dietary Guidelines for Americans and risk of major chronic disease in men. Am J Clin Nutr. 2000 Nov;72(5):1223-31. PubMed PMID: 11063453.

12 Feinman RD, Fine EJ. "A calorie is a calorie" violates the second law of thermodynamics. Nutr J. 2004 Jul 28;3:9. PubMed PMID: 15282028; PubMed Central PMCID: PMC506782.

13 Fine EJ, Feinman RD. Thermodynamics of weight loss diets. Nutr Metab (Lond).2004 Dec 8;1(1):15. PubMed PMID: 15588283; PubMed Central PMCID: PMC543577.

14 Garrow, J.S.. Energy Balance and Obesity in Man. 2nd ed. New York: Elsevier Science Ltd, 1978. Print. & Keesey RE, Powley TL. The regulation of body weight. Annu Rev Psychol. 1986;37:109-33. PubMed PMID: 3963779.

Chapter 8

1   Feinman RD, Fine EJ. "A calorie is a calorie" violates the second law of thermodynamics. Nutr J. 2004 Jul 28;3:9.

2   Manninen AH. Is a calorie really a calorie? Metabolic advantage of low-carbohydrate diets. J Int Soc Sports Nutr. 2004 Dec 31;1(2):21-6. PubMed PMID: 18500946; PubMed Central PMCID: PMC2129158.

3   Ludwig DS. The glycemic index: physiological mechanisms relating to obesity, diabetes, and cardiovascular disease. JAMA. 2002 May 8;287(18):2414-23. Review. PubMed PMID: 11988062. & Miller WC. Diet composition, energy intake, and nutritional status in relation to obesity in men and women. Med Sci Sports Exerc. 1991 Mar;23(3):280-4. Review. PubMed PMID: 2020264.

4   Bailes JR, Strow MT, Werthammer J, McGinnis RA, Elitsur Y. Effect of low-carbohydrate, unlimited calorie diet on the treatment of childhood obesity: a prospective controlled study. Metab Syndr Relat Disord. 2003 Sep;1(3):221-5. PubMed PMID: 18370665.

5   Powell JJ, Tucker L, Seafooder AG, Wilcox K. The effects of different percentages of dietary fat intake, exercise, and calorie restriction on body composition and body weight in obese females. Am J Health Promot. 1994 Jul-Aug;8(6):442-8. PubMed PMID: 10161100. & Kekwick A, Pawan GL. Calorie intake in relation to body-weight changes in the obese. Lancet. 1956 Jul 28;271(6935):155-61. PubMed PMID: 13347103.

6   Fuhrman, Joel. Eat to Live: The Revolutionary Formula for Fast and Sustained Weight Loss. London: Little, Brown and Company, 2005. Print.

7   Krieger JW, Sitren HS, Daniels MJ, Langkamp-Henken B. Effects of variation in protein and carbohydrate intake on body mass and composition during energy restriction: a meta-regression 1. Am J Clin Nutr. 2006 Feb;83(2):260-74. PubMed PMID: 16469983.

8   Young CM, Scanlan SS, Im HS, Lutwak L. Effect of body composition and other parameters in obese young men of carbohydrate level of reduction diet. Am J Clin Nutr. 1971 Mar;24(3):290-6. PubMed PMID: 5548734.

9 Benoit FL, Martin RL, Watten RH. Changes in body composition during weight reduction in obesity. Balance studies comparing effects of fasting and a ketogenic diet. Ann Intern Med. 1965 Oct;63(4):604-12. PubMed PMID: 5838326.

10 A sampling of supporting data:

- Fine EJ, Feinman RD. Thermodynamics of weight loss diets. Nutr Metab (Lond).2004 Dec 8;1(1):15. PubMed PMID: 15588283; PubMed Central PMCID: PMC543577.
- Rabast U, Kasper H, Schonborn J: Comparative studies in obese subjects fed carbohydrate-restricted and high carbohydrate 1,000-calorie formula diets. Nutr Metab 1978, 22:269-77.
- Rabast U, Hahn A, Reiners C, Ehl M: Thyroid hormone changes in obese subjects during fasting and a very-low-calorie diet. Int J Obes 1981, 5:305-11.
- Golay A, Eigenheer C, Morel Y, Kujawski P, Lehmann T, de Tonnac N: Weight-loss with low or high carbohydrate diet? Int J Obes Relat Metab Disord 1996, 20:1067-72.
- Golay A, Allaz AF, Morel Y, de Tonnac N, Tankova S, Reaven G: Similar weight loss with low- or high-carbohydrate diets. Am J Clin Nutr 1996, 63:174-8.
- ML Piatti PM, Magni F, Fermo I, Baruffaldi L, Nasser R, Santambrogia G, Librenti MC, Galli-Kienle M, Pontiroli AE, Pozza G: Hypocaloric High-Protein Diet Improves Glucose Oxidation and Spares Lean Body Mass: Comparison to High-Carbohydrate Diet. Metabolism 1994, 43:1481-87.
- Layman DK, Boileau RA, Erickson DJ, Painter JE, Shiue H, Sather C, Christou DD: A reduced ratio of dietary carbohydrate to protein improves body composition and blood lipid profiles during weight loss in adult women. J Nutr 2003, 133:411-7.
- Lean ME, Han TS, Prvan T, Richmond PR, Avenell A: Weight loss with high and low carbohydrate 1200 kcal diets in free living women. Eur J Clin Nutr 1997, 51:243-8.
- Baba NH, Sawaya S, Torbay N, Habbal Z, Azar S, Hashim SA: High protein vs high carbohydrate hypoenergetic diet for the treatment of obese hyperinsulinemic subjects. Int J Obes Relat Metab Disord 1999, 23:1202-6.
- Young CM, Scanlan SS, Im HS, Lutwak L: Effect of body composition and other parameters in obese young men of carbohydrate level of reduction diet. Am J Clin Nutr 1971, 24:290-6.
- Greene P, Willett W, Devecis J, Skaf A: Pilot 12-Week Feeding Weight-Loss Comparison: Low-Fat vs Low-Carbohydrate (Ketogenic) Diets. Obesity Research 2003, 11:A23.

Chapter 9

1 Weigle DS. Human obesity. Exploding the myths. West J Med. 1990 Oct;153(4):421-8. Review. PubMed PMID: 2244378; PubMed Central PMCID: PMC1002573.

2 A sampling of research supporting that a calorie is not a calorie when it comes to filling you up and keeping you full:

- Holt SH, Miller JC, Petocz P, Farmakalidis E. A satiety index of common foods. Eur J Clin Nutr. 1995 Sep;49(9):675-90. PubMed PMID: 7498104.
- Anderson, G.H., and Woodend, D., "Effect of glycemic carbohydrates on short-term satiety and food intake," Nutr Rev 2003; 61(5): 17-26
- Araya, H., et al., "Short-term satiety in preschool children: a comparison between high protein meal and a high complex carbohydrate meal," Int J Food Sci Nutr 2000; 51(2): 119-124
- Blundell, J.E., and MacDiarmid, J.I., "Fat as a risk factor for overconsumption: satiation, satiety, and patterns of eating," J Am Diet Assoc 1997 97(7): S63-S69
- Bell, E.A., et al., "Sensory-specific satiety is affected more by volume than by energy content of a liquid food," Phys Behav 2003; 78(4): 593-600
- Green, S.M., et al., "Effect of fat- and sucrose-containing foods on the size of eating episodes and energy intake in lean males: potential for causing overconsumption," Eur J Clin Nutr 1994; 48(8): 547-555

- Guinard, J-X, and Brun, P., "Sensory-specific satiety: comparison of taste and texture effects," Appetite 1998; 31(2): 141-157
- Holt, S.H., et al., "A satiety index of common foods," Eur J Clin Nutr 1995 Sep; 49(9): 675-690
- Holt, S.A., et al., "The effects of equal-energy portions of different breads on blood glucose levels, feelings of fullness and subsequent food intake," J Am Diet Assoc 2001; 101(7): 767-773
- Marmonier, C., et al., "Effects of macronutrient content and energy density of snacks consumed in a satiety state on the onset of the next meal," Appetite 2000; 34(2): 161-168
- Pasman, W.J., et al., "Effect of one week of fiber supplementation on hunger and satiety ratings and energy intake," Appetite 29(1): 77-87
- Porrini, M., et al., "Effects of physical and chemical characteristics of food on specific and general satiety," Phys Behav 1995; 57(3): 461-468
- Porrini, M., et al., "Evaluation of satiety sensations and food intake after different preloads," Appetite 1995; 25(1): 17-30
- Rigaud, D., et al., "Effects of a moderate dietary fiber supplement on hunger rating, energy input and faecal energy output in young, healthy volunteers. A randomized, double-blind, cross-over trial," Int J Obes 1987; 11(1): 73-78
- Rolls, B.J., and Roe, L.S., "Effect of the volume of liquid food infused intragastrically on satiety in women," Phys Behav 2002; 76(4): 623-631
- Blundell John E., Stubbs R. James. Diet Composition and the Control of Food Intake in Humans In: Bray GA, Couchard d, James WP, eds. Handbook of Obesity. New York: Marcel Dekker, 1997: 243-272.

3   Boden G, Sargrad K, Homko C, Mozzoli M, Stein TP. Effect of a low-carbohydrate diet on appetite, blood glucose levels, and insulin resistance in obese patients with type 2 diabetes. Ann Intern Med. 2005 Mar 15;142(6):403-11. PubMed PMID: 15767618.

4   "Dietary fiber: Essential for a healthy diet—MayoClinic.com." Mayo Clinic. N.p., n.d. Web. 21 Jan. 2011. <http://www.mayoclinic.com/health/fiber/NU00033>.

5   Smith GP, Gibbs J. The effect of gut peptides on hunger, satiety, and food intake in humans. Ann N Y Acad Sci. 1987;499:132-6. Review. PubMed PMID: 3300478. & Harvey RF. Gut peptides and the control of food intake. Br Med J (Clin Res Ed). 1983 Nov 26;287(6405):1572-4. PubMed PMID: 6416508; PubMed Central PMCID: PMC1549802.

6   http://www.wisegeek.com/what-does-200-calories-look-like.htm

7   Halton TL, Hu FB. The effects of high protein diets on thermogenesis, satiety and weight loss: a critical review. J Am Coll Nutr. 2004 Oct;23(5):373-85. Review. PubMed PMID: 15466943.

8   Weigle DS, Breen PA, Matthys CC, Callahan HS, Meeuws KE, Burden VR, Purnell JQ. A high-protein diet induces sustained reductions in appetite, ad libitum caloric intake, and body weight despite compensatory changes in diurnal plasma leptin and ghrelin concentrations. Am J Clin Nutr. 2005 Jul;82(1):41-8. PubMed PMID: 16002798.

9   Booth DA, Chase A, Campbell AT. Relative effectiveness of protein in the late stages of appetite suppression in man. Physiol Behav. 1970 Nov;5(11):1299-302.PubMed PMID: 5524514.

10 Hill AJ, Blundell JE: Macronutrients and satiety; the effects of a high protein or high carbohydrate meal on subjective motivation to eat and food preferences. Nutr Behav3 :133 –144,1986 .

11 Barkeling B, Rössner S, Björvell H. Effects of a high-protein meal (meat) and a high-carbohydrate meal (vegetarian) on satiety measured by automated computerized monitoring of subsequent food intake, motivation to eat and food preferences. Int J Obes. 1990 Sep;14(9):743-51. PubMed PMID: 2228407.

12 Westerterp-Plantenga MS. The significance of protein in food intake and body weight regulation. Curr Opin Clin Nutr Metab Care. 2003 Nov;6(6):635-8. Review. PubMed PMID: 14557793.

13 Weigle DS, Breen PA, Matthys CC, Callahan HS, Meeuws KE, Burden VR, Purnell JQ. A high-protein diet induces sustained reductions in appetite, ad libitum caloric intake, and body weight despite compensatory changes in diurnal plasma leptin and ghrelin concentrations. Am J Clin Nutr. 2005

Jul;82(1):41-8. PubMed PMID: 16002798.

14 Blundell John E., Stubbs R. James. Diet Composition and the Control of Food Intake in Humans In: Bray GA, Couchard d, James WP, eds. Handbook of Obesity. New York: Marcel Dekker, 1997: 243-272.

15 Schoeller DA, Buchholz AC. Energetics of obesity and weight control: does diet composition matter? J Am Diet Assoc. 2005 May;105(5 Suppl 1):S24-8. Review. PubMed PMID: 15867892.

16 Stubbs RJ, van Wyk MC, Johnstone AM, Harbron CG. Breakfasts high in protein, fat or carbohydrate: effect on within-day appetite and energy balance. Eur J Clin Nutr. 1996 Jul;50(7):409-17. PubMed PMID: 8862476. & Paddon-Jones D, Westman E, Mattes RD, Wolfe RR, Astrup A, Westerterp-Plantenga M. Protein, weight management, and satiety. Am J Clin Nutr. 2008 May;87(5):1558S-1561S. Review. PubMed PMID: 18469287.

Chapter 10

1 Taubes, Gary. Good Calories, Bad Calories: Fats, Carbohydrates, and the Controversial Science of Diet and Health (Vintage). New York: Anchor, 2008. Print.

2 Colagiuri S, Brand Miller J. The 'carnivore connection'--evolutionary aspects of insulin resistance. Eur J Clin Nutr. 2002 Mar;56 Suppl 1:S30-5. Review. PubMed PMID: 11965520.

3 Buchholz AC, Schoeller DA. Is a calorie a calorie? Am J Clin Nutr. 2004 May;79(5):899S-906S. Review. PubMed PMID: 15113737.

4 "Glycemic index and glycemic load for 100+ foods—Harvard Health Publications." Health Information and Medical Information—Harvard Health Publications. N.p., n.d. Web. 16 June 2010. <http://www.health.harvard.edu/newsweek/Glycemic_index_and_glycemic_load_for_100_foods.htm>.

5 A sampling of supporting research:
   • Cordain L, Eaton SB, Sebastian A, Mann N, Lindeberg S, Watkins BA, O'Keefe JH, Brand-Miller J. Origins and evolution of the Western diet: health implications for the 21st century. Am J Clin Nutr. 2005 Feb;81(2):341-54. Review. PubMed PMID: 15699220.
   • Foster-Powell K, Holt SH, Brand-Miller JC. International table of glycemic index and glycemic load values: 2002. Am J Clin Nutr. 2002 Jul;76(1):5-56. PubMed PMID: 12081815.
   • Haber GB, Heaton KW, Murphy D, Burroughs LF. (1977). Depletion and disruption of dietary fibre. Effects on satiety, plasma-glucose, and serum-insulin. Lancet, 2: 679-682.
   • Leathwood P, Pollet P. (1988). Effects of slow release carbohydrates in the form of bean flakes on the evolution of hunger and satiety in man. Appetite, 10: 1-11.
   • Rodin J, Reed D, Jamner L. (1988). Metabolic effects of fructose and glucose: implications for food intake. Am. J. Clin. Nutr., 47: 683-689.
   • Holt S, Brand J, Soveny C, Hansky J. (1992). Relationship of satiety to postprandial glycaemic, insulin and cholecystokinin responses. Appetite, 18: 129-141.
   • Holt SH, Miller JB. (1994). Particle size, satiety and the glycaemic response. Eur. J. Clin. Nutr., 48: 496-502.
   • van Amelsvoort JM, Weststrate JA. (1992). Amylose-amylopectin ratio in a meal affects postprandial variables in male volunteers. Am. J. Clin. Nutr., 55: 712-718.
   • Liljeberg HG, Akerberg AK, Bjorck IM. (1999). Effect of the glycemic index and content of indigestible carbohydrates of cereal-based breakfast meals on glucose tolerance at lunch in healthy subjects. Am. J. Clin. Nutr., 69: 647-655.
   • Ludwig DS, Majzoub JA, Al-Zahrani A, Dallal GE, Blanco I, Roberts SB. High glycemic index foods, overeating, and obesity. Pediatrics. 1999 Mar;103(3):E26. PubMed PMID: 10049982.
   • Roberts SB. High-glycemic index foods, hunger, and obesity: is there a connection? Nutr Rev. 2000 Jun;58(6):163-9. Review. PubMed PMID: 10885323.
   • Obesity and leanness. Basic aspects. Stock, M., Rothwell, N., Author Affiliation: Dep. Physiology, St. George's Hospital Medical School, London Univ., London, UK.

- Jenkins DJ, Jenkins AL. Dietary fiber and the glycemic response. Proc Soc Exp Biol Med. 1985;180:422-431.
- Potter JG, Coffman KP, Reid RL, Krall JM, Apoundrink MJ. Effect of test meals of varying dietary fiber content on plasma insulin and glucose response. Am J Clin Nutr. 1981;34:328-334.
- Chandalia M, Garg A, Lutjohann D, von Bergmann K, Grundy SM, Brinkley LJ. Beneficial effects of high dietary fiber intake in patients with type 2 diabetes mellitus. N Engl J Med. 2000 May 11;342(19):1392-8. PubMed PMID: 10805824.
- Augustin LS, Franceschi S, Jenkins DJ, Kendall CW, La Vecchia C. Glycemic index in chronic disease: a review. Eur J Clin Nutr. 2002 Nov;56(11):1049-71.Review. PubMed PMID: 12428171.
- Welch IM, Bruce C, Hill SE, Read NW. (1987). Duodenal and ileal lipid suppresses postprandial blood glucose and insulin responses in man: possible implications for the dietary management of diabetes mellitus. Clin. Sci. (Lond), 72: 209-216.
- Trout DL, Behall KM, Osilesi O. Prediction of glycemic index for starchy foods. Am J Clin Nutr. 1993;58:873-878.
- Holt SH, Miller JC, Petocz P. An insulin index of foods: The insulin demand generated by 1000-kJ portions of common foods. Am J Clin Nutr. 1997 Nov;66(5):1264-76. PubMed PMID: 9356547.

6 A sampling of supporting research:
- O'Keefe JH Jr, Cordain L. Cardiovascular disease resulting from a diet and lifestyle at odds with our Paleolithic genome: how to become a 21st-century hunter-gatherer. Mayo Clin Proc 2004 Jan;79(1):101-8.
- Ford ES, Liu S. Glycemic index and serum high-density lipoprotein cholesterol concentration among U.S. adults. Arch Intern Med. 2001;161:572-576.
- Leeds AR. Glycemic index and heart disease. Am J Clin Nutr.2002;76:286S-289S.
- Ludwig DS. The glycemic index: physiological mechanisms relating to obesity, diabetes, and cardiovascular disease. JAMA. 2002; 287:2414-2423.
- Lamarche B, Tchernof A, Mauriege P, et al. Fasting insulin and apolipoprotein B levels and low-density lipoprotein particle size as risk factors for ischemic heart disease. JAMA. 1998;279:1955-1961.
- Augustin LS, Franceschi S, Jenkins DJ, Kendall CW, La Vecchia C. Glycemic index in chronic disease: a review. Eur J Clin Nutr. 2002 Nov;56(11):1049-71.Review. PubMed PMID: 12428171.
- Salmeron J, Ascherio A, Rimm EB et al. (1997a). Dietary fiber, glycemic load, and risk of NIDDM in men. Diabetes Care, 20: 545-550.
- Salmeron J, Manson JE, Stampfer MJ, Colditz GA, Wing AL, Willett WC. (1997b). Dietary fiber, glycemic load, and risk of non-insulin-dependent diabetes mellitus in women. JAMA, 277: 472-477.
- Liu S, Willett WC, Stampfer MJ, Hu FB, Franz M, Sampson L, Hennekens CH, Manson JE. A prospective study of dietary glycemic load, carbohydrate intake, and risk of coronary heart disease in U.S. women. Am J Clin Nutr. 2000 Jun;71(6):1455-61. PubMed PMID: 10837285.
- Jenkins DJ, Wolever TM, Collier GR, Ocana A, Rao AV, Buckley G, Lam Y, Mayer A, Thompson LU. Metabolic effects of a low-glycemic-index diet. Am J Clin Nutr.

Chapter 11

1 Willett WC. Is dietary fat a major determinant of body fat? Am J Clin Nutr. 1998 Mar;67(3 Suppl):556S-562S. Review. Erratum in: Am J Clin Nutr 1999 Aug;70(2):304. PubMed PMID: 9497170.
2 Nestle, Marion. What to Eat. 1 ed. New York: North Point Press, 2007. Print.
3 USDA SR-21
4 Drewnowski A. Concept of a nutritious food: Toward a nutrient density score. Am J Clin Nutr. 2005 Oct;82(4):721-32. PubMed PMID: 16210699.
5 Cordain, Loren, and Joe Friel. The Paleo diet for athletes: a nutritional formula for peak athletic performance. Emmaus, Pa.: Rodale, 2005. Print.

6   Cordain L, Eaton SB, Sebastian A, Mann N, Lindeberg S, Watkins BA, O'Keefe JH, Brand-Miller J. Origins and evolution of the Western diet: health implications for the 21st century. Am J Clin Nutr. 2005 Feb;81(2):341-54. Review. PubMed PMID: 15699220. Note: My addition of sweets is considering sweets such as soda and hard candy which contain no vitamins nor minerals.
7   http://www.nal.usda.gov/fnic/foodcomp/search/
8   A sampling of supporting research:
   • Rolls BJ, Bell EA, Castellanos VH, Chow M, Pelkman CL, Thorwart ML. Energy density but not fat content of foods affected energy intake in lean and obese women. Am J Clin Nutr. 1999 May;69(5):863-71. PubMed PMID: 10232624.
   • Bell EA, Rolls BJ. Energy density of foods affects energy intake across multiple levels of fat content in lean and obese women. Am J Clin Nutr. 2001 Jun;73(6):1010-8. PubMed PMID: 11382653.
   • Drewnowski A. The role of energy density. Lipids. 2003 Feb;38(2):109-15. Review. PubMed PMID: 12733741.
   • Layman DK. Dietary Guidelines should reflect new understandings about adult protein needs. Nutr Metab (Lond). 2009 Mar 13;6:12. PubMed PMID: 19284668; PubMed Central PMCID: PMC2666737.

Chapter 12

1   Feinman RD, Fine EJ. "A calorie is a calorie" violates the second law of thermodynamics. Nutr J. 2004 Jul 28;3:9. PubMed PMID: 15282028; PubMed Central PMCID: PMC506782.
2   A sampling of supporting research:
   • Johnston CS, Day CS, Swan PD. Postprandial thermogenesis is increased 100% on a high-protein, low-fat diet versus a high-carbohydrate, low-fat diet in healthy, young women. J Am Coll Nutr. 2002 Feb;21(1):55-61. PubMed PMID: 11838888.
   • Schutz Y, Jequier E. Resting Energy Expenditure, thermic Effect of Food, and Total Energy Expenditure In: Bray GA, Couchard d, James WP, eds. Handbook of Obesity. New York: Marcel Dekker, 1997: 379-396.
   • Halton TL, Hu FB. The effects of high protein diets on thermogenesis, satiety and weight loss: a critical review. J Am Coll Nutr. 2004 Oct;23(5):373-85. Review. PubMed PMID: 15466943.
   • Feinman RD, Fine EJ. "A calorie is a calorie" violates the second law of thermodynamics. Nutr J. 2004 Jul 28;3:9. PubMed PMID: 15282028; PubMed Central PMCID: PMC506782.
   • FAO/OMS/UNU. Necessidades de energia e proteína: Série de relatos técnicos 724. Genebra: Organização Mundial da Saúde, 1998.
3   A sampling of supporting research:
   • Jéquier E. Pathways to obesity. Int J Obes Relat Metab Disord. 2002 Sep;26 Suppl 2:S12-7. Review. PubMed PMID: 12174324.
   • Jéquier E, Acheson K, Schutz Y. Assessment of energy expenditure and fuel utilization in man. Annu Rev Nutr. 1987;7:187-208. Review. PubMed PMID: 3300732.
   • Tappy L, Jéquier E. Fructose and dietary thermogenesis. Am J Clin Nutr. 1993 Nov;58(5 Suppl):766S-770S. Review. PubMed PMID: 8213608.
   • Keesey RE, Powley TL. The regulation of body weight. Annu Rev Psychol.1986;37:109-33. PubMed PMID: 3963779.
   • Fine EJ, Feinman RD. Thermodynamics of weight loss diets. Nutr Metab (Lond).2004 Dec 8;1(1):15. PubMed PMID: 15588283
   • Schutz Y, Jequier E. Resting Energy Expenditure, thermic Effect of Food, and Total Energy Expenditure In: Bray GA, Couchard d, James WP, eds. Handbook of Obesity. New York: Marcel Dekker, 1997: 443-456.
   • Paddon-Jones D, Westman E, Mattes RD, Wolfe RR, Astrup A, Westerterp-Plantenga M. Protein, weight management, and satiety. Am J Clin Nutr. 2008 May;87(5):1558S-1561S. Review. PubMed

PMID: 18469287.

- Obesity and leanness. Basic aspects. Stock, M., Rothwell, N., Author Affiliation: Dep. Physiology, St. George's Hospital Medical School, London Univ., London, UK.

4 A sampling of supporting research:
- Hellerstein MK. De novo lipogenesis in humans: metabolic and regulatory aspects. Eur J Clin Nutr. 1999 Apr;53 Suppl 1:S53-65. Review. PubMed PMID:10365981.
- Cox, Michael M., Apoundert L. Lehninger, and David L. Nelson. Principles of Biochemistry. 3rd ed. New York: W.H. Freeman & Company, 2000. Print.
- Veldhorst MA, Westerterp-Plantenga MS, Westerterp KR. Gluconeogenesis and energy expenditure after a high-protein, carbohydrate-free diet. Am J Clin Nutr. 2009 Sep;90(3):519-26. Epub 2009 Jul 29. PubMed PMID: 19640952.

5 A sampling of supporting research:
- Flatt JP. Conversion of carbohydrate to fat in adipose tissue: an energy-yielding and, therefore, self-limiting process. J Lipid Res. 1970 Mar;11(2):131-43. PubMed PMID: 4392141.
- Acheson KJ, Schutz Y, Bessard T, Anantharaman K, Flatt JP, Jéquier E. Glycogen storage capacity and de novo lipogenesis during massive carbohydrate overfeeding in man. Am J Clin Nutr. 1988 Aug;48(2):240-7. PubMed PMID: 3165600.
- Hue L. Regulation of gluconeogenesis in liver: In Handbook of Physiology—Section 7: The Endocrine System—Volume II: The Endocrine Pancreas and Regulation of Metabolism. Oxford: Oxford University Press, pp. 649-657, 2001.

6 Feinman RD, Fine EJ. "A calorie is a calorie" violates the second law of thermodynamics. Nutr J. 2004 Jul 28;3:9. PubMed PMID: 15282028; PubMed Central PMCID: PMC506782. & Flatt JP. Energetics of intermediary metabolism. In: Garrow JS, Halliday D, eds. Substrate and Energy Metabolism in Man. London: Libbey, 1985: 58.

7 the graph assumed the calories not coming from protein are equally divided between fat and carbohydrates.

8 Taubes, Gary. Good Calories, Bad Calories: Fats, Carbohydrates, and the Controversial Science of Diet and Health (Vintage). New York: Anchor, 2008. Print.

9 Mayes PA. Intermediary metabolism of fructose. Am J Clin Nutr. 1993 Nov;58(5 Suppl):754S-765S. Review. PubMed PMID: 8213607.

10 A sampling of supporting research:
- Havel PJ. Dietary fructose: implications for dysregulation of energy homeostasis and lipid/carbohydrate metabolism. Nutr Rev. 2005 May;63(5):133-57.Review. PubMed PMID: 15971409.
- Whitehead, Saffron A.; Nussey, Stephen (2001). Endocrinology: an integrated approach. Oxford: BIOS. pp. 122. ISBN 1-85996-252-1.
- http://en.wikipedia.org/wiki/Glyceraldehyde_3-phosphate
- http://en.wikipedia.org/wiki/Dihydroxyacetone_phosphate
- http://en.wikipedia.org/wiki/Fructose_1,6-bisphosphate
- Elliott SS, Keim NL, Stern JS, Teff K, Havel PJ. Fructose, weight gain, and the insulin resistance syndrome. Am J Clin Nutr. 2002 Nov;76(5):911-22. Review. PubMed PMID: 12399260.
- Advanced Nutrition and Human Metabolism, James L. Groff, and Sareen S. Gropper

Chapter 13

1 Lindeberg S, Jönsson T, Granfeldt Y, Borgstrand E, Soffman J, Sjöström K, Ahrén B. A Palaeolithic diet improves glucose tolerance more than a Mediterranean-like diet in individuals with ischaemic heart disease. Diabetologia. 2007 Sep;50(9):1795-807. Epub 2007 Jun 22. PubMed PMID: 17583796.

2 A sampling of supporting research:
- Layman DK, Boileau RA, Erickson DJ, Painter JE, Shiue H, Sather C, Christou DD. A reduced ratio

of dietary carbohydrate to protein improves body composition and blood lipid profiles during weight loss in adult women. J Nutr. 2003 Feb;133(2):411-7.

- Farnsworth E, Luscombe ND, Noakes M, Wittert G, Argyiou E, Clifton PM. Effect of a high-protein, energy-restricted diet on body composition, glycemic control, and lipid concentrations in overweight and obese hyperinsulinemic men and women.Am J Clin Nutr. 2003 Jul;78(1):31-9.

- McAuley KA, Hopkins CM, Smith KJ, McLay RT, Williams SM, Taylor RW, Mann JI. Comparison of high-fat and high-protein diets with a high-carbohydrate diet in insulin-resistant obese women. Diabetologia. 2005 Jan;48(1):8-16.

- Nuttall FQ, Gannon MC. The metabolic response to a high-protein, low-carbohydrate diet in men with type 2 diabetes mellitus. Metabolism. 2006 Feb;55(2):243-51.

- Nuttall FQ, Gannon MC. Metabolic response of people with type 2 diabetes to a high protein diet. Nutr Metab (Lond). 2004 Sep 13;1(1):652.

- McAuley KA, Smith KJ, Taylor RW, McLay RT, Williams SM, Mann JI. Long-term effects of popular dietary approaches on weight loss and features of insulin resistance. Int J Obes (Lond). 2006 Feb;30(2):342-9.

- Brand-Miller J. Diets with a low glycemic index: From theory to practice. Nutrition Today. 1999;34:64–72.

- Gannon MC, Nuttall FQ, Saeed A, Jordan K, Hoover H. An increase in dietary protein improves the blood glucose response in persons with type 2 diabetes. Am J Clin Nutr. 2003 Oct;78(4):734-41. PubMed PMID: 14522731.

- Børsheim E, Bui Q-UT, Tissier S, Kobayashi H, Ferrando AA, Wolfe RR. Effect of amino acid supplementation in insulin sensitivity in elderly. Fed Proc (in press).

- Frost G, Keogh B, Smith D, Akinsanya K, Leeds A. (1996). The effect of low-glycemic carbohydrate on insulin and glucose response in vivo and in vitro in patients with coronary heart disease. Metabolism, 45: 669-672.

- Noakes M, Keogh JB, Foster PR, Clifton PM. Effect of an energy-restricted, high-protein, low-fat diet relative to a conventional high-carbohydrate, low-fat diet on weight loss, body composition, nutritional status, and markers of cardiovascular health in obese women. Am J Clin Nutr. 2005 Jun;81(6):1298-306.

- Weigle DS, Breen PA, Matthys CC, Callahan HS, Meeuws KE, Burden VR, Purnell JQ. A high-protein diet induces sustained reductions in appetite, ad libitum caloric intake, and body weight despite compensatory changes in diurnal plasma leptin and ghrelin concentrations. Am J Clin Nutr. 2005 Jul;82(1):41-8

- Skov AR, Toubro S, Rønn B, Holm L, Astrup A. Randomized trial on protein vs carbohydrate in ad libitum fat reduced diet for the treatment of obesity. Int J Obes Relat Metab Disord. 1999 May;23(5):528-36. PubMed PMID: 10375057.

- Lasker DA, Evans EM, Layman DK. Moderate carbohydrate, moderate protein weight loss diet reduces cardiovascular disease risk compared to high carbohydrate, low protein diet in obese adults: A randomized clinical trial. Nutr Metab (Lond). 2008 Nov 7;5:30. PubMed PMID: 18990242; PubMed Central PMCID: PMC2585565.

- Wolfe RR. The underappreciated role of muscle in health and disease. Am J Clin Nutr. 2006 Sep;84(3):475-82. Review. PubMed PMID: 16960159.

- Westerterp-Plantenga MS, Lejeune MP, Nijs I, van Ooijen M, Kovacs EM. High protein intake sustains weight maintenance after body weight loss in humans. Int J Obes Relat Metab Disord. 2004 Jan;28(1):57-64.

- Lejeune MP, Kovacs EM, Westerterp-Plantenga MS. Additional protein intake limits weight regain after weight loss in humans. Br J Nutr. 2005 Feb;93(2):281-9. PubMed PMID: 15788122.

- Baba NH, Sawaya S, Torbay N, Habbal Z, Azar S, Hashim SA: High protein vs high carbohydrate hypoenergetic diet for the treatment of obese hyperinsulinemic subjects. Int J Obes23 :1202 –1206,1999

- Brehm BJ, Seeley RJ, Daniels SR, D'Alessio DA: A randomized trial comparing a very low carbo-hydrate diet and a calorie restricted low fat diet on body weight and cardiovascular risk factors in healthy women. J Clin Endocrinol Metab88 :1617 –1623,2003
- Foster GD, Wyatt HR, Hill JO, McGuckin BG, Brill C, Mohammed S: A randomized trial of a low-carbohydrate diet. N Eng J Med348 :2082 –2090,2003
- Samaha FF, Iqbal N, Seshadri P, Chicano KL, Daily D, Mcgrory J: A low carbohydrate as compared with a low fat diet in severe obesity. N Eng J Med348 :2074 –2081,2003 .
- Worthington BS, Taylor LE: Balanced low calorie vs high protein, low carbohydrate reducing diets. J Am Diet Assoc64 :47 –51,1974 .
- Yancy Jr WS, Olsen MK, Guyton JR, Bakst RP, Westman EC: A low-carbohydrate, ketogenic diet versus a low-fat diet to treat obesity and hyperlipidemia. Ann Intern Med140 :769 –777,2004

3   A sampling of supporting research:
- Ha E, Zemel MB. Functional properties of whey, whey components, and essential amino ac-ids: mechanisms underlying health benefits for active people (review). J Nutr Biochem. 2003 May;14(5):251-8. Review. PubMed PMID: 12832028.
- Krissansen GW. Emerging health properties of whey proteins and their clinical implications. J Am Coll Nutr. 2007 Dec;26(6):713S-23S. Review. PubMed PMID: 18187438.
- Luhovyy BL, Akhavan T, Anderson GH. Whey proteins in the regulation of food intake and satiety. J Am Coll Nutr. 2007 Dec;26(6):704S-12S. Review. PubMed PMID:18187437.
- Yalçin AS. Emerging therapeutic potential of whey proteins and peptides. Curr Pharm Des. 2006;12(13):1637-43. Review. PubMed PMID: 16729875.

Chapter 14

1   Wertheimer, E., and Shapiro, B., the physiology of adipose tissue, Physiol. Rev., 1948, 28, 451.

2   From Research to Practice/The Art and Science of Obesity Management: Betsy B. Dokken and Tsu-Shuen Tsao the Physiology of Body Weight Regulation: Are We Too Efficient for Our Own Good? Diabe-tes Spectrum July 2007 20:166-170; doi:10.2337/diaspect.20.3.166

3   Goldberg M, Gordon E. Energy Metabolism In Human Obesity. Plasma Free Fatty Acid, Glucose, And Glycerol Response To Epinephrine. JAMA. 1964 Aug 24;189:616-23. PubMed PMID: 14162576.

4   A sampling of supporting research:
- Woods SC, Figlewicz Lattemann DP, Schwartz MW, Porte D Jr. A re-assessment of the regulation of adiposity and appetite by the brain insulin system. Int J Obes.1990;14 Suppl 3:69-73; discussion 74-6. Review. PubMed PMID: 2086517.
- Porte D Jr, Woods SC. Regulation of food intake and body weight in insulin. Diabetologia. 1981 Mar;20 Suppl:274-80. PubMed PMID: 7014326.
- Woods SC, Benoit SC, Clegg DJ, Seeley RJ. Clinical endocrinology and metabolism. Regulation of energy homeostasis by peripheral signals. Best Pract Res Clin Endocrinol Metab. 2004 Dec;18(4):497-515. Review. PubMed PMID: 15533772.

5   A sampling of supporting research:
- Harris RB, Martin RJ. Specific depletion of body fat in parabiotic partners of tube-fed obese rats. Am J Physiol. 1984 Aug;247(2 Pt 2):R380-6. PubMed PMID: 6431831.
- Harris RB, Martin RJ. Influence of diet on the production of a "lipid-depleting" factor in obese para-biotic rats. J Nutr. 1986 Oct;116(10):2013-27. PubMed PMID: 3772528.
- Obesity and leanness. Basic aspects. Stock, M., Rothwell, N., Author Affiliation: Dep. Physiology, St. George's Hospital Medical School, London Univ., London, UK.
- Harris RB, Martin RJ. Metabolic response to a specific lipid-depleting factor in parabiotic rats. Am J Physiol. 1986 Feb;250(2 Pt 2):R276-86. PubMed PMID: 3511738.
- Havel PJ. Update on adipocyte hormones: regulation of energy balance and carbohydrate/lipid me-

tabolism. Diabetes. 2004 Feb;53 Suppl 1:S143-51. Review. PubMed PMID: 14749280.

- Parameswaran SV, Steffens AB, Hervey GR, de Ruiter L. Involvement of a humoral factor in regulation of body weight in parabiotic rats. Am J Physiol. 1977 May;232(5):R150-7. PubMed PMID: 324294.

6 Chen HC, Jensen DR, Myers HM, Eckel RH, Farese RV Jr. Obesity resistance and enhanced glucose metabolism in mice transplanted with white adipose tissue lacking acyl CoA:diacylglycerol acyltransferase 1. J Clin Invest. 2003 Jun;111(11):1715-22. PubMed PMID: 12782674; PubMed Central PMCID: PMC156099.

7 Kraemer FB, Shen WJ. Hormone-sensitive lipase knockouts. Nutr Metab (Lond). 2006 Feb 10;3:12. PubMed PMID: 16472389; PubMed Central PMCID: PMC1391915.

8 Polak P, Cybulski N, Feige JN, Auwerx J, Rüegg MA, Hall MN. Adipose-specific knockout of raptor results in lean mice with enhanced mitochondrial respiration. Cell Metab. 2008 Nov;8(5):399-410. PubMed PMID: 19046571. & Havel PJ. Update on adipocyte hormones: regulation of energy balance and carbohydrate/lipid metabolism. Diabetes. 2004 Feb;53 Suppl 1:S143-51. Review. PubMed PMID: 14749280.

9 A sampling of supporting research:
- Drent M. Obesity and Endocrine Funtion. In: Bray GA, Couchard d, James WP, eds. Handbook of Obesity. New York: Marcel Dekker, 1997: 697-707.
- Kopelman P. Endocrine Determinants of Obesity In: Bray GA, Couchard d, James WP, eds. Handbook of Obesity. New York: Marcel Dekker, 1997: 475-490.
- Flatt, Jen-Pierre. Tremblay, Angelo. Energy Expenditure and Substrate Oxidation. In: Bray GA, Couchard d, James WP, eds. Handbook of Obesity. New York: Marcel Dekker, 1997: 513-538.
- Obesity and Leanness: Basic Aspects. London: John Libbey & Co Ltd, 1982. Print.
- Goldberg M, Gordon E. Energy Metabolism In Human Obesity. Plasma Free Fatty Acid, Glucose, And Glycerol Response To Epinephrine. JAMA. 1964 Aug 24;189:616-23. PubMed PMID: 14162576.
- From Research to Practice/The Art and Science of Obesity Management: Betsy B. Dokken and Tsu-Shuen Tsao the Physiology of Body Weight Regulation: Are We Too Efficient for Our Own Good? Diabetes Spectrum July 2007 20:166-170; doi:10.2337/diaspect.20.3.166
- Westman EC, Feinman RD, Mavropoulos JC, Vernon MC, Volek JS, Wortman JA, Yancy WS, Phinney SD. Low-carbohydrate nutrition and metabolism. Am J Clin Nutr. 2007 Aug;86(2):276-84. Review. PubMed PMID: 17684196.
- Le Magnen J. Is regulation of body weight elucidated. Neurosci Biobehav Rev. 1984 Winter;8(4):515-22. Review. PubMed PMID: 6392951.
- Drent M. Effects of Obesity on Endocrine Function In: Bray GA, Couchard d, James WP, eds. Handbook of Obesity. New York: Marcel Dekker, 1997: 753-773.
- Murray I, Havel PJ, Sniderman AD, Cianflone K. Reduced body weight, adipose tissue, and leptin levels despite increased energy intake in female mice lacking acylation-stimulating protein. Endocrinology. 2000 Mar;141(3):1041-9. PubMed PMID: 10698180.
- Whitehead, Saffron A.; Nussey, Stephen (2001). Endocrinology: an integrated approach. Oxford: BIOS. pp. 122. ISBN 1-85996-252-1.
- Nielsen JV, Jonsson E, Nilsson AK: Lasting improvement of hyperglycaemia and bodyweight: low-carbohydrate diet in type 2 diabetes—a brief report. Ups J Med Sci 2005, 110(1):69-73.
- Accurso A, Bernstein RK, Dahlqvist A, Draznin B, Feinman RD, Fine EJ, Gleed A, Jacobs DB, Larson G, Lustig RH, Manninen AH, McFarlane SI, Morrison K, Nielsen JV, Ravnskov U, Roth KS, Silvestre R, Sowers JR, Sundberg R, Volek JS, Westman EC, Wood RJ, Wortman J, Vernon MC. Dietary carbohydrate restriction in type 2 diabetes mellitus and metabolic syndrome: Time for a critical appraisal. NutrMetab (Lond). 2008 Apr 8;5:9. PubMed PMID: 18397522; PubMed Central PMCID: PMC2359752.

10 A sampling of supporting research:

- Havel PJ. Peripheral signals conveying metabolic information to the brain: short-term and long-term regulation of food intake and energy homeostasis. Exp Biol Med (Maywood). 2001 Dec;226(11):963-77. Review. PubMed PMID: 11743131.
- Havel PJ. Dietary fructose: implications for dysregulation of energy homeostasis and lipid/carbohydrate metabolism. Nutr Rev. 2005 May;63(5):133-57.Review. PubMed PMID: 15971409.
- Murphy KG, Dhillo WS, Bloom SR. Gut peptides in the regulation of food intake and energy homeostasis. Endocr Rev. 2006 Dec;27(7):719-27. Epub 2006 Oct 31. Review. PubMed PMID: 17077190.
- Hameed S, Dhillo WS, Bloom SR. Gut hormones and appetite control. Oral Dis. 2009 Jan;15(1):18-26. Epub 2008 Oct 17. Review. PubMed PMID: 18939959.

11 A sampling of supporting research:
- Papoushek C. The "glitazones": rosiglitazone and pioglitazone. J Obstet Gynaecol Can. 2003 Oct;25(10):853-7. Review. Erratum in: J Obstet Gynaecol Can. 2003 Nov;25(11):907. PubMed PMID: 14532954.
- Sinha A, Formica C, Tsalamandris C, Panagiotopoulos S, Hendrich E, DeLuise M, Seeman E, Jerums G. Effects of insulin on body composition in patients with insulin-dependent and non-insulin-dependent diabetes. Diabet Med. 1996 Jan;13(1):40-6. PubMed PMID: 8741811.
- Laville M, Andreelli F. [Mechanisms for weight gain during blood glucose normalization]. Diabetes Metab. 2000 Jun;26 Suppl 3:42-5. Review. French. PubMed PMID: 10945152.
- Carlson MG & Campbell PJ. Intensive insulin therapy and weight gain in IDDM. Diabetes 1993 42 1700–1707.
- Joslin, Elliott Proctor, C. Ronald. Kahn, and Gordon C. Weir. Joslin's Diabetes Mellitus. Philadelphia: Lea & Febiger, 1994. Print.
- MacKay, Eaton M., Callaway, James W., Barnes, Richard H. Hyperalimentation in Normal Animals Produced by Protamine Insulin: Three Figures J. Nutr. 1940 20: 59-66
- Hoebel BG, Teitepoundaum P. Weight regulation in normal and hypothalamic hyperphagic rats. J Comp Physiol Psychol. 1966 Apr;61(2):189-93. PubMed PMID: 5909295.
- Havel PJ. Update on adipocyte hormones: regulation of energy balance and carbohydrate/lipid metabolism. Diabetes. 2004 Feb;53 Suppl 1:S143-51. Review. PubMed PMID: 14749280.
- Rosenbaum M, Vandenborne K, Goldsmith R, Simoneau JA, Heymsfield S, Joanisse DR, Hirsch J, Murphy E, Matthews D, Segal KR, Leibel RL. Effects of experimental weight perturbation on skeletal muscle work efficiency in human subjects. Am J Physiol Regul Integr Comp Physiol. 2003 Jul;285(1):R183-92. Epub 2003 Feb 27. PubMed PMID: 12609816.

12 Kersten S. Mechanisms of nutritional and hormonal regulation of lipogenesis. EMBO Rep. 2001 Apr;2(4):282-6. Review. PubMed PMID: 11306547; PubMed Central PMCID: PMC1083868.

13 A sampling of supporting research:
- York DA, Bray GA. Dependence of hypothalamic obesity on insulin, the pituitary and the adrenal gland. Endocrinology. 1972 Apr;90(4):885-94. PubMed PMID:4258778.
- Wilcox G. Insulin and insulin resistance. Clin Biochem Rev. 2005 May;26(2):19-39. PubMed PMID: 16278749; PubMed Central PMCID: PMC1204764.
- Goldberg M, Gordon E. Energy Metabolism In Human Obesity. Plasma Free Fatty Acid, Glucose, And Glycerol Response To Epinephrine. JAMA. 1964 Aug 24;189:616-23. PubMed PMID: 14162576.
- Obesity and leanness. Basic aspects. Stock, M., Rothwell, N., Author Affiliation: Dep. Physiology, St. George's Hospital Medical School, London Univ., London, UK.
- Blüher M, Michael MD, Peroni OD, Ueki K, Carter N, Kahn BB, Kahn CR. Adipose tissue selective insulin receptor knockout protects against obesity and obesity-related glucose intolerance. Dev Cell. 2002 Jul;3(1):25-38. PubMed PMID: 12110165.
- Flatt, Jen-Pierre. Tremblay, Angelo. Energy Expenditure and Substrate Oxidation. In: Bray GA, Couchard d, James WP, eds. Handbook of Obesity. New York: Marcel Dekker, 1997: 513-538.
- E.A. Newsholme and C. Start. Regulation of Metabolism. 173 ISBN: 0471635308

- Havel PJ. Update on adipocyte hormones: regulation of energy balance and carbohydrate/lipid metabolism. Diabetes. 2004 Feb;53 Suppl 1:S143-51. Review. PubMed PMID: 14749280.

14 Newsholme, E. A., and C. Start. Regulation in metabolism . London: Wiley, 1973. Print.

15 A sampling of supporting research:
- Ludwig DS. The glycemic index: physiological mechanisms relating to obesity, diabetes, and cardiovascular disease. JAMA. 2002 May 8;287(18):2414-23. Review. PubMed PMID: 11988062.
- Schenk S, Saberi M, Olefsky JM. Insulin sensitivity: modulation by nutrients and inflammation. J Clin Invest. 2008 Sep;118(9):2992-3002. Review. PubMed PMID: 18769626; PubMed Central PMCID: PMC2522344.
- Whitehead, Saffron A.; Nussey, Stephen (2001). Endocrinology: an integrated approach. Oxford: BIOS. pp. 122. ISBN 1-85996-252-1.
- York DA, Hansen B. Animal models of obesity. In: Bray GA, Couchard d, James WP, eds. Handbook of Obesity. New York: Marcel Dekker, 1997: 191-221

16 Cordain, Loren, and Joe Friel. The Paleo Diet for Athletes: A Nutritional Formula for Peak Athletic Performance. Emmaus, Pa.: Rodale Books, 2005. Print.

17 "Diabetes mellitus." Belinda Rowland., Teresa G. Odle., and Tish Davidson, A. M. The Gale Encyclopedia of Alternative Medicine. Ed. Laurie Fundukian. 3rd ed. Detroit: Gale, 2009. 4 vols.

18 A sampling of supporting research:
- Caro JF. Clinical review 26: Insulin resistance in obese and nonobese man. J Clin Endocrinol Metab. 1991 Oct;73(4):691-5. Review. PubMed PMID: 1890146.
- DeFronzo RA, Ferrannini E. Insulin resistance. A multifaceted syndrome responsible for NIDDM, obesity, hypertension, dyslipidemia, and atherosclerotic cardiovascular disease. Diabetes Care. 1991 Mar;14(3):173-94. Review. PubMed PMID: 2044434.
- Kissebah AH, Peiris AN. Biology of regional body fat distribution: relationship to non-insulin-dependent diabetes mellitus. Diabetes Metab Rev. 1989 Mar;5(2):83-109. Review. PubMed PMID: 2647436.
- Apoundu J. Pi-Sunyer F. Obesity and Diabetes In: Bray GA, Couchard d, James WP, eds. Handbook of Obesity. New York: Marcel Dekker, 1997: 697-707.
- Lamarche B, Tchernof A, Mauriege P, et al. Fasting insulin and apolipoprotein B levels and low-density lipoprotein particle size as risk factors for ischemic heart disease. JAMA. 1998;279:1955-1961.
- Cordain L, Eaton SB, Sebastian A, Mann N, Lindeberg S, Watkins BA, O'Keefe JH, Brand-Miller J. Origins and evolution of the Western diet: health implications for the 21st century. Am J Clin Nutr. 2005 Feb;81(2):341-54. Review. PubMed PMID: 15699220.
- Knowler WC, Pettitt DJ, Savage PJ, Bennett PH. Diabetes incidence in Pima indians: contributions of obesity and parental diabetes. Am J Epidemiol. 1981

19 Haskell WL, Lee IM, Pate RR, Powell KE, Blair SN, Franklin BA, Macera CA, Heath GW, Thompson PD, Bauman A; American College of Sports Medicine; American Heart Association. Physical activity and public health: updated recommendation for adults from the American College of Sports Medicine and the American Heart Association. Circulation. 2007 Aug 28;116(9):1081-93. Epub 2007 Aug 1. PubMed PMID: 17671237.

20 Bruch, Hilde. The Importance of Overweight. New York: Norton, 1957. Print.

21 "Diabetes Epidemic out of Control." International Diabetes Federation | IDF. Web. 12 Apr. 2010. <http://www.idf.org/diabetes-epidemic-out-control>.

22 A sampling of supporting research:
- Narayan KM, Boyle JP, Thompson TJ, Sorensen SW, Williamson DF. Lifetime risk for diabetes mellitus in the United States. JAMA. 2003 Oct 8;290(14):1884-90. PubMed PMID: 14532317.
- Warram JH, Martin BC, Krolewski AS, Soeldner JS, Kahn CR. Slow glucose removal rate and hyperinsulinemia precede the development of type II diabetes in the offspring of diabetic parents. Ann Intern Med. 1990 Dec 15;113(12):909-15. PubMed PMID: 2240915.
- Kannel WB, McGee DL. Diabetes and cardiovascular disease: The Framingham study. JAMA

1979;241:2035-2058.

- Stamler J, Vaccaro O, Neaton JD, Wentworth D. Diabetes, other risk factors, and 12-yr cardiovascular mortality for men screened in the Multiple Risk Factor Intervention Trial. Diabetes Care. 1993;16:434-444.
- "CDC—Diabetes Public Health Resources—Diabetes Projects—Children and Diabetes—More Information." Centers for Disease Control and Prevention. N.p., n.d. Web. 21 Dec. 2010. <http://www.cdc.gov/diabetes/projects/cda2.htm>.
- Gu K, Cowie CC, Harris MI. Mortality in adults with and without diabetes in a national cohort of the U.S. population, 1971-1993. Diabetes Care 1998;21:1138-1145.
- Haffner SM, Lehto S, Rönnemaa T, Pyörälä K, Laakso M. Mortality from coronary heart disease in subjects with type 2 diabetes and in nondiabetic subjects with and without prior myocardial infarction. N Engl J Med. 1998;339:229-234.

23 A sampling of supporting research:
- The Principles and Practice of Medicine, William Osler, M.D. Fourth Edition
- "Diabetes mellitus." Belinda Rowland., Teresa G. Odle., and Tish Davidson, A. M. The Gale Encyclopedia of Alternative Medicine. Ed. Laurie Fundukian. 3rd ed. Detroit: Gale, 2009. 4 vols.
- Popkin, Barry. The World is Fat: The Fads, Trends, Policies, and Products That Are Fattening the Human Race. New York: Avery, 2008. Print.

24 World Health Organization: Definition, Diagnosis, and Classification of Diabetes Mellitus and its Complications: Report of a WHO Consultation. Geneva, World Health Org., 1999

25 A sampling of supporting research:
- Westman EC, Yancy WS Jr, Haub MD, Volek JS: Insulin Resistance from a Low-Carbohydrate, High Fat Diet Perspective. Metabolic Syndrome and Related Disorders 2005, 3:3-7.
- Boden G, Sargrad K, Homko C, Mozzoli M, Stein TP: Effect of a low-carbohydrate diet on appetite, blood glucose levels, and insulin resistance in obese patients with type 2 diabetes. Ann Intern Med 2005, 142(6):403-411
- Nielsen JV, Jönsson EA: Low-carbohydrate diet in type 2 diabetes. Stable improvement of bodyweight and glycaemic control during 22 months follow-up. Nutr Metab (Lond) 2006, 3(1):22.
- Eaton SB, Cordain L, Sparling PB. Evolution, body composition, insulin receptor competition, and insulin resistance. Prev Med. 2009 Oct;49(4):283-5. Epub 2009 Aug 15. PubMed PMID: 19686772.
- Craig BW, Everhart J, Brown R. The influence of high-resistance training on glucose tolerance in young and elderly subjects. Mech Ageing Dev. 1989 Aug;49(2):147-57. Review. PubMed PMID: 2677535.
- Miller WJ, Sherman WM, Ivy JL. Effect of strength training on glucose tolerance and post-glucose insulin response. Med Sci Sports Exerc. 1984 Dec;16(6):539-43. PubMed PMID: 6392812.

Chapter 15

1 Nestle, Marion. Food Politics: How the Food Industry Influences Nutrition, and Health, Revised and Expanded Edition (California Studies in Food and Culture).

2 Ottoboni A, Ottoboni F. The Food Guide Pyramid: will the defects be corrected? J Am Phys Surg 2004;9:109-113.

3 A sampling of supporting research:
- Agriculture started about 12,000 years ago. Our ancestors débuted about 5,000,000. Early food processing—canning etc—started about 200 years ago. Low-calorie food engineering started about 60 years ago. All of human evolution = 5,000,000 divided by 24 hours in a day = 208,333.33. A day has 86,400 seconds in it. One second is .0016% of a day. Smallest increment needed = 60 years...which is 0.0012% of all of human evolution. .0012% of a day is 86,400 seconds times .000012 is about 1 second. 12,000 years is .024% of human evolution. 0.24% of a day is .0024 times 86,400 seconds which

is about 207 seconds, or 3 and a half minutes. 200 is 0.004% of all of human evolution. .00004 times 86,400 seconds is about 3.5 seconds.

- 195,000 years of human history. Agriculture emerged 10,000 years ago. http://www.newscientist. com/article/dn7020--oldest-known-humans-just-got-older.html
- O'Keefe JH Jr, Cordain L. Cardiovascular disease resulting from a diet and lifestyle at odds with our Paleolithic genome: how to become a 21st-century hunter-gatherer. Mayo Clin Proc 2004 Jan;79(1):101-8.
- Wood B. Hominid revelations from Chad. Nature. 2002 Jul 11;418(6894):133-5. PubMed PMID: 12110870.
- http://www.ajcn.org/content/81/2/341/F1.large.jpg
- Macaulay V, Richards M, Hickey E, et al. The emerging tree of West Eurasian mtDNAs: a synthesis of control-region sequences and RFLPs. Am J Hum Genet. 1999;64:232-249.
- Eaton SB, Konner M. Paleolithic nutrition. A consideration of its nature and current implications. N Engl J Med. 1985 Jan 31;312(5):283-9. Review. PubMed PMID: 2981409.

4   Eaton SB, Eaton SB 3rd, Konner MJ. Paleolithic nutrition revisited: a twelve-year retrospective on its nature and implications. Eur J Clin Nutr. 1997 Apr;51(4):207-16. Review. PubMed PMID: 9104571.

5   A sampling of supporting research:
- Diamond, Jared M.. Guns, germs, and steel: The fates of human societies. New York: W.W. Norton & Co., 1998. Print.
- Cordain L, Eaton SB, Sebastian A, Mann N, Lindeberg S, Watkins BA, O'Keefe JH, Brand-Miller J. Origins and evolution of the Western diet: health implications for the 21st century. Am J Clin Nutr. 2005 Feb;81(2):341-54. Review. PubMed PMID: 15699220.
- O'Keefe JH Jr, Cordain L. Cardiovascular disease resulting from a diet and lifestyle at odds with our Paleolithic genome: how to become a 21st-century hunter-gatherer. Mayo Clin Proc 2004 Jan;79(1):101-8.

6   Lee, R.B. (1968) What hunters do for a living, or how to make out on scarce resources, in Man the Hunter (Lee, R.B. & DeVore, I., eds), p.30 Aldine, Chicago & Boyd, S., Melvin Konner, Marjorie Shostak, and M.D. Eaton. The Paleolithic Prescription: A Program of Diet & Exercise and a Design for Living. New York: HarperCollins, 1989. Print.

7   A sampling of supporting research:
- Truswell AS. Diet and nutrition of hunter-gatherers. Ciba Found Symp. 1977;(49):213-21. PubMed PMID: 244410.
- Truswell, A. S. & Hansen, J. D. 1976 Medical research among the !Kung. In Kalahari hunter-gatherers. Studies of the !Kung San and their neighbors (ed. R. B. Lee & I. DeVore), pp. 168–195. Cambridge, MA: Harvard University Press.
- Arthaud JB. Cause of death in 339 Alaskan natives as determined by autopsy. Arch Pathol. 1970 Nov;90(5):433-8. PubMed PMID: 5476239.
- Popkin, Barry. The World is Fat: The Fads, Trends, Policies, and Products That Are Fattening the Human Race. New York: Avery, 2008. Print.
- Boyd, S., Melvin Konner, Marjorie Shostak, and M.D. Eaton. The Paleolithic Prescription: A Program of Diet & Exercise and a Design for Living. New York: HarperCollins, 1989. Print.

8   Eaton SB, Konner M. Paleolithic nutrition. A consideration of its nature and current implications. N Engl J Med. 1985 Jan 31;312(5):283-9. Review. PubMed PMID: 2981409. & Moodie PM. Aboriginal health. Canberra, Austrlia: Australian National University Press, 1973:92.

9   A sampling of supporting research:
- P.J. Skerrett, and W.C. Willett. Eat, Drink, and Be Healthy: The Harvard Medical School Guide to Healthy Eating. Free Press Trade Pbk. Ed ed. New York City: Free Press, 2005. Print.
- Weinberg SL. The diet-heart hypothesis: a critique. J Am Coll Cardiol. 2004 Mar 3;43(5):731-3. Review. PubMed PMID: 14998608.

- Jacobson, Michael F.. Nutrition Scoreboard. New York: Avon Books, 1975. Print.

10 A sampling studies documenting the starch's role on diabetes are provided below.
- Coulston AM, Hollenbeck CB, Swislocki AL, Chen YD, Reaven GM. Deleterious metabolic effects of high-carbohydrate, sucrose-containing diets in patients with non-insulin-dependent diabetes mellitus. Am J Med 1987;82:213-20.
- Parillo M, Coulston A, Hollenbeck C, Reaven G. Effect of a low fat diet on carbohydrate metabolism in patients with hypertension. Hypertension 1988;11:244-8.
- Coulston AM, Hollenbeck CB, Swislocki AL, Reaven GM. Persistence of hypertriglyceridemic effect of low-fat high-carbohydrate diets in NIDDM patients. Diabetes Care 1989;12:94-101.
- Fuh MM, Lee MM, Jeng CY, Ma F, Chen YD, Reaven GM.. Effect of low fat, high carbohydrate diets in hypertensive patients with non-insulin-dependent diabetes mellitus. Am J Hypertension 1990; 3: 527-32.
- Rasmussen OW, Thomsen C, Hansen KW, Vesterlund M, Winther E, Hermansen K. Effects on blood pressure, glucose, and lipid levels of a high-monounsaturated fat diet compared with a high-carbohydrate diet in NIDDM subjects. Diabetes Care 1993;16:1565-71
- Campbell LV, Marmot PE, Dyer JA, Borkman M, Storlien LH. The high-monounsaturated fat diet as a practical alternative for NIDDM. Diabetes Care 1994;17:177-82
- Garg A, Bantle JP, Henry RR, Coulston AM, Griver KA, Raatz SK et al. Effects of varying carbohydrate content of diet in patients with non-insulin-dependent diabetes mellitus. JAMA 1994; 271: 1421-8.
- Parillo M, Giacco R, Ciardullo AV, Rivellese AA, Riccardi G. Does a high-carbohydrate diet have different effects in NIDDM patients treated with diet alone or hypoglycemic drugs? Diabetes Care 1996;19:498-500.
- Low CC, Grossman EB, Gumbiner B. Potentiation of effects of weight loss by monounsaturated fatty acids in obese NIDDM patients. Diabetes 1996;45:569-75.
- Gutierrez M, Akhavan M, Jovanovic L, Peterson CM. Utility of a short-term 25% carbohydrate diet on improving glycemic control in type 2 diabetes mellitus. J Am Coll Nutr 1998;17:595-600.
- Hays JH, Gorman RT, Shakir KM. Results of use of metformin and replacement of starch with saturated fat in diets of patients with type 2 diabetes. Endocr Pract 2002;8:177-83
- Gannon MC, Nuttall FQ, Saeed A, Jordan K, Hoover H An increase in dietary protein improves the blood glucose response in persons with type 2 diabetes. Am J Clin Nutr 2003;78:734-41.
- Samaha FF, Iqbal N, Seshadri P, Chicano KL, Daily DA, McGrory J, Williams et al. A low-carbohydrate as compared with a low-fat diet in severe obesity. N Engl J Med 2003;348:2074-81
- Vernon MC, Mavropoulos J, Transue M, Yancy WS, Westman EC. Clinical Experience of a carbohydrate-restricted diet: Effect on diabetes mellitus. Metabolic Syndrome and Related Disorders 2003;1:233-7.
- Yancy WS, Vernon MC, Westman EC. A Pilot Trial of a Low-Carbohydrate, Ketogenic Diet in Patients with Type 2 Diabetes. Metabolic Syndrome and Related Disorders 2003;1:239-43.
- Gannon MC, Nuttall FQ. Effect of a high-protein, low-carbohydrate diet on blood glucose control in people with type 2 diabetes. Diabetes 2004;53:2375-82.
- Shah M, Adams-Huet B, Grundy SM, Garg A. Effect of a high-carbohydrate vs a high-cis-monounsaturated fat diet on lipid and lipoproteins in individuals with and without type 2 diabetes. Nutr Res 2004;24:969-79
- Stern L, Iqbal N, Seshadri P, Chicano KL, Daily DA, McGrory J. The effects of low-carbohydrate versus conventional weight loss diets in severely obese adults: one-year follow-up of a randomized trial. Ann Intern Med 2004;140:778-85.
- Boden G, Sargrad K, Homko C, Mozzoli M, Stein TP.Effect of a low-carbohydrate diet on appetite, blood glucose levels, and insulin resistance in obese patients with type 2 diabetes. Ann Intern Med 2005;142:403-11.

- Yancy WS Jr, Foy M, Chalecki AM, Vernon MC, Westman EC. A low-carbohydrate, ketogenic diet to treat type 2 diabetes. Nutr Metab 2005;2:34-40.
- Daly ME, Paisey R, Paisey R, Millward BA, Eccles C, Williams K. Short-term effects of severe dietary carbohydrate-restriction advice in Type 2 diabetes--a randomized controlled trial. Diabet Med 2006;23:15-20.
- Nielsen JV, Joensson E . Low-carbohydrate diet in type 2 diabetes. Stable improvement of body-weight and glycemic control during 22 months follow-up. Nutr Metabol 2006;3:22.
- A sampling studies documenting the starch's role on obesity are provided below.
- Rabast U, Kasper H, Schonborn J: Comparative studies in obese subjects fed carbohydrate-restricted and high carbohydrate 1,000-calorie formula diets. Nutr Metab 1978, 22:269-77.
- Rabast U, Hahn A, Reiners C, Ehl M: Thyroid hormone changes in obese subjects during fasting and a very-low-calorie diet. Int J Obes 1981, 5:305-11.
- Golay A, Eigenheer C, Morel Y, Kujawski P, Lehmann T, de Tonnac N: Weight-loss with low or high carbohydrate diet? Int J Obes Relat Metab Disord 1996, 20:1067-72.
- Golay A, Allaz AF, Morel Y, de Tonnac N, Tankova S, Reaven G: Similar weight loss with low- or high-carbohydrate diets. Am J Clin Nutr 1996, 63:174-8.
- ML Piatti PM, Magni F, Fermo I, Baruffaldi L, Nasser R, Santambrogia G, Librenti MC, Galli-Kienle M, Pontiroli AE, Pozza G: Hypocaloric High-Protein Diet Improves Glucose Oxidation and Spares Lean Body Mass: Comparison to High-Carbohydrate Diet. Metabolism 1994, 43:1481-87.
- Layman DK, Boileau RA, Erickson DJ, Painter JE, Shiue H, Sather C, Christou DD: A reduced ratio of dietary carbohydrate to protein improves body composition and blood lipid profiles during weight loss in adult women. J Nutr 2003, 133:411-7.
- Lean ME, Han TS, Prvan T, Richmond PR, Avenell A: Weight loss with high and low carbohydrate 1200 kcal diets in free living women. Eur J Clin Nutr 1997, 51:243-8.
- Baba NH, Sawaya S, Torbay N, Habbal Z, Azar S, Hashim SA: High protein vs high carbohydrate hypoenergetic diet for the treatment of obese hyperinsulinemic subjects. Int J Obes Relat Metab Disord 1999, 23:1202-6.
- Young CM, Scanlan SS, Im HS, Lutwak L: Effect of body composition and other parameters in obese young men of carbohydrate level of reduction diet. Am J Clin Nutr 1971, 24:290-6.
- Greene P, Willett W, Devecis J, Skaf A: Pilot 12-Week Feeding Weight-Loss Comparison: Low-Fat vs Low-Carbohydrate (Ketogenic) Diets. Obesity Research 2003, 11:A23.
- P.J. Skerrett, and W.C. Willett. Eat, Drink, and Be Healthy: The Harvard Medical School Guide to Healthy Eating. Free Press Trade Pbk. Ed ed. New York City: Free Press, 2005. Print.

11 A sampling of supporting research:
- 2005 U.S.DA Dietary Guidelines: http://www.cnpp.usda.gov/Publications/DietaryGuidelines/2005/2005DGPolicyDocument.pdf
- 2000 U.S.DA DietaryGuidelines: http://www.cnpp.usda.gov/Publications/DietaryGuidelines/2000/2000DGProfessionalBooklet.pdf
- http://www.cnpp.usda.gov/Publications/DietaryGuidelines/2005/2005DGMessageFromSecretary.pdf
- http://www.cnpp.usda.gov/DGAs2010-PolicyDocument.htm
- Nestle, Marion. Food politics: how the food industry influences nutrition and health. Berkeley: University of California Press, 2002. Print.

Chapter 16

1   P.J. Skerrett, and W.C. Willett. Eat, Drink, and Be Healthy: The Harvard Medical School Guide to Healthy Eating. Free Press Trade Pbk. Ed ed. New York City: Free Press, 2005. Print.
2   P.J. Skerrett, and W.C. Willett. Eat, Drink, and Be Healthy: The Harvard Medical School Guide to

Healthy Eating. Free Press Trade Pbk. New York City: Free Press, 2005. & Ottoboni A, Ottoboni F. The Food Guide Pyramid: will the defects be corrected? J Am Phys Surg 2004;9:109-113. & U.S. Senate Select Committee on Nutrition and Human Needs. Dietary goals for the United States. 2nd ed. Washington, DC: U.S. Government Printing office, 1977.

3 A sampling of supporting research:
- German JB, Dillard CJ. Saturated fats: what dietary intake? Am J Clin Nutr. 2004 Sep;80(3):550-9. Review. PubMed PMID: 15321792.
- Carter, James P. Eating in America; Dietary Goals for the United States; Report of the Select Committee on Nutrition and Human Needs, U.S. Senate: MIT Press, Cambridge, Massachusetts. 1977. No price Am J Trop Med Hyg 1978 27: 369-b-370
- U.S. Senate Select Committee on Nutrition and Human Needs. Dietary goals for the United States. 2nd ed. Washington, DC: U.S. Government Printing office, 1977.
- "APPENDIX I: HISTORY OF DIETARY GUIDELINES FOR AMERICANS." Health.gov | Your Portal to Health Information from the U.S. Government. N.p., n.d. Web. 8 Dec. 2010. <http://www.health.gov/dietaryguidelines/dga95/12dietap.htm>.

4 A sampling of supporting research:
- Sanders TA. High- versus low-fat diets in human diseases. Curr Opin Clin Nutr Metab Care. 2003 Mar;6(2):151-5. Review. PubMed PMID: 12589184.
- Truswell AS. Evolution of dietary recommendations, goals, and guidelines. Am J Clin Nutr. 1987 May;45(5 Suppl):1060-72. Review. PubMed PMID: 3554965.
- Harper AE. Dietary goals-a skeptical view. Am J Clin Nutr. 1978 Feb;31(2):310-21. Review. PubMed PMID: 341685.
- Dietary goals for the United States: statement of the American Medical Association to the Select Committee on Nutrition and Human Needs, United States Senate. R I Med J. 1977 Dec;60(12):576-81. PubMed PMID: 272018.

5 Council for Responsible Nutrition . Resolution endorsing dietary goals for the United States presented to members of the Senate Select Committee on Nutrition and Human Needs. May 12, 1977. Comm. Nutr. Inst. Weekly Report 7, No. 21 , p.4, 1977.

6 http://www.cdc.gov/brfss/

7 Jane Brody's Nutrition Book: A Lifetime Guide to Good Eating for Better Health and Weight Control by the Award-Winning Columnist of the New York Times

8 Keys A, Anderson JT, Grande F. Prediction of serum-cholesterol responses of man to changes in the diet. Lancet: 1957;273:959–66.

9 Keys A. Atherosclerosis: a problem in newer public health. J Mt Sinai Hosp N Y 1953;20:118-139.

10 Yerushalmy J, Hilleboe He. Fat in the diet and mortality from heart disease; a methodologic note. N Y State J Med. 1957 Jul 15;57(14):2343-54. PubMed PMID:13441073.

11 Fallon, Mary G.(Author) ;, and Sally(Author) Enig. Eat Fat, Lose Fat: The Healthy Alternative to Trans Fats [EAT FAT LOSE FAT] [Paperback]. Nashville Tennessee: Plume Books, 2006. Print.

12 Elmadfa I, Kornsteiner M. Fats and fatty acid requirements for adults. Ann Nutr Metab. 2009;55(1-3):56-75. Epub 2009 Sep 15. Review. PubMed PMID: 19752536.

13 P.J. Skerrett, and W.C. Willett. Eat, Drink, and Be Healthy: The Harvard Medical School Guide to Healthy Eating. Free Press Trade Pbk. Ed ed. New York City: Free Press, 2005. Print.

14 Siri-Tarino PW, Sun Q, Hu FB, Krauss RM. Meta-analysis of prospective cohort studies evaluating the association of saturated fat with cardiovascular disease. Am J Clin Nutr. 2010 Jan 13. [Epub ahead of print] PubMed PMID: 20071648.

15 Multiple risk factor intervention trial. Risk factor changes and mortality results. Multiple Risk Factor Intervention Trial Research Group. JAMA. 1982 Sep 24;248(12):1465-77. PubMed PMID: 7050440.

16 Howard BV, Van Horn L, Hsia J, Manson JE, Stefanick ML, Wassertheil-Smoller S, Kuller LH, LaCroix AZ, Langer RD, Lasser NL, Lewis CE, Limacher MC, Margolis KL, Mysiw WJ, Ockene JK, Parker LM,

Perri MG, Phillips L, Prentice RL, Robbins J, Rossouw JE, Sarto GE, Schatz IJ, Snetselaar LG, Stevens VJ, Tinker LF, Trevisan M, Vitolins MZ, Anderson GL, Assaf AR, Bassford T, Beresford SA, Black HR, Brunner RL, Brzyski RG, Caan B, Chlebowski RT, Gass M, Granek I, Greenland P, Hays J, Heber D, Heiss G, Hendrix SL, Hubbell FA, Johnson KC, Kotchen JM. Low-fat dietary pattern and risk of cardiovascular disease: The Women's Health Initiative Randomized Controlled Dietary Modification Trial. JAMA. 2006 Feb 8;295(6):655-66. PubMed PMID: 16467234.

17   Tuomilehto J, Kuulasmaa K. WHO MONICA Project: assessing CHD mortality and morbidity. Int J Epidemiol. 1989;18(3 Suppl 1):S38-45. PubMed PMID: 2807706.

18   Willett W. Challenges for public health nutrition in the 1990s. Am J Public Health. 1990 Nov;80(11):1295-8. PubMed PMID: 2240291; PubMed Central PMCID: PMC1404889.

19   Leosdottir M, Nilsson PM, Nilsson JA, Månsson H, Berglund G. Dietary fat intake and early mortality patterns--data from the Malmö Diet and Cancer Study. JIntern Med. 2005 Aug;258(2):153-65. PubMed PMID: 16018792.

20   Ascherio A, Rimm EB, Giovannucci EL, Spiegelman D, Stampfer M, Willett WC. Dietary fat and risk of coronary heart disease in men: cohort follow up study in the United States. BMJ. 1996 Jul 13;313(7049):84-90. PubMed PMID: 8688759; PubMed Central PMCID: PMC2351515.

21   Hu FB, Manson JE, Willett WC. Types of dietary fat and risk of coronary heart disease: a critical review. J Am Coll Nutr. 2001 Feb;20(1):5-19. Review.

22   McCullough ML, Feskanich D, Rimm EB, Giovannucci EL, Ascherio A, Variyam JN, Spiegelman D, Stampfer MJ, Willett WC. Adherence to the Dietary Guidelines for Americans and risk of major chronic disease in men. Am J Clin Nutr. 2000 Nov;72(5):1223-31. PubMed PMID: 11063453. & Willett WC, Leibel RL. Dietary fat is not a major determinant of body fat. Am J Med. 2002 Dec 30;113 Suppl 9B:47S-59S. Review. PubMed PMID: 12566139.

Chapter 17

1   Ravnskov, Uffe. Fat and Cholesterol Are Good for You. S.l.: GP, 2009. Print.

2   Leosdottir M, Nilsson PM, Nilsson JA, Månsson H, Berglund G. Dietary fat intake and early mortality patterns--data from the Malmö Diet and Cancer Study. J Intern Med. 2005 Aug;258(2):153-65. PubMed PMID: 16018792.

3   Diet and Health: Implications for Reducing Chronic Disease Risk. Washington, D.C.: National Academy, 1989. Print. & P.J. Skerrett, and W.C. Willett. Eat, Drink, and Be Healthy: The Harvard Medical School Guide to Healthy Eating. Free Press Trade Pbk. Ed ed. New York City: Free Press, 2005. Print.

4   Hu FB, Willett WC. Optimal diets for prevention of coronary heart disease. JAMA. 2002 Nov 27;288(20):2569-78. Review. PubMed PMID: 12444864.

5   A sampling of supporting research:

   • Drewnowski A. The role of energy density. Lipids. 2003 Feb;38(2):109-15. Review. PubMed PMID: 12733741.

   • Ludwig DS, Pereira MA, Kroenke CH, Hilner JE, Van Horn L, Slattery ML, Jacobs DR Jr. Dietary fiber, weight gain, and cardiovascular disease risk factors in young adults. JAMA. 1999 Oct 27;282(16):1539-46. PubMed PMID: 10546693.

   • Levine AS, Billington CJ. Dietary fiber: does it affect food intake and body weight? In: Fernstrom JD, Miller GD, eds. Appetite and body weight regulation: sugar, fat, and macronutrient substitutes. Boca Raton, FL: CRC Press, 1994:191–200.

   • Rolls BJ, Bell EA, Castellanos VH, Chow M, Pelkman CL, Thorwart ML. Energy density but not fat content of foods affected energy intake in lean and obese women. Am J Clin Nutr. 1999 May;69(5):863-71. PubMed PMID: 10232624.

   • Bell EA, Rolls BJ. Energy density of foods affects energy intake across multiple levels of fat content in lean and obese women. Am J Clin Nutr. 2001 Jun;73(6):1010-8. PubMed PMID: 11382653.

- Obesity and leanness. Basic aspects. Stock, M., Rothwell, N., Author Affiliation: Dep. Physiology, St. George's Hospital Medical School, London Univ., London, UK.

6   Economic Research Service (ERS), U.S. Department of Agriculture (USDA). Food Availability (Per Capita) Data System. http://www.ers.usda.gov/Data/FoodConsumption.

7   http://www.cdc.gov/nchs/data/hestat/overweight/overweight_adult.htm

8   A sampling of supporting research:

- Flegal KM, Carroll MD, Ogden CL, Curtin LR. Prevalence and trends in obesity among U.S. adults, 1999-2008. JAMA. 2010 Jan 20;303(3):235-41. Epub 2010 Jan 13. PubMed PMID: 20071471.
- Data Source: Centers for Disease Control and Prevention, National Center for Health Statistics, Division of Health Interview Statistics, data from the National Health Interview Survey. U.S. Bureau of the Census, census of the population and population estimates. Data computed by the Division of Diabetes Translation, National Center for Chronic Disease Prevention and Health Promotion, Centers for Disease Control and Prevention.http://www.cdc.gov/diabetes/statistics/prev/national/tnumage.htm. http://www.cdc.gov/diabetes/pubs/pdf/ndfs_2007.pdf. http://www.cdc.gov/diabetes/statistics/slides/long_term_trends.pdf
- Based on NHANES data. MMWR 2004;53:80-82. Diabetes Care 2004;27:2806.
- Based on NHANES data. Int J Obes 1998;22:39-47. JAMA 2002;288:1723. MMWR 2004;53:80-82.
- Ogden CL, Carroll MD, Curtin LR, McDowell MA, Tabak CJ, Flegal KM. Prevalence of overweight and obesity in the United States, 1999-2004. JAMA 2006;295:1549-1555.
- Hedley AA, Ogden CL, Johnson CL, Carroll MD, Curtin LR, Flegal KM. Prevalence of overweight and obesity among U.S. children, adolescents, and adults, 1999-2002. JAMA 2004;291:2847-2850.
- Flegal KM, Carroll MD, Ogden CL, Johnson CL. Prevalence and trends in obesity among U.S. adults, 1999-2000. JAMA 2002;288:1723-7.
- National Institutes of Health. Clinical guidelines on the identification, evaluation, and treatment of overweight and obesity in adults--the evidence report. Obes Res 1998;6(Suppl 2):51S-209S.

9   Data Source: Centers for Disease Control and Prevention, National Center for Health Statistics, Division of Health Interview Statistics, data from the National Health Interview Survey. U.S. Bureau of the Census, census of the population and population estimates. Data computed by the Division of Diabetes Translation, National Center for Chronic Disease Prevention and Health Promotion, Centers for Disease Control and Prevention. http://www.cdc.gov/diabetes/statistics/prev/national/tnumage.htm

- http://www.cdc.gov/diabetes/pubs/pdf/ndfs_2007.pdf. http://www.cdc.gov/diabetes/statistics/slides/long_term_trends.pdf

10   Centers for Disease Control and Prevention (CDC). Trends in intake of energy and macronutrients--United States, 1971-2000. MMWR Morb Mortal Wkly Rep. 2004 Feb 6;53(4):80-2. PubMed PMID: 14762332.   &   What if It is All Been a Big Fat Lie? Gary Taubes.http://www.nytimes.com/2002/07/07/magazine/what-if-it-s-all-been-a-big-fat-lie.html

11   2010 U.S.DA Dietary Guidelines: http://www.cnpp.usda.gov/DGAs2010-PolicyDocument.htm & 2005 U.S.DA Dietary Guidelines: http://www.cnpp.usda.gov/Publications/DietaryGuidelines/2005/2005DGPolicyDocument.pdf & 2000 U.S.DA DietaryGuidelines: http://www.cnpp.usda.gov/Publications/DietaryGuidelines/2000/2000DGProfessionalBooklet.pdf

12   A sampling of supporting research:

- Carey, Anne R., and Paul Trap. "Stretching the Truth." USA Today 13 Jan. 2011, sec. USA Today Snapshots: 1. Print.
- 2000 U.S.DA DietaryGuidelines: http://www.cnpp.usda.gov/Publications/DietaryGuidelines/2000/2000DGProfessionalBooklet.pdf
- GaryTaubes. Good Calories, Bad Calories ,Challenging the Conventional Wisdom on Diet, Weight Control, &Disease 2007 publication. New York: Alfred A Knopf,2007, 2007. Print.
- Parks EJ, Hellerstein MK. Carbohydrate-induced hypertriacylglycerolemia: historical perspective and review of biological mechanisms. Am J Clin Nutr. 2000 Feb;71(2):412-33. Review. PubMed

PMID: 10648253.

- Macaulay V, Richards M, Hickey E, et al. The emerging tree of West Eurasian mtDNAs: a synthesis of control-region sequences and RFLPs. Am J Hum Genet. 1999;64:232-249.
- Cordain, Loren. The Paleo diet: lose weight and get healthy by eating the food you were designed to eat. New York: J. Wiley, 2002. Print.

13 St Jeor ST, Howard BV, Prewitt TE, Bovee V, Bazzarre T, Eckel RH; Nutrition Committee of the Council on Nutrition, Physical Activity, and Metabolism of the American Heart Association. Dietary protein and weight reduction: a statement for healthcare professionals from the Nutrition Committee of the Council on Nutrition, Physical Activity, and Metabolism of the American Heart Association. Circulation. 2001 Oct 9;104(15):1869-74. PubMed PMID: 11591629.

14 Cordain, Loren. The Paleo Diet: Lose Weight and Get Healthy by Eating the Food You Were Designed to Eat. New Ed ed. New York, NY: Wiley, 2002. Print. & U.S. Department of Agriculture, Agricultural Research Service. 2007. Nutrient Intakes from Food: Mean Amounts and Percentages of Calories from Protein, Carbohydrate, Fat, and Alcohol, One Day, 2003-2004. Available: www.ars.usda.gov/ba/bhnrc/fsrg.

15 A sampling of supporting research:

- St Jeor ST, Howard BV, Prewitt TE, Bovee V, Bazzarre T, Eckel RH; Nutrition Committee of the Council on Nutrition, Physical Activity, and Metabolism of the American Heart Association. Dietary protein and weight reduction: a statement for healthcare professionals from the Nutrition Committee of the Council on Nutrition, Physical Activity, and Metabolism of the American Heart Association. Circulation. 2001 Oct 9;104(15):1869-74. PubMed PMID: 11591629.
- Parks EJ, Hellerstein MK. Carbohydrate-induced hypertriacylglycerolemia: historical perspective and review of biological mechanisms. Am J Clin Nutr. 2000 Feb;71(2):412-33. Review. PubMed PMID: 10648253.
- Macaulay V, Richards M, Hickey E, et al. The emerging tree of West Eurasian mtDNAs: a synthesis of control-region sequences and RFLPs. Am J Hum Genet. 1999;64:232-249.
- St Jeor ST, Howard BV, Prewitt TE, Bovee V, Bazzarre T, Eckel RH; Nutrition Committee of the Council on Nutrition, Physical Activity, and Metabolism of the American Heart Association. Dietary protein and weight reduction: a statement for healthcare professionals from the Nutrition Committee of the Council on Nutrition, Physical Activity, and Metabolism of the American Heart Association. Circulation. 2001 Oct 9;104(15):1869-74. PubMed PMID: 11591629.

Chapter 18

1 Coulston AM, Hollenbeck CB, Swislocki AL, Reaven GM. Persistence of hypertriglyceridemic effect of low-fat high-carbohydrate diets in NIDDM patients.Diabetes Care. 1989 Feb;12(2):94-101. PubMed PMID: 2539286.

2 Frost G, Leeds AA, Dore' CJ, Madeiros S, Brading S, Dornhorst A. (1999). Glycaemic index as a determinant of serum HDL-cholesterol concentration. Lancet, 353: 1045-1048. & Ford ES, Liu S. (2001). Glycemic index and serum high-density lipoprotein cholesterol concentration among U.S. adults. Arch. Intern. Med., 161: 572-576.

3 Status of Articles offered to the General Public for the Control or Reduction of Blood Cholesterol Levels and for the Prevention and Treatment of Heart and Artery Disease Under the Federal Food, Drug, and Cosmetic Act. Federal Register. 1959, December 12.

4 German JB, Dillard CJ. Saturated fats: what dietary intake? Am J Clin Nutr. 2004 Sep;80(3):550-9. Review. PubMed PMID: 15321792. & Gordon T, Castelli WP, Hjortland MC, Kannel WB, Dawber TR. High density lipoprotein as a protective factor against coronary heart disease. The Framingham Study. Am J Med 1977;62:707-714.

5 Ravnskov U. Cholesterol lowering trials in coronary heart disease: frequency of citation and outcome.

BMJ. 1992 Jul 4;305(6844):15-9. Erratum in: BMJ 1992 Aug 29;305(6852):505. PubMed PMID: 1638188; PubMed Central PMCID: PMC1882525.

6   A sampling of supporting research:

- Sondike SB, Copperman N, Jacobson MS. Effects of a low-carbohydrate diet on weight loss and cardiovascular risk factor in overweight adolescents. J Pediatr 2003;142:253–8.
- Hays JH, DiSabatino A, Gorman RT, Vincent S, Stillabower ME. Effect of a high saturated fat and no-starch diet on serum lipid subfractions in patients with documented atherosclerotic cardiovascular disease. Mayo Clin Proc 2003;78:1331–6.
- Meckling KA, O'Sullivan C, Saari D. Comparison of a low-fat diet to a low-carbohydrate diet on weight loss, body composition, and risk factors for diabetes and cardiovascular disease in free-living, overweight men and women. J Clin Endocrinol Metab 2004;89:2717–23.
- Sharman MJ, Gomez AL, Kraemer WJ, Volek JS. Very low-carbohydrate and low-fat diets affect fasting lipids and postprandial lipemia differently in overweight men. J Nutr 2004;134:880–5.
- Ravnskov U. Saturated fat doesn't affect blood cholesterol. Am J Clin Nutr. 2006 Dec;84(6):1550-1; author reply 1551-2. PubMed PMID: 17158443.
- Ravnskov U. High cholesterol may protect against infections and atherosclerosis. QJM. 2003 Dec;96(12):927-34. Review. PubMed PMID: 14631060.
- Scientific steering committee on behalf of the Simon Broome Register group. Risk of fatal coronary heart disease in familial hypercholesterolaemia. Br Med J 1991; 303:893–6.
- Anderson KM, Castelli WP, Levy D. Cholesterol and mortality. 30 years of follow-up from the Framingham study. JAMA 1987; 257:2176–80.
- Siegel D, Kuller L, Lazarus NB, Black D, Feigal D, Hughes G, Schoenberger JA, Hulley SB. Predictors of cardiovascular events and mortality in the Systolic Hypertension in the Elderly Program pilot project. Am J Epidemiol 1987; 126:385–9.
- Forette B, Tortrat D, Wolmark Y. Cholesterol as risk factor for mortality in elderly women. Lancet 1989; 1:868–70.
- Zimetbaum P, Frishman WH, Ooi WL, Derman MP, Aronson M, Gidez LI, Eder HA. Plasma lipids and lipoproteins and the incidence of cardiovascular disease in the very elderly. The Bronx aging study. Arterioscl Thromb 1992; 12:416–23.
- Krumholz HM, Seeman TE, Merrill SS, Mendes de Leon CF, Vaccarino V, Silverman DI, Tsukahara R, Ostfeld AM, Berkman LF. Lack of association between cholesterol and coronary heart disease mortality and morbidity and all-cause mortality in persons older than 70 years. JAMA 1994; 272:1335–40.
- Weverling-Rijnsburger AW, Blauw GJ, Lagaay AM, Knook DL, Meinders AE, Westendorp RG. Total cholesterol and risk of mortality in the oldest old. Lancet 1997; 350:1119–23.
- Jonsson A, Sigvaldason H, Sigfusson N. Total cholesterol and mortality after age 80 years. Lancet 1997; 350:1778–9.
- Räihä I, Marniemi J, Puukka P, Toikka T, Ehnholm C, Sourander L. Effect of serum lipids, lipoproteins, and apolipoproteins on vascular and nonvascular mortality in the elderly. Arterioscler Thromb Vasc Biol 1997; 17:1224–32.
- Fried LP, Kronmal RA, Newman AB, Bild DE, Mittelmark MB, Polak JF, Robbins JA, Gardin JM. Risk factors for 5-year mortality in older adults: The Cardiovascular Health Study. JAMA 1998; 279:585–92.
- Chyou PH, Eaker ED. Serum cholesterol concentrations and all-cause mortality in older people. Age Ageing 2000; 29:69–74.
- Menotti A, Mulder I, Nissinen A, Feskens E, Giampaoli S, Tervahauta M, Kromhout D. Cardiovascular risk factors and 10-year all-cause mortality in elderly European male populations; the FINE study. Eur Heart J 2001; 22:573–9.
- Schatz IJ, Masaki K, Yano K, Chen R, Rodriguez BL, Curb JD. Cholesterol and all-cause mortality in

elderly people from the Honolulu Heart Program: a cohort study. Lancet 2001; 358:351–5.

- Yudkin J. Diet and coronary thrombosis hypothesis and fact. Lancet. 1957 Jul 27;273(6987):155-62. PubMed PMID: 13450357.
- German JB, Dillard CJ. Saturated fats: what dietary intake? Am J Clin Nutr. 2004 Sep;80(3):550-9. Review. PubMed PMID: 15321792.

7   A sampling of supporting research:
- Wood, Philip A.. How fat works. Cambridge: Harvard University Press, 2006. Print.
- "Cholesterol : LIPID MAPS--Nature Lipidomics Gateway." Home : LIPID MAPS--Nature Lipidomics Gateway. N.p., n.d. Web. 3 Jan. 2011. <http://www.lipidmaps.org/update/2009/090501/full/lipidmaps.2009.3.html>.
- http://www.idf.org/webdata/docs/IDF_Meta_def_final.pdf
- [Grundy SM, Cleeman JI, Daniels SR, Donato KA, Eckel RH, Franklin BA, Gordon DJ, Krauss RM, Savage PJ, Smith SC, Jr, Spertus JA Costa F. Diagnosis and Management of the Metabolic Syndrome: An American Heart Association/National Heart, Lung, and Blood Institute Scientific Statement. Circulation 2005, 112:2735-2752: originally published online September 12, 2005; doi: 10.1161/CIR-CULATIONAHA.105.169404].

8   A sampling of supporting research:
- Castelli WP. Cholesterol and lipids in the risk of coronary artery disease--the Framingham Heart Study. Can J Cardiol 1988;4:5A-10A.
- Gordon T, Castelli WP, Hjortland MC, Kannel WB, Dawber TR. High density lipoprotein as a protective factor against coronary heart disease. The Framingham Study. Am J Med 1977;62:707-714.
- Gordon DJ, Probstfield JL, Garrison RJ, et al. High-density lipoprotein cholesterol and cardiovascular disease. Four prospective American studies. Circulation 1989;79:8-15.
- Sharrett AR, Ballantyne CM, Coady SA, et al. Coronary heart disease prediction from lipoprotein cholesterol levels, triglycerides, lipoprotein(a), apolipoproteins A-I and B, and HDL density subfractions: The Atherosclerosis Risk in Communities (ARIC) Study. Circulation 2001;104:1108-1113.

9   Lee-Han H, Cousins M, Beaton M, McGuire V, Kriukov V, Chipman M, Boyd N. Compliance in a randomized clinical trial of dietary fat reduction in patientswith breast dysplasia. Am J Clin Nutr. 1988 Sep;48(3):575-86. PubMed PMID: 3046298. & Willett W. Challenges for public health nutrition in the 1990s. Am J Public Health. 1990 Nov;80(11):1295-8. PubMed PMID: 2240291; PubMed Central PMCID: PMC1404889.

10 Mensink RP, Zock PL, Kester AD, Katan MB. Effects of dietary fatty acids and carbohydrates on the ratio of serum total to HDL cholesterol and on serum lipids and apolipoproteins: a meta-analysis of 60 controlled trials. Am J Clin Nutr. 2003 May;77(5):1146-55. PubMed PMID: 12716665.

11 Despres JP. Krauss R. Obesity and Lipoprotein Metabolism In: Bray GA, Couchard d, James WP, eds. Handbook of Obesity. New York: Marcel Dekker, 1997: 651-675.

12 A sampling of supporting research:
- Mensink RPM, Katan MB. Effect of dietary trans fatty acids on highdensity and low-density lipoprotein cholesterol levels in healthy subjects. N Engl J Med 1990;323:439–45.
- Willett WC, Stampfer MJ, Manson JE, et al. Intake of trans fatty acids and risk of coronary heart disease among women. Lancet 1993;341:581–5.
- Hu FB, Stampfer MJ, Manson JE, et al. Dietary fat intake and the risk of coronary heart disease in women. N Engl J Med 1997;337:1491–9.
- Sharman MJ, Kraemer WJ, Love DM, Avery NG, Gómez AL, Scheett TP, Volek JS. A ketogenic diet favorably affects serum biomarkers for cardiovascular disease in normal-weight men. J Nutr. 2002 Jul;132(7):1879-85. PubMed PMID: 12097663.
- German JB, Dillard CJ. Saturated fats: what dietary intake? Am J Clin Nutr. 2004 Sep;80(3):550-9. Review. PubMed PMID: 15321792.
- Hu FB, Manson JE, Willett WC. Types of dietary fat and risk of coronary heart disease: a critical

review. J Am Coll Nutr. 2001 Feb;20(1):5-19. Review. PubMed PMID: 11293467.

- Willett W. Challenges for public health nutrition in the 1990s. Am J Public Health. 1990 Nov;80(11):1295-8. PubMed PMID: 2240291; PubMed Central PMCID: PMC1404889.
- Parks EJ, Hellerstein MK. Carbohydrate-induced hypertriacylglycerolemia: historical perspective and review of biological mechanisms. Am J Clin Nutr. 2000 Feb;71(2):412-33. Review. PubMed PMID: 10648253.
- Augustin LS, Franceschi S, Jenkins DJ, Kendall CW, La Vecchia C. Glycemic index in chronic disease: a review. Eur J Clin Nutr. 2002 Nov;56(11):1049-71. Review. PubMed PMID: 12428171.
- Ravnskov U. The questionable role of saturated and polyunsaturated fatty acids in cardiovascular disease. J Clin Epidemiol. 1998 Jun;51(6):443-60. Review. PubMed PMID: 9635993.

13 Mozaffarian D. Effects of dietary fats versus carbohydrates on coronary heart disease: a review of the evidence. Curr Atheroscler Rep. 2005 Nov;7(6):435-45.Review. PubMed PMID: 16256001 & Garg A, Bantle JP, Henry RR, Coulston AM, Griver KA, Raatz SK, Brinkley L, Chen YD, Grundy SM, Huet BA, et al. Effects of varying carbohydrate content of diet in patients with non-insulin-dependent diabetes mellitus. JAMA. 1994 May 11;271(18):1421-8. PubMed PMID: 7848401.

14 A sampling of supporting research:
- Mensink RP, Zock PL, Kester AD, Katan MB. Effects of dietary fatty acids and carbohydrates on the ratio of serum total to HDL cholesterol and on serum lipids and apolipoproteins: a meta-analysis of 60 controlled trials. Am J Clin Nutr. 2003 May;77(5):1146-55. PubMed PMID: 12716665.
- Mensink RP, Katan MB. Effect of monounsaturated fatty acids versus complex carbohydrates on high-density lipoproteins in healthy men and women. Lancet. 1987 Jan 17;1(8525):122-5. PubMed PMID: 2879969.
- Sacks FM, Katan M. Randomized clinical trials on the effects of dietary fat and carbohydrate on plasma lipoproteins and cardiovascular disease. Am J Med. 2002 Dec 30;113 Suppl 9B:13S-24S. Review. PubMed PMID: 12566134.
- Gardner CD, Kiazand A, Alhassan S, Kim S, Stafford RS, Balise RR, Kraemer HC, King AC. Comparison of the Atkins, Zone, Ornish, and LEARN diets for change in weight and related risk factors among overweight premenopausal women: The A TO Z Weight Loss Study: a randomized trial. JAMA. 2007 Mar 7;297(9):969-77. Erratum in: JAMA. 2007 Jul 11;298(2):178. PubMed PMID: 17341711.
- Apoundert CM, Campos H, Stampfer MJ, et al. Blood levels of long-chain n-3 fatty acids and the risk of sudden death. N Engl J Med 2002;346:1113-1118.
- Apoundert CM, Gaziano JM, Willett WC, Manson JE. Nut consumption and decreased risk of sudden cardiac death in the Physicians' Health Study. Arch Intern Med. 2002;162:1382-1387.
- Marchioli R, Barzi F, Bomba E, et al, GISSI-Prevenzione Investigators. Early protection against sudden dealth by n-3 polyunsaturated fatty acids after myocardial infarction: Time-course analysis of the results of the Gruppo Italiano per lo Studio della Sopravvivenza nell'Infarto Miocardico (GISSI)-Prevenzione. Circulation. 2002;105:1897-1903.
- Siscovick DS, Raghunathan TE, King I, Weinmann S, Wicklund KG, Apoundright J, Bovbjerg V, Arbogast P, Smith H, Kushi LH, Cobb LA, Copass MK, Psaty BM, Lemaitre R, Retzlaff B, Childs M, Knopp RH. Dietary intake and cell membrane levels of long-chain n-3 polyunsaturated fatty acids and the risk of primary cardiac arrest. JAMA 1995;274:1363-1367.

15 Coulston AM, Hollenbeck CB, Swislocki AL, Reaven GM. Persistence of hypertriglyceridemic effect of low-fat high-carbohydrate diets in NIDDM patients. Diabetes Care. 1989 Feb;12(2):94-101. PubMed PMID: 2539286.

16 Arefhosseini SR, Edwards CA, Malkova D, Higgins S. Effect of advice to increase carbohydrate and reduce fat intake on dietary profile and plasma lipid concentrations in healthy postmenopausal women. Ann Nutr Metab. 2009;54(2):138-44. Epub 2009 Apr 1. PubMed PMID: 19339775.

17 A sampling of supporting research:

- Haskell WL, Lee IM, Pate RR, Powell KE, Blair SN, Franklin BA, Macera CA, Heath GW, Thompson PD, Bauman A; American College of Sports Medicine; American Heart Association. Physical activity and public health: updated recommendation for adults from the American College of Sports Medicine and the American Heart Association. Circulation. 2007 Aug 28;116(9):1081-93. Epub 2007 Aug 1. PubMed PMID: 17671237.
- Kersten S. Mechanisms of nutritional and hormonal regulation of lipogenesis. EMBO Rep. 2001 Apr;2(4):282-6. Review. PubMed PMID: 11306547; PubMed Central PMCID: PMC1083868.
- Jump DB, Clarke SD, thelen A, Liimatta M. Coordinate regulation of glycolytic and lipogenic gene expression by polyunsaturated fatty acids. J Lipid Res. 1994 Jun;35(6):1076-84. PubMed PMID: 8077846.
- Lopez-Garcia E, Schulze MB, Manson JE, Meigs JB, Apoundert CM, Rifai N, Willett WC, Hu FB. Consumption of (n-3) fatty acids is related to plasma biomarkers of inflammation and endothelial activation in women. J Nutr. 2004 Jul;134(7):1806-11. PubMed PMID: 15226473.
- Sands SA, Reid KJ, Windsor SL, Harris WS. The impact of age, body mass index, and seafood intake on the EPA and DHA content of human erythrocytes. Lipids 2005;40:343-347.
- Hu FB, Manson JE, Willett WC. Types of dietary fat and risk of coronary heart disease: a critical review. J Am Coll Nutr. 2001 Feb;20(1):5-19. Review. PubMed PMID: 11293467.
18 http://www.nal.usda.gov/fnic/foodcomp/search/
19 McCullough ML, Feskanich D, Stampfer MJ, Rosner BA, Hu FB, Hunter DJ, Variyam JN, Colditz GA, Willett WC. Adherence to the Dietary Guidelines for Americans and risk of major chronic disease in women. Am J Clin Nutr. 2000 Nov;72(5):1214-22. PubMed PMID: 11063452.
20 A sampling of supporting research:
- Simopoulos AP. Essential fatty acids in health and chronic disease. Am J Clin Nutr. 1999 Sep;70(3 Suppl):560S-569S. Review. PubMed PMID: 10479232.
- Simopoulos AP. The importance of the ratio of omega-6/omega-3 essential fatty acids. Biomed Pharmacother. 2002 Oct;56(8):365-79. Review. PubMed PMID: 12442909.
- Mori TA, Beilin LJ. Omega-3 fatty acids and inflammation. Curr Atheroscler Rep. 2004 Nov;6(6):461-7. Review. PubMed PMID: 15485592.
- Pirozzo S, Summerbell C, Cameron C, Glasziou P. Should we recommend low-fat diets for obesity? Obes Rev. 2003 May;4(2):83-90. Review. Erratum in: Obes Rev. 2003 Aug;4(3):185. PubMed PMID: 12760443.
21 Boyd, S., Melvin Konner, Marjorie Shostak, and M.D. Eaton. The Paleolithic Prescription: A Program of Diet & Exercise and a Design for Living. New York: HarperCollins, 1989. Print.
22 195,000 years of human history. Agriculture emerged 10,000 years ago. http://www.newscientist.com/article/dn7020--oldest-known-humans-just-got-older.html & Cordain L, Eaton SB, Sebastian A, Mann N, Lindeberg S, Watkins BA, O'Keefe JH, Brand-Miller J. Origins and evolution of the Western diet: health implications for the 21st century. Am J Clin Nutr. 2005 Feb;81(2):341-54. Review. PubMed PMID: 15699220

Chapter 19

1 Friedman JM. Modern science versus the stigma of obesity. Nat Med. 2004 Jun;10(6):563-9. Review. PubMed PMID: 15170194.
2 Weis W. Academy of Health Care Management Journal, 2005. http://www.alliedacademies.org/public/journals/JournalDetails.aspx?jid=20
3 Hendrickson, M. and Heffernan, W. (2007) Concentration of Agricultural Markets April 2007. Greenwood Village, CO: National Farmers Union (http://www.nfu.org/wp-content/2007-heffernanreport.pdf).
4 "Lobbying Spending Database | OpenSecrets." OpenSecrets.org: Money in Politics -- See Who's Giving & Who's Getting. N.p., n.d. Web. <http://www.opensecrets.org/lobby/top.php?indexType=c>.

5   A sampling of supporting research:
  • Brownell, Kelly, and Katherine Battle Horgen. Food Fight. 1 ed. New York: McGraw-Hill, 2004. Print.
  • http://www.gmabrands.com/publicpolicy/docs/Correspondence.cfm?DocID=1123&
  • Hays CL, McNeil Jr. DG. Putting Africa on Coke's map. New York Times. May 26, 1998.P. D1.
6   A sampling of supporting research:
  • Cannon G. The Politics of Food. London: Century Hutchinson, 1987.
  • Cauchon D. FDA Advisers Tied to Industry. USA Today, Sept. 25, 2000.
  • The National Institutes of Health: Public Servant or Private Marketer?—Los Angeles Times." Featured Articles From the Los Angeles Times. N.p., n.d. Web. 28 Apr. 2010. <http://articles.latimes.com/2004/dec/22/nation/na-nih22>.
  • The National Institutes of Health: Public Servant or Private Marketer?—Los Angeles Times." Featured Articles From the Los Angeles Times. N.p., n.d. Web. 28 Apr. 2010. <http://articles.latimes.com/2004/dec/22/nation/na-nih22>.
7   Nestle, Marion. Food politics: how the food industry influences nutrition and health. Berkeley: University of California Press, 2002. Print.
8   A sampling of supporting research:
  • Nestle, Marion. Food Politics: How the Food Industry Influences Nutrition, and Health, Revised and Expanded Edition (California Studies in Food and Culture).
  • Sugarman C, Gladwell M. U.S. drops new food chart. Washington Post, April 27, 1991: A1, A10.
  • Cannon G. The Politics of Food. London: Century Hutchinson, 1987.
  • Cauchon D. FDA Advisers Tied to Industry. USA Today, Sept. 25, 2000.
9   Nestle, Marion. Food Politics: How the Food Industry Influences Nutrition, and Health, Revised and Expanded Edition (California Studies in Food and Culture). & Simon, Michele. Appetite for Profit: How the food industry undermines our health and how to fight back. New York City, New York: Nation Books, 2006. Print.

Chapter 20

1   Yudkin, John. Sweet and Dangerous. Washington D.C.: Natl Health Federation, 1978. Print.
2   http://www.cspinet.org/new/pdf/liquid_candy_final_w_new_supplement.pdf
3   Johnson RJ, Segal MS, Sautin Y, Nakagawa T, Feig DI, Kang DH, Gersch MS, Benner S, Sánchez-Lozada LG. Potential role of sugar (fructose) in the epidemic of hypertension, obesity and the metabolic syndrome, diabetes, kidney disease, and cardiovascular disease. Am J Clin Nutr. 2007 Oct;86(4):899-906. Review. PubMed PMID: 17921363.
4   Johnson RJ, Segal MS, Sautin Y, Nakagawa T, Feig DI, Kang DH, Gersch MS, Benner S, Sánchez-Lozada LG. Potential role of sugar (fructose) in the epidemic of hypertension, obesity and the metabolic syndrome, diabetes, kidney disease, and cardiovascular disease. Am J Clin Nutr. 2007 Oct;86(4):899-906. Review. PubMed PMID: 17921363.
5   Popkin, Barry. The World is Fat: The Fads, Trends, Policies, and Products That Are Fattening the Human Race. New York: Avery, 2008. Print.
6   A sampling of supporting research:
  • Marion Nestle, quoted in : J.M. Hirsch, "Food Industry a Targe in Obesity Fight," March 19, 2006. www.forbes.com/feeds/ap/2006/03/18/ap2605096.html.
  • Malik VS, Schulze MB, Hu FB. Intake of sugar-sweetened beverages and weight gain: a systematic review. Am J Clin Nutr. 2006 Aug;84(2):274-88. Review. PubMed PMID: 16895873.
  • Nielsen SJ, Siega-Riz AM, Popkin BM. Trends in energy intake in U.S. between 1977 and 1996: similar shifts seen across age groups. Obes Res. 2002 May;10(5):370-8. PubMed PMID: 12006636.
  • The Principles and Practice of Medicine, William Osler, M.D. Fourth Edition
  • "Diabetes mellitus." Belinda Rowland., Teresa G. Odle., and Tish Davidson, A. M. The Gale Encyclopedia of Alternative Medicine. Ed. Laurie Fundukian. 3rd ed. Detroit: Gale, 2009. 4 vols.

7   Johnson, Richard J., and Timothy Gower. The sugar fix: The high-fructose fallout that is making you fat and sick. Emmaus, Pa.: Rodale, 2008. Print. & Stanhope KL, Griffen SC, Bair BR, Swarbrick MM, Keim NL, Havel PJ. Twenty-four-hour endocrine and metabolic profiles following consumption of high-fructose corn syrup-, sucrose-, fructose-, and glucose-sweetened beverages with meals. Am J Clin Nutr. 2008 May;87(5):1194-203. PubMed PMID: 18469239.

8   Bray GA, Nielsen SJ, Popkin BM. Consumption of high-fructose corn syrup in beverages may play a role in the epidemic of obesity. Am J Clin Nutr. 2004 Apr;79(4):537-43. Review. Erratum in: Am J Clin Nutr. 2004 Oct;80(4):1090. PubMed PMID: 15051594.

9   Cordain L, Eaton SB, Sebastian A, Mann N, Lindeberg S, Watkins BA, O'Keefe JH, Brand-Miller J. Origins and evolution of the Western diet: health implications for the 21st century. Am J Clin Nutr. 2005 Feb;81(2):341-54. Review. PubMed PMID: 15699220.

10 A sampling of supporting research:

- Anderson JW, Story LJ, Zettwoch NC, Gustafson NJ, Jefferson BS. Metabolic effects of fructose supplementation in diabetic individuals. Diabetes Care. 1989 May;12(5):337-44. PubMed PMID: 2721342.
- Bocarsly ME, Powell ES, Avena NM, Hoebel BG. High-fructose corn syrup causes characteristics of obesity in rats: Increased body weight, body fat and triglyceride levels. Pharmacol Biochem Behav. 2010 Feb 26. [Epub ahead of print] PubMed PMID: 20219526.
- Bray GA, Nielsen SJ, Popkin BM. Consumption of high-fructose corn syrup in beverages may play a role in the epidemic of obesity. Am J Clin Nutr. 2004 Apr;79(4):537-43. Review. Erratum in: Am J Clin Nutr. 2004 Oct;80(4):1090. PubMed PMID: 15051594.
- DiMeglio DP, Mattes RD. Liquid versus solid carbohydrate: effects on food intake and body weight. Int J Obes Relat Metab Disord. 2000 Jun;24(6):794-800. PubMed PMID: 10878689. & Malik VS, Schulze MB, Hu FB. Intake of sugar-sweetened beverages and weight gain: a systematic review. Am J Clin Nutr. 2006 Aug;84(2):274-88. Review. PubMed PMID: 16895873.
- Elliott SS, Keim NL, Stern JS, Teff K, Havel PJ. Fructose, weight gain, and the insulin resistance syndrome. Am J Clin Nutr. 2002 Nov;76(5):911-22. Review. PubMed PMID: 12399260.
- Email correspondence on August 11, 2010. Referencing his work in: Bocarsly ME, Powell ES, Avena NM, Hoebel BG. High-fructose corn syrup causes characteristics of obesity in rats: Increased body weight, body fat and triglyceride levels. Pharmacol Biochem Behav. 2010 Feb 26. [Epub ahead of print] PubMed PMID: 20219526.
- Havel PJ. Dietary fructose: implications for dysregulation of energy homeostasis and lipid/carbohydrate metabolism. Nutr Rev. 2005 May;63(5):133-57. Review. PubMed PMID: 15971409.
- Jürgens H, Haass W, Castañeda TR, Schürmann A, Koebnick C, Dombrowski F, Otto B, Nawrocki AR, Scherer PE, Spranger J, Ristow M, Joost HG, Havel PJ, Tschöp MH. Consuming fructose-sweetened beverages increases body adiposity in mice. Obes Res. 2005 Jul;13(7):1146-56. PubMed PMID: 16076983.
- Raben A, Vasilaras TH, Møller AC, Astrup A. Sucrose compared with artificial sweeteners: different effects on ad libitum food intake and body weight after 10 wk of supplementation in overweight subjects. Am J Clin Nutr. 2002 Oct;76(4):721-9. PubMed PMID: 12324283.
- Stanhope KL, Havel PJ. Endocrine and metabolic effects of consuming beverages sweetened with fructose, glucose, sucrose, or high-fructose corn syrup. Am J Clin Nutr. 2008 Dec;88(6):1733S-1737S. Review. PubMed PMID: 19064538.
- Stanhope KL, Havel PJ. Fructose consumption: considerations for future research on its effects on adipose distribution, lipid metabolism, and insulinsensitivity in humans. J Nutr. 2009 Jun;139(6):1236S-1241S. Epub 2009 Apr 29. PubMed PMID: 19403712.
- Stanhope KL, Havel PJ. Fructose consumption: potential mechanisms for its effects to increase visceral adiposity and induce dyslipidemia and insulinresistance. Curr Opin Lipidol. 2008 Feb;19(1):16-24. Review. PubMed PMID: 18196982.

- Stanhope KL, Havel PJ. Fructose consumption: recent results and their potential implications. Ann N Y Acad Sci. 2010 Mar;1190(1):15-24. Review. PubMed PMID: 20388133.
- Stanhope KL, Schwarz JM, Keim NL, Griffen SC, Bremer AA, Graham JL, Hatcher B, Cox CL, Dyachenko A, Zhang W, McGahan JP, Seibert A, Krauss RM, Chiu S, Schaefer EJ, Ai M, Otokozawa S, Nakajima K, Nakano T, Beysen C, Hellerstein MK, Berglund L, Havel PJ. Consuming fructose-sweetened, not glucose-sweetened, beverages increases visceral adiposity and lipids and decreases insulin sensitivity in overweight/obese humans. J Clin Invest. 2009 May;119(5):1322-34. doi:10.1172/JCI37385. Epub 2009 Apr 20. PubMed PMID: 19381015; PubMed Central PMCID: PMC2673878.
- Tordoff MG, Alleva AM. Effect of drinking soda sweetened with aspartame or high-fructose corn syrup on food intake and body weight. Am J Clin Nutr. 1990 Jun;51(6):963-9. PubMed PMID: 2349932.
- Vrána A, Fábry P. Metabolic effects of high sucrose or fructose intake. World Rev Nutr Diet. 1983;42:56-101. Review. PubMed PMID: 6375162.

11 Colantuoni C, Rada P, McCarthy J, Patten C, Avena NM, Chadeayne A, Hoebel BG. Evidence that intermittent, excessive sugar intake causes endogenous opioid dependence. Obes Res. 2002 Jun;10(6):478-88. PubMed PMID: 12055324. & Email correspondence on August 11, 2010. Referencing his work in: Avena NM, Rada P, Hoebel BG. Evidence for sugar addiction: behavioral and neurochemical effects of intermittent, excessive sugar intake. Neurosci Biobehav Rev. 2008;32(1):20-39. Epub 2007 May 18. Review. PubMed PMID: 17617461; PubMed Central PMCID: PMC2235907. & Avena NM, Rada P, Hoebel BG. Sugar and fat bingeing have notable differences in addictive-like behavior. J Nutr. 2009 Mar;139(3):623-8. Epub 2009 Jan 28. Review. PubMed PMID: 19176748; PubMed Central PMCID: PMC2714381.

12 Beck J. Teen suspended from school for wearing Pepsi T-shirt on Coke Day. Chicago Tribune, April 1, 1998.

13 Nestle, Marion. Food Politics: How the Food Industry Influences Nutrition, and Health, Revised and Expanded Edition (California Studies in Food and Culture). 2 ed. Berkeley: University of California Press, 2007. Print.

14 Ali H. Mokdad; James S. Marks; Donna F. Stroup; Julie L. Gerberding Actual Causes of Death in the United States, 2000 JAMA. 2004;291(10):1238-1245.

15 "Tobacco CEO's Statement to Congress." UCSF Academic Senate. N.p., n.d. Web. 18 July 2010. <http://senate.ucsf.edu/tobacco/executives1994congress.html>.

16 National Soft Drink Association web site. Available at http://www.nsda.org/softdrinks/CSDHealth/Index.html.

17 "Daily Doc: Lorillard, Aug 30, 1978: 'The base of our business is the high school student'." Tobacco.org : Welcome. N.p., n.d. Web. 18 July 2010. <http://www.tobacco.org/Documents/dd/ddbasebusiness.html>.

18 Horovitz B. McDonald's rediscovers its future with kids. USA Today, Apr. 18, 1997.

19 "Jan. 4, 1954: TIRC Announced." Tobacco.org : Welcome. N.p., n.d. Web. 18 July 2010. <http://www.tobacco.org/History/540104frank.html>.

20 "Jan. 4, 1954: TIRC Announced." Tobacco.org : Welcome. N.p., n.d. Web. 18 July 2010. <http://www.tobacco.org/History/540104frank.html>.

21 Hays CL, McNeil Jr. DG. Putting Africa on Coke's map. New York Times. May 26, 1998.P. D1.

22 National Soft Drink Association web site. Available at http://www.nsda.org/softdrinks/CSDHealth/Index.html.

23 Simon, Michele. Appetite for Profit: How the food industry undermines our health and how to fight back. New York City, New York: Nation Books, 2006. Print.

24 Brownell, Kelly, and Katherine Battle Horgen. Food Fight. 1 ed. New York: McGraw-Hill, 2004. Print. & Donohue, T, Meyer T, Henke L. Black and White Children: Perceptions of TV Commercials. The Journal of Marketing, Vol. 42, No. 4 (Oct., 1978), pp. 34-40.

25 Taubes, Gary. Good calories, bad calories: challenging the conventional wisdom on diet, weight control, and disease. New York: Knopf, 2007. Print.

Chapter 21

1 Lindeberg S, Jönsson T, Granfeldt Y, Borgstrand E, Soffman J, Sjöström K, Ahrén B. A Palaeolithic diet improves glucose tolerance more than a Mediterranean-like diet in individuals with ischaemic heart disease. Diabetologia. 2007 Sep;50(9):1795-807. Epub 2007 Jun 22. PubMed PMID: 17583796.

2 A sampling of supporting research:
  - Diamond, Jared M.. Guns, germs, and steel: The fates of human societies. New York: W.W. Norton & Co., 1998. Print.
  - Cordain L, Eaton SB, Sebastian A, Mann N, Lindeberg S, Watkins BA, O'Keefe JH, Brand-Miller J. Origins and evolution of the Western diet: health implications for the 21st century. Am J Clin Nutr. 2005 Feb;81(2):341-54. Review. PubMed PMID: 15699220.
  - O'Keefe JH Jr, Cordain L. Cardiovascular disease resulting from a diet and lifestyle at odds with our Paleolithic genome: how to become a 21st-century hunter-gatherer. Mayo Clin Proc 2004 Jan;79(1):101-8.

3 Cordain, Loren. The Paleo Diet: Lose Weight and Get Healthy by Eating the Food You Were Designed to Eat. New Ed ed. New York, NY: Wiley, 2002. Print.   &   U.S. Department of Agriculture, Agricultural Research Service. 2007. Nutrient Intakes from Food: Mean Amounts and Percentages of Calories from Protein, Carbohydrate, Fat, and Alcohol, One Day, 2003-2004. Available: www.ars.usda.gov/ba/bhnrc/fsrg.

4 Boyd, S., Melvin Konner, Marjorie Shostak, and M.D. Eaton. The Paleolithic Prescription: A Program of Diet & Exercise and a Design for Living. New York: HarperCollins, 1989. Print.   &   Yudkin, John. Sweet and Dangerous. Washington D.C.: Natl Health Federation, 1978. Print.

5 A sampling of supporting research:
  - Garg A, Bantle JP, Henry RR, Coulston AM, Griver KA, Raatz SK, Brinkley L, Chen YD, Grundy SM, Huet BA, et al. Effects of varying carbohydrate content of diet in patients with non-insulin-dependent diabetes mellitus. JAMA. 1994 May 11;271(18):1421-8. PubMed PMID: 7848401.
  - Haimoto H, Sasakabe T, Wakai K, Umegaki H. Effects of a low-carbohydrate diet on glycemic control in outpatients with severe type 2 diabetes. Nutr Metab (Lond). 2009 May 6;6:21. PubMed PMID: 19419563; PubMed Central PMCID: PMC2690585.
  - Westman EC, Yancy WS Jr, Mavropoulos JC, Marquart M, McDuffie JR. The effect of a low-carbohydrate, ketogenic diet versus a low-glycemic index diet on glycemic control in type 2 diabetes mellitus. Nutr Metab (Lond). 2008 Dec 19;5:36. PubMed PMID: 19099589; PubMed Central PMCID: PMC2633336.Daniel M, Rowley KG, McDermott R, Mylvaganam A, O'Dea K. Diabetes incidence in an Australian aboriginal population: an 8-year follow-up study. Diabetes Care. 1999;22:1993-1998.
  - Ebbesson SO, Schraer CD, Risica PM, et al. Diabetes and impaired glucose tolerance in three Alaskan Eskimo populations: The Alaska-Siberia Project. Diabetes Care. 1998;21:563-569.
  - Gutierrez M, Akhavan M, Jovanovic L, Peterson CM. Utility of a short-term 25% carbohydrate diet on improving glycemic control in type 2 diabetes mellitus. J Am Coll Nutr. 1998 Dec;17(6):595-600. PubMed PMID: 9853539.
  - O'Dea K. Marked improvement in carbohydrate and lipid metabolism in diabetic Australian aborigines after temporary reversion to traditional lifestyle. Diabetes. 1984 Jun;33(6):596-603. PubMed PMID: 6373464.
  - Lindeberg S, Jonsson T, Granfeldt Y, Borgstrand E, Soffman J, Sjostrom K, Ahren B: A Palaeolithic diet improves glucose tolerance more than a Mediterranean-like diet in individuals with ischaemic heart disease. Diabetologia 2007, 50(9):1795-1807.
  - Osterdahl M, Kocturk T, Koochek A, Wandell PE: Effects of a short-term intervention with a paleolithic diet in healthy volunteers. Eur J Clin Nutr 2008, 62(5):682-685.
  - Frassetto LA, Schloetter M, Mietus-Synder M, Morris RC, Jr., Sebastian A: Metabolic and physiologic improvements from consuming a paleolithic, hunter-gatherer type diet. Eur J Clin Nutr 2009.

- Jönsson T, Granfeldt Y, Ahrén B, Branell UC, Pålsson G, Hansson A, Söderström M, Lindeberg S. Beneficial effects of a Paleolithic diet on cardiovascular risk factors in type 2 diabetes: a randomized cross-over pilot study. Cardiovasc Diabetol. 2009;8:35

6   Boyd, S., Melvin Konner, Marjorie Shostak, and M.D. Eaton. The Paleolithic Prescription: A Program of Diet & Exercise and a Design for Living. New York: HarperCollins, 1989. Print.

Chapter 22

1   Friedman JM. Modern science versus the stigma of obesity. Nat Med. 2004 Jun;10(6):563-9. Review. PubMed PMID: 15170194.

2   A sampling of supporting research:
- Weigle DS. Human obesity. Exploding the myths. West J Med. 1990 Oct;153(4):421-8. Review. PubMed PMID: 2244378; PubMed Central PMCID: PMC1002573.
- Westman EC, Feinman RD, Mavropoulos JC, Vernon MC, Volek JS, Wortman JA, Yancy WS, Phinney SD. Low-carbohydrate nutrition and metabolism. Am J Clin Nutr. 2007 Aug;86(2):276-84. Review. PubMed PMID: 17684196
- Rose, Geoffrey, and K. T. Khaw. Rose's Strategy of Preventive Medicine the Complete Original Text. Oxford [etc.]: Oxford UP, 2008. Print.
- Miller WC. Diet composition, energy intake, and nutritional status in relation to obesity in men and women. Med Sci Sports Exerc. 1991 Mar;23(3):280-4. Review. PubMed PMID: 2020264.

3   Cordain, Loren. The Paleo Diet: Lose Weight and Get Healthy by Eating the Food You Were Designed to Eat. New Ed ed. New York, NY: Wiley, 2002. Print.

4   Eaton SB, Konner MJ, Cordain L. Diet-dependent acid load, Paleolithic nutrition, and evolutionary health promotion. Am J Clin Nutr. 2010 Feb;91(2):295-7. Epub 2009 Dec 30. PubMed PMID: 20042522. & Eaton SB, Eaton SB 3rd, Konner MJ. Paleolithic nutrition revisited: a twelve-year retrospective on its nature and implications. Eur J Clin Nutr. 1997 Apr;51(4):207-16. Review. PubMed PMID: 9104571.

5   Boyd, S., Melvin Konner, Marjorie Shostak, and M.D. Eaton. The Paleolithic Prescription: A Program of Diet and Exercise and a Design for Living. 1st ed ed. New York: HarperCollins, 1988. Print.

6   Taubes, Gary. Good calories, bad calories: challenging the conventional wisdom on diet, weight control, and disease. New York: Knopf, 2007. Print.

Chapter 23

1   Schoeller DA, Buchholz AC. Energetics of obesity and weight control: does diet composition matter? J Am Diet Assoc. 2005 May;105(5 Suppl 1):S24-8. Review. PubMed PMID: 15867892.

Chapter 24

1   Halton TL, Hu FB. The effects of high protein diets on thermogenesis, satiety and weight loss: a critical review. J Am Coll Nutr. 2004 Oct;23(5):373-85. Review. PubMed PMID: 15466943.

2   A sampling of supporting research:
- Layman DK. Dietary Guidelines should reflect new understandings about adult protein needs. Nutr Metab (Lond). 2009 Mar 13;6:12. PubMed PMID: 19284668; PubMed Central PMCID: PMC2666737.
- Layman DK, Boileau RA, Erickson DJ, et al. A reduced ratio of dietary carbohydrate to protein improves body composition and blood lipid profiles during weight loss in adult women. J Nutr 2003;133:411–7.
- Farnsworth E, Luscombe ND, Noakes M, Wittert G, Argyiou E, Clifton PM. Effect of a high-protein, energy-restricted diet on body composition, glycemic control, and lipid concentrations in overweight and obese hyperinsulinemic men and women. Am J Clin Nutr 2003;78:31–9.

- Paddon-Jones D, Westman E, Mattes RD, Wolfe RR, Astrup A, Westerterp-Plantenga M. Protein, weight management, and satiety. Am J Clin Nutr. 2008 May;87(5):1558S-1561S. Review. PubMed PMID:18469287.

3 Manninen AH. High-protein weight loss diets and purported adverse effects: where is the evidence? Sports Nutr Rev J 2004; 1: 45–51. & Halton TL, Hu FB. The effects of high protein diets on thermogenesis, satiety and weight loss: a critical review. J Am Coll Nutr. 2004 Oct;23(5):373-85.Review. PubMed PMID: 15466943.

4 A sampling of supporting research:
- Wolfe RR. The underappreciated role of muscle in health and disease. Am J Clin Nutr. 2006 Sep;84(3):475-82. Review. PubMed PMID: 16960159.
- Westerterp-Plantenga MS. Protein intake and energy balance. Regul Pept. 2008 Aug 7;149(1-3):67-9. Epub 2008 Mar 25. Review. PubMed PMID: 18448177.
- Paddon-Jones D, Westman E, Mattes RD, Wolfe RR, Astrup A, Westerterp-Plantenga M. Protein, weight management, and satiety. Am J Clin Nutr. 2008 May;87(5):1558S-1561S. Review. PubMed PMID: 18469287.
- Manninen, A.H. (2002) Protein metabolism in exercising humans with special reference to protein supplementation. Master thesis. Department of Physiology, Faculty of Medicine, University of Kuopio, Finland.
- Wolfe BM, Piché LA. Replacement of carbohydrate by protein in a conventional-fat diet reduces cholesterol and triglyceride concentrations in healthy normolipidemic subjects. Clin Invest Med. 1999 Aug;22(4):140-8. PubMedPMID: 10497712.
- The Evolutionary Basis for the therapeutic Effects of High Protein Diets: http://cathletics.com/articles/proteinDebate.pdf

5 Eaton SB, Eaton SB 3rd, Konner MJ. Paleolithic nutrition revisited: a twelve-year retrospective on its nature and implications. Eur J Clin Nutr. 1997 Apr;51(4):207-16. Review. PubMed PMID: 9104571.

6 P.J. Skerrett, and W.C. Willett. Eat, Drink, and Be Healthy: The Harvard Medical School Guide to Healthy Eating. Free Press Trade Pbk. Ed ed. New York City: Free Press, 2005. Print.

7 McCullough ML, Feskanich D, Stampfer MJ, Giovannucci EL, Rimm EB, Hu FB, Spiegelman D, Hunter DJ, Colditz GA, Willett WC. Diet quality and major chronic disease risk in men and women: moving toward improved dietary guidance. Am J Clin Nutr. 2002 Dec;76(6):1261-71. PubMed PMID: 12450892.

8 Rudman D, DiFulco TJ, Galambos JT, Smith RB 3rd, Salam AA, Warren WD. Maximal rates of excretion and synthesis of urea in normal and cirrhotic subjects. J Clin Invest. 1973 Sep;52(9):2241-9. PubMed PMID: 4727456; PubMed Central PMCID: PMC333026. & The Evolutionary Basis for the therapeutic Effects of High Protein Diets: http://www.cathletics.com/articles/proteinDebate.pdf

9 Skov AR, Toubro S, Bülow J, Krabbe K, Parving HH, Astrup A. Changes in renal function during weight loss induced by high vs low-protein low-fat diets in overweight subjects. Int J Obes Relat Metab Disord. 1999 Nov;23(11):1170-7. PubMed PMID: 10578207. & Eisenstein J, Roberts SB, Dallal G, Saltzman E: High protein weight loss diets: are they safe and do they work? A review of the experimental and epidemiologic data. Nutr Rev60 :189 –200,2002 .

10 A sampling of supporting research:
- Skov AR, Toubro S, Bülow J, Krabbe K, Parving HH, Astrup A. Changes in renal function during weight loss induced by high vs low-protein low-fat diets in overweight subjects. Int J Obes Relat Metab Disord. 1999 Nov;23(11):1170-7.PubMed PMID: 10578207.
- Cordain L, Eaton SB, Brand Miller J, Mann N, Hill K. The paradoxical nature of hunter-gatherer diets: Meat based, yet non-atherogenic. Eur J Clin Nutr 2002; 56 (suppl 1):S42-S52.
- Cordain L. The nutritional characteristics of a contemporary diet based upon Paleolithic food groups. J Am Nutraceut Assoc 2002; 5:15-24.
- O'Dea K. Marked improvement in carbohydrate and lipid metabolism in diabetic Australian aborigines after temporary reversion to traditional lifestyle.Diabetes. 1984 Jun;33(6):596-603. PubMed

PMID: 6373464.

- Samaha FF, Iqbal N, Seshadri P, Chicano KL, Daily D, Mcgrory J: A low carbohydrate as compared with a low fat diet in severe obesity. N Eng J Med348 :2074 –2081,2003

- Skov AR, Toubro S, Ronn B, Holm L, Astrup A: Randomized trial on protein vs carbohydrate in ad libitum fat reduced diet for the treatment of obesity. Int J Obes23 :528 –536,1999

- Farnsworth E, Luscombe ND, Noakes M, Wittert G, Argyiou E, Clifton PM: Effect of a high protein, energy restricted diet on body composition, glycemic control and lipid concentrations in overweight and obese hyperinsulinemic men and women. Am J Clin Nut78 :31 –39,2003

- Parker B, Noakes M, Luscombe N, Clifton P: Effect of a high protein, high monounsaturated fat weight loss diet on glycemic control and lipid levels in type-2 diabetes. Diabetes Care25 :425 –430,2002

- Wolfe BM: Potential role of raising dietary protein intake for reducing risk of atherosclerosis. Can J Cardiol11(Supp G) :127 g –131 g,1995 .

- Wolfe BM, Giovannetti PM. Short term effects of substituting protein for carbohydrate in the diets of moderately hypercholesterolemic human subjects. Metabolism. 1991;40:338-343.

- Layman DK, Boileau RA, Erickson DJ, Painter JE, Shiue H, Sather C, Christou DD. A reduced ratio of dietary carbohydrate to protein improves body composition and blood lipid profiles during weight loss in adult women. J Nutr. 2003 Feb;133(2):411-7.

- Noakes M, Keogh JB, Foster PR, Clifton PM. Effect of an energy-restricted, high-protein, low-fat diet relative to a conventional high-carbohydrate, low-fat diet on weight loss, body composition, nutritional status, and markers of cardiovascular health in obese women. Am J Clin Nutr. 2005 Jun;81(6):1298-306.

- Farnsworth E, Luscombe ND, Noakes M, Wittert G, Argyiou E, Clifton PM. Effect of a high-protein, energy-restricted diet on body composition, glycemic control, and lipid concentrations in overweight and obese hyperinsulinemic men and women.Am J Clin Nutr. 2003 Jul;78(1):31-9.

- Luscombe-Marsh ND, Noakes M, Wittert GA, Keogh JB, Foster P, Clifton PM.Carbohydrate-restricted diets high in either monounsaturated fat or protein are equally effective at promoting fat loss and improving blood lipids. Am J Clin Nutr. 2005 Apr;81(4):762-72

- Aude YW, Agatston AS, Lopez-Jimenez F, Lieberman EH, Marie Almon, Hansen M, Rojas G, Lamas GA, Hennekens CH. The national cholesterol education program diet vs a diet lower in carbohydrates and higher in protein and monounsaturated fat: a randomized trial. Arch Intern Med. 2004 Oct 25;164(19):2141-6.

- McAuley KA, Hopkins CM, Smith KJ, McLay RT, Williams SM, Taylor RW, Mann JI. Comparison of high-fat and high-protein diets with a high-carbohydrate diet in insulin-resistant obese women. Diabetologia. 2005 Jan;48(1):8-16.

- Appel LJ, Sacks FM, Carey VJ, Obarzanek E, Swain JF, Miller ER 3rd, Conlin PR, Erlinger TP, Rosner BA, Laranjo NM, Charleston J, McCarron P, Bishop LM; OmniHeart Collaborative Research Group. Effects of protein, monounsaturated fat, and carbohydrate intake on blood pressure and serum lipids: results of the OmniHeart randomized trial. JAMA. 2005 Nov 16;294(19):2455-64.

- Hu FB, Stampfer MJ, Manson JE, Rimm E, Colditz GA, Speizer FE, Hennekens CH, Willett WC. Dietary protein and risk of ischemic heart disease in women. Am J Clin Nutr. 1999;70:221-227.

- Iso H, Stampfer MJ, Manson JE, Rexrode K, Hu FB, Hennekens CH, Colditz GA: Prospective study of fat and protein intake and risk of intraparenchymal hemorrhage in women. Circulation103 :856 –863,2001

- Komachi Y, Iida M, Shimamoto T: Geographic and occupational comparisons of risk factors in cardiovascular diseases in Japan. Jpn Circ J35 :189 –207,1971

- Shimamoto T, Komachi Y, Inada H: Trends of coronary heart disease and stroke and their risk factors in Japan. Circulation79 :503 –513,1989

- Halton TL, Hu FB. The effects of high protein diets on thermogenesis, satiety and weight loss: a critical review. J Am Coll Nutr. 2004 Oct;23(5):373-85. Review. PubMed PMID: 15466943.

11 A sampling of supporting research:
- Cordain L, Miller JB, Eaton SB, Mann N, Holt SH, Speth JD. Plant-animal subsistence ratios and macronutrient energy estimations in worldwide hunter-gatherer diets. Am J Clin Nutr. 2000 Mar;71(3):682-92. PubMed PMID:10702160.
- Hu FB, Willett WC. Optimal diets for prevention of coronary heart disease. JAMA. 2002 Nov 27;288(20):2569-78. Review. PubMed PMID: 12444864.
- Yudkin J. Lancet 2, 155-162, 1957.

12 A sampling of supporting research
- Slattery ML, Randall DE. Trends in coronary heart disease mortality and food consumption in the United States between 1909 and 1980. Am J Clin Nutr. 1988 Jun;47(6):1060-7. PubMed PMID: 3376904.Davidson MH, Hunninghake D, Maki KC, Kwiterovich PO Jr, Kafonek S. Comparison of the effects of lean red meat vs lean white meat on serum lipid levels among free-living persons with hypercholesterolemia: a long-term, randomized clinical trial. Arch Intern Med. 1999 Jun 28;159(12):1331-8. PubMed PMID: 10386509.
- O'Keefe JH Jr, Cordain L. Cardiovascular disease resulting from a diet and lifestyle at odds with our Paleolithic genome: how to become a 21st-century hunter-gatherer. Mayo Clin Proc 2004 Jan;79(1):101-8.
- Cordain L, Eades MR, Eades MD. Hyperinsulinemic diseases of civilization: more than just Syndrome X. Comp Biochem Physiol A Mol Integr Physiol. 2003;136:95-112.
- O'Dea K, Traianedes K, Chisholm K, Leyden H, Sinclair AJ. Cholesterol-lowering effect of a low-fat diet containing lean beef is reversed by the addition of beef fat. Am J Clin Nutr. 1990;52:491-494.
- Arciero PJ, Gentile CL, Pressman R, Everett M, Ormsbee MJ, Martin J, Santamore J, Gorman L, Fehling PC, Vukovich MD, Nindl BC. Moderate protein intake improves total and regional body composition and insulin sensitivity in overweight adults. Metabolism. 2008 Jun;57(6):757-65. PubMed PMID: 18502257.

13 A sampling of supporting research:
- Eaton SB, Eaton SB 3rd, Konner MJ. Paleolithic nutrition revisited: a twelve-year retrospective on its nature and implications. Eur J Clin Nutr. 1997 Apr;51(4):207-16. Review. PubMed PMID: 9104571.
- Committee on Diet and Health, Natiional Research Council (1989): Diet and Health. Washington, D.C.: National Academy Press, pp 15, 58, 59, 263-265.
- Hunt JR, Gallagher SK, Johnson LK, Lykken GI. High- versus low-meat diets: effects on zinc absorption, iron status, and calcium, copper, iron, magnesium, manganese, nitrogen, phosphorus, and zinc balance in postmenopausal women. Am J Clin Nutr. 1995 Sep;62(3):621-32. PubMed PMID: 7661125.
- Spencer H, Kramer L, Osis D, Norris C. Effect of a high protein (meat) intake on calcium metabolism in man. Am J Clin Nutr. 1978 Dec;31(12):2167-80. PubMedPMID: 727162.
- Pannemans DL, Schaafsma G, Westerterp KR. Calcium excretion, apparent calcium absorption and calcium balance in young and elderly subjects: influence of protein intake. Br J Nutr. 1997 May;77(5):721-9.
- Kerstetter JE, O'Brien KO, Insogna KL. Dietary protein affects intestinal calcium absorption. Am J Clin Nutr. 1998 Oct;68(4):859-65. PubMed PMID: 9771863.
- Dawson-Hughes B, Harris SS, Rasmussen H, Song L, Dallal GE. Effect of dietary protein supplements on calcium excretion in healthy older men and women. J Clin Endocrinol Metab. 2004 Mar;89(3):1169-73
- Kerstetter JE, O'Brien KO, Caseria DM, Wall DE, Insogna KL. The impact of dietary protein on calcium absorption and kinetic measures of bone turnover in women. J Clin Endocrinol Metab. 2005 Jan;90(1):26-31.
- Kerstetter JE, Wall DE, O'Brien KO, Caseria DM, Insogna KL. Meat and soy protein affect calcium homeostasis in healthy women. J Nutr. 2006 Jul;136(7):1890-5

14 Westerterp-Plantenga MS, Nieuwenhuizen A, Tomé D, Soenen S, Westerterp KR. Dietary protein, weight loss, and weight maintenance. Annu Rev Nutr. 2009;29:21-41. Review. PubMed PMID: 19400750.

15 Spencer H, Kramer L, Osis D. Do protein and phosphorus cause calcium loss? J Nutr. 1988 Jun;118(6):657-60. Review. PubMed PMID: 3286844.

16 http://www.nal.usda.gov/fnic/foodcomp/search

Chapter 25

1 Hu FB, Willett WC. Optimal diets for prevention of coronary heart disease. JAMA. 2002 Nov 27;288(20):2569-78. Review. PubMed PMID: 12444864.

2 A sampling of supporting research:
  - Apoundert CM, Campos H, Stampfer MJ, et al. Blood levels of long-chain n-3 fatty acids and the risk of sudden death. N Engl J Med 2002;346:1113-1118.
  - Siscovick DS, Raghunathan TE, King I, Weinmann S, Wicklund KG, Apoundright J, Bovbjerg V, Arbogast P, Smith H, Kushi LH, Cobb LA, Copass MK, Psaty BM, Lemaitre R, Retzlaff B, Childs M, Knopp RH. Dietary intake and cell membrane levels of long-chain n-3 polyunsaturated fatty acids and the risk of primary cardiac arrest. JAMA 1995;274:1363-1367.
  - Hu FB, Manson JE, Willett WC. Types of dietary fat and risk of coronary heart disease: a critical review. J Am Coll Nutr. 2001 Feb;20(1):5-19. Review. PubMed PMID: 11293467.

3 Wood, Philip A.. How fat works. Cambridge: Harvard University Press, 2006. Print

4 A sampling of supporting research
  - Willett WC. Is dietary fat a major determinant of body fat? Am J Clin Nutr. 1998 Mar;67(3 Suppl):556S-562S. Review. Erratum in: Am J Clin Nutr 1999 Aug;70(2):304. PubMed PMID: 9497170.
  - Willett WC. Dietary fat plays a major role in obesity: no. Obes Rev. 2002 May;3(2):59-68. Review. PubMed PMID: 12120421.
  - Willett WC, Leibel RL. Dietary fat is not a major determinant of body fat. Am J Med. 2002 Dec 30;113 Suppl 9B:47S-59S. Review. PubMed PMID: 12566139.
  - McCullough ML, Feskanich D, Stampfer MJ, Rosner BA, Hu FB, Hunter DJ, Variyam JN, Colditz GA, Willett WC. Adherence to the Dietary Guidelines for Americans and risk of major chronic disease in women. Am J Clin Nutr. 2000 Nov;72(5):1214-22. PubMed PMID: 11063452
  - Hu FB, Manson JE, Willett WC. Types of dietary fat and risk of coronary heart disease: a critical review. J Am Coll Nutr. 2001 Feb;20(1):5-19. Review. PubMed PMID: 11293467.

Chapter 26

1 Wolfe BM, Piché LA. Replacement of carbohydrate by protein in a conventional-fat diet reduces cholesterol and triglyceride concentrations in healthy normolipidemic subjects. Clin Invest Med. 1999 Aug;22(4):140-8. PubMedPMID: 10497712.

2 A sampling of supporting research:
  - Brownell, Kelly, and Katherine Battle Horgen. Food Fight. 1 ed. New York: McGraw-Hill, 2004. Print.
  - Abbasi F, Brown BW Jr, Lamendola C, McLaughlin T, Reaven GM. Relationship between obesity, insulin resistance, and coronary heart disease risk. J Am Coll Cardiol. 2002 Sep 4;40(5):937-43. PubMed PMID: 12225719.
  - Saltzman E. Benotti P. The Effects of Obesity on the Cardiovascular System In: Bray GA, Couchard d, James WP, eds. Handbook of Obesity. New York: Marcel Dekker, 1997: 637-649.
  - On obesity and depression:
  - Simon GE, Von Korff M, Saunders K, Miglioretti DL, Crane PK, van Belle G, Kessler RC. Association between obesity and psychiatric disorders in the U.S. adult population. Arch Gen Psychiatry. 2006 Jul;63(7):824-30. PubMed PMID: 16818872; PubMed Central PMCID: PMC1913935.

- Luppino FS, de Wit LM, Bouvy PF, Stijnen T, Cuijpers P, Penninx BW, Zitman FG. Overweight, obesity, and depression: a systematic review and meta-analysis of longitudinal studies. Arch Gen Psychiatry. 2010 Mar;67(3):220-9. Review. PubMed PMID: 20194822.
- Ma J, Xiao L. Obesity and depression in U.S. women: results from the 2005-2006 National Health and Nutritional Examination Survey. Obesity (Silver Spring). 2010 Feb;18(2):347-53. Epub 2009 Jul 9. PubMed PMID: 19590500.
- On the discrimination of obese people:
- Amy NK, Aapoundorg A, Lyons P, Keranen K. Barriers to routing gynecological cancer screening for White and African-American obese women. In J Obes. 2006; 30: 147-155.
- Brownell KD, Puhl R, Schwartz MB, Rudd L, eds. Weight Bias: Nature, Consequences, and Remedies. New York: Guilford Publications; 2005
- Latner JD, Stunkard AJ. Getting worse: The stigmatization of obese children. Obes Res. 2003; 11: 452-456.
- Neumark-Sztainer D, Story M., Faibisch L. Perceived stigmatization among overweight African-American and Caucasian adolescent girls. J Adolesc Health. 1998; 23: 264-270
- Neumark-Sztainer D, Story M, Harris T. Beliefs and attitudes about obesity among teachers and school health care providers working with adolescents. J Nutr Education. 1999; 31: 3-9.
- Puhl R, Brownell KD. Bias, discrimination, and obesity. Obes Res. 2001;9:788-805.
- Roehling MV. Weight-based discrimination in employment: Psychological and legal aspects. Pers Psychol. 1999; 52: 969-1017.
- Schwartz MB, O'Neal H, Brownell KD, Blair S, Billington C. Weight bias among health professionals specializing in obesity. Obes Res. 2003;11:1033-1039.

3 Wood, Philip A.. How fat works. Cambridge: Harvard University Press, 2006. Print. & Yudkin, John. Sweet and Dangerous. Washington D.C.: Natl Health Federation, 1978. Print.

4 P.J. Skerrett, and W.C. Willett. Eat, Drink, and Be Healthy: The Harvard Medical School Guide to Healthy Eating. Free Press Trade Pbk. Ed ed. New York City: Free Press, 2005. Print.

5 Layman DK. Dietary Guidelines should reflect new understandings about adult protein needs. Nutr Metab (Lond). 2009 Mar 13;6:12. PubMed PMID: 19284668; PubMed Central PMCID: PMC2666737.

6 A sampling of supporting research:
- Keller U, Szinnai G, Bilz S, Berneis K. Effects of changes in hydration on protein, glucose and lipid metabolism in man: impact on health. Eur J Clin Nutr. 2003 Dec;57 Suppl 2:S69-74. PubMed PMID: 14681716.
- Bilz S, Ninnis R, Keller U. Effects of hypoosmolality on whole-body lipolysis in man. Metabolism. 1999 Apr;48(4):472-6. PubMed PMID: 10206440.
- Berneis K, Ninnis R, Häussinger D, Keller U. Effects of hyper- and hypoosmolality on whole body protein and glucose kinetics in humans. Am J Physiol. 1999 Jan;276(1 Pt 1):E188-95. PubMed PMID: 9886966.
- Boschmann M, Steiniger J, Hille U, Tank J, Adams F, Sharma AM, Klaus S, Luft FC, Jordan J. Water-induced thermogenesis. J Clin Endocrinol Metab. 2003 Dec;88(12):6015-9. PubMed PMID: 14671205.
- Jordan J. Acute effect of water on blood pressure. What do we know? Clin Auton Res. 2002 Aug;12(4):250-5. Review. PubMed PMID: 12357278.
- Stookey JD, Constant F, Popkin BM, Gardner CD. Drinking water is associated with weight loss in overweight dieting women independent of diet and activity. Obesity (Silver Spring). 2008 Nov;16(11):2481-8. Epub 2008 Sep 11. PubMed PMID: 18787524.
- Dennis EA, Flack KD, Davy BM. Beverage consumption and adult weight management: A review. Eat Behav. 2009 Dec;10(4):237-46. Epub 2009 Jul 16. Review. PubMed PMID: 19778754; PubMed Central PMCID: PMC2864136.
- Malik VS, Schulze MB, Hu FB. Intake of sugar-sweetened beverages and weight gain: a systematic

review. Am J Clin Nutr. 2006 Aug;84(2):274-88. Review. PubMed PMID: 16895873.

- Popkin BM, Armstrong LE, Bray GM, Caballero B, Frei B, Willett WC. A new proposed guidance system for beverage consumption in the United States. Am J Clin Nutr. 2006 Mar;83(3):529-42. Erratum in: Am J Clin Nutr. 2007 Aug;86(2):525. PubMed PMID: 16522898.
- Popkin BM, Nielsen SJ. The sweetening of the world's diet. Obes Res. 2003 Nov;11(11):1325-32. PubMed PMID: 14627752.
- Almiron-Roig E, Drewnowski A. Hunger, thirst, and energy intakes following consumption of caloric beverages. Physiol Behav 2003;79:767–773.
- Beridot-Therond ME, Arts I, Fantino M, De La Gueronniere V. Short-term effects of the flavour of drinks on ingestive behaviours in man. Appetite 1998;31:67–81.
- DellaValle DM, Roe LS, Rolls BJ. Does the consumption of caloric and non-caloric beverages with a meal affect energy intake? Appetite 2005;44:187–193.
- Engell D. Effects of beverage consumption and hydration status on caloric intake. In: Marriott BM (ed). Committee on Military Nutrition Research Food and Nutrition Board, Institute of Medicine. Institute of Medicine: Washington, DC, 1995, pp 217–238.
- Hagg A, Jacobson T, Nordlund G, Rossner S. Effects of milk or water on lunch intake in preschool children. Appetite 1998;31:83–92.
- Ludwig DS, Peterson KE, Gortmaker SL. Relation between consumption of sugar-sweetened drinks and childhood obesity: a prospective observational analysis. Lancet 2001;357:505–508.
- Mattes RD. Dietary compensation by humans for supplemental energy provided as ethanol or carbohydrate in fluids. Physiol Behav 1996;59: 179–187.
- Poppitt SD, Eckhardt JW, McGonagle J, Murgatroyd PR, Prentice AM. Short-term effects of alcohol consumption on appetite and energy intake. Physiol Behav 1996;60:1063–1070.
- Van Wymepoundeke V, Béridot-Thérond ME, de La Guéronnière V, Fantino M. Influence of repeated consumption of beverages containing sucrose or intense sweeteners on food intake. Eur J Clin Nutr 2004;58:154–161.
- De Castro JM. The effects of the spontaneous ingestion of particular foods or beverages on the meal pattern and overall nutrient intake of humans. Physiol Behav 1993;53:1133–1144.
- Canty DJ, Chan MM. Effects of consumption of caloric vs noncaloric sweet drinks on indices of hunger and food consumption in normal adults. Am J Clin Nutr 1991;53:1159–1164.

7 Stookey JD, Constant F, Popkin BM, Gardner CD. Drinking water is associated with weight loss in overweight dieting women independent of diet and activity. Obesity (Silver Spring). 2008 Nov;16(11):2481-8. Epub 2008 Sep 11. PubMed PMID: 18787524.

8 A sampling of supporting research:

- Lee KW, Lee HJ, Lee CY. Antioxidant activity of black tea vs. green tea. J Nutr. 2002 Apr;132(4):785; author reply 786. PubMed PMID: 11925478.
- Cabrera C, Artacho R, Giménez R. Beneficial effects of green tea--a review. J Am Coll Nutr. 2006 Apr;25(2):79-99. Review. PubMed PMID: 16582024.
- Chung FL, Schwartz J, Herzog CR, Yang YM: Tea and cancer prevention: Studies in animals and humans. J Nutr133 :3268 –3274,2003 .
- Lambert JD, Yang CS: Mechanisms of cancer prevention by tea constituents. J Nutr133 :3262 –3267,2003 .
- Mittal A, Pate MS, Wylie RC, Tollesfsbol TO, Katiyar SK: EGCG down regulates telomerase in human breast carcinoma MCF-7 cells, leading to suppression of cell viability and induction of apoptosis. Int J Oncol24 :703 –710,2004 .[Medline]
- Laurie SA, Miller VA, Grant SC, Kris MG: Phase I study of green tea extract in patients with advanced lung cancer. Cancer Chemother Pharmacol55 :33 –38,2005 .[Medline]
- Siddiqui IA, Afaq F, Adhami VM, Ahmad N, Mukhtar H: Antioxidants of the beverage tea in promotion of human health. Antioxid Redox Signal6 :571 –582,2004 .[Medline]

- D'Alessandro T, Prasain J, Benton MR, Botting N, Moore R, Darley-Usmar V, Patel R, Barnes S: Polyphenols, inflammatory response, and cancer prevention: Chlorination of isoflavones by human neutrophils. J Nutr133 :3773 –3777,2003 .
- Chen J, Han C: The protective effect of tea on cancer: Human evidence. In Bidlach WR, Omaye ST, Meshin MS, Topham DK (eds): "Phytochemicals as Bioactive Agents." Lancaster: Technomic, pp131 –150,2000 .
- Hoshiyama Y, Kawaguchi T, Miura Y, Mizou T, Tokui N, Yatsuya H, Sakata K, Kondo T, Kikuchi S, Toyoshima H, Hayakawa N, Tamakoshi A, Ohno Y, Yoshimura T: A nested case-control study of stomach cancer in relation to green tea consumption in Japan. Br J Cancer90 :135 –138,2004 .[Medline]
- Rosengren RJ: Catechins and the treatment of breast cancer: Possible utility and mechanistic targets. Drugs6 :1073 –1078,2003 .
- Wu AH, Yu MC, Tseng CC, Hankin J, Pike MC: Green tea and risk of breast cancer in Asian Americans. Int J Cancer106 :574 –579,2003 .[Medline]
- Zhang M, Binns CV, Lee AH: Tea consumption and ovarian cancer risk: A case-control study in China. Cancer Epidemiol Biomarkers Prev11 :713 –718,2002 .[Abstract/Free Full Text]
- Jian L, Xie LP, Lee AH, Binns CW: Protective effect of green tea against prostate cancer: A case-control study in southeast China. Int J Cancer108 :130 –135,2004 .[Medline]
- Borrelli F, Capasso R, Russo A, Ernst E: Systematic review: green tea and gastrointestinal cancer risk. Aliment Pharmacol ther19 :497 –510,2004 .[Medline]
- Arab L, Il'yasova D: The epidemiology of tea consumption and colorectal cancer incidence. J Nutr133 :3310 –3318,2003 .
- Yang YC, Lu FH, Wu JS, Wu CH, Chang CJ: The protective effect of habitual tea consumption on hypertension. Arch Intern Med164 :1534 –1540,2004 .[Abstract/Free Full Text]
- Hodgson JM, Devine A, Puddey IB, Chan SY, Beilin LJ, Prince RL: Tea intake is inversely related to blood pressure in older women. J Nutr133 :2883 –2886,2003 .[Abstract/Free Full Text]
- Geleijnse J, Launer L, Hofman A, Pols H, Witteman J: Tea flavonoids may protect against atherosclerosis: The Rotterdam Study. Arch Intern Med159 :2170 –2174,1999 .[Abstract/Free Full Text]
- Sasazuki S, Kodama H, Yoshimasu K, Liu Y, Washio M, Tanaka K, Tokunaga S, Kono S, Arai H, Doy Y, Kawano T, Nakagaki O, Takada K, Koyanagi S, Hiyamuta K, Nii T, Shirai K, Ideishi M, Arakawa K, Mohri M, Takeshita A: Relation between green tea consumption and the severity of coronary atherosclerosis among Japanese men and women. Ann Epidemiol10 :401 –408,2000 .[Medline]
- "Green tea." University of Maryland Medical Center. N.p., n.d. Web. 24 Dec. 2010. <http://www.umm.edu/altmed/articles/green-tea-000255.htm>.
- Nakachi K, Matsuyama S, Miyake S, Suganuma M, Imai K: Preventive effects of drinking green tea on cancer and cardiovascular disease: Epidemiological evidence for multiple targeting prevention. Biofactors13 :49 –54,2000 .[Medline]
- Trevisanato S, Kim Y: Tea and health. Nutr Rev58 :1 –10,2000 .[Medline]
- Sesso H, Gaziano J, Buring J, Hennekens C: Coffee and tea intake and the risk of myocardial infarction. Am J Epidemiol149 :162 –169,1999 .[Abstract/Free Full Text]
- Peters U, Poole C, Arab L: Does tea affect cardiovascular disease? A meta-analysis. Am J Epidemiol154 :495 –503,2001 .[Abstract/Free Full Text]
- Hirano R, Momiyama Y, Takahashi R, Taniguchi H, Kondo K, Nakamura H, Ohusuzu F: Comparison of green tea intake in Japanese patients with and without angiographic coronary artery disease. Am J Cardiol90 :1150 –1153,2002 .[Medline]
- Hertog M, Sweetnam P, Fehily A, Elwood P, Kromhout D: Antioxidant flavonols and ischemic heart disease in a Welsh population of men: The Caerphilly study. Am J Clin Nutr65 :1489 –1494,1997 .[Abstract/Free Full Text]
- Mitscher LA, Jung M, Shankel D: Chemoprotection: a review of the potential therapeutic antioxi-

dant properties of green tea (Camellia sinensis) and certain of its constituents. Med Res Rev17 :327 −332,1997 .[Medline]

- Otake S, Makimura M, Kuroki T: Anticaries effects of polyphenolic compounds from Japanese green tea. Caries Res25 :438 −442,1991 .[Medline]
- Zhang J, Kashket S: Inhibition of salivary amylase by black and green teas and their effects on the intraoral hydrolysis of starch. Caries Res32 :233 −236,1998 .[Medline]
- Simpson A, Shaw L, Smith AJ: The bio-availability of fluoride from black tea. J Dent29 :15 −21,2001 .[Medline]
- Elmets CA, Singh D, Tubesing K, Matsui M, Katiyar S, Mukhtar H: Cutaneous photoprotection from ultraviolet injury by green tea polyphenols. J Am Acad Dermatol44 :425 −432,2001 .[Medline]
- Dulloo AG, Duret C, Rohrer D, Girardier L, Mensi N, Fathi M, Chantre P, Vandermander J: Efficacy of a green tea extract rich in catechin polyphenols and caffeine in increasing 24-h energy expenditure and fat oxidation in humans. Am J Clin Nutr70 :1040 −1045,1999 .[Abstract/Free Full Text]
- Zheng G, Sayama K, Okubo T, Junefa LR, Oguni I: Anti-obesity effects of three major components of green tea, catechins, caffeine and theanine in mice. In vivo18 :55 −62,2004 .[Abstract/Free Full Text]
- Juhel C, Armand M, Pafumi Y, Rosier C, Vandermander J, Larson D: Green tea extract (AR25°) inhibits lipolysis of triglycerides in gastric and duodenal medium in vitro. J Nutr Biochem11 :45 −51,2000 .[Medline]
- Chantre P, Lairon D: Recent findings of green tea extract AR25° (exolise) and its activity for the treatment of obesity. Phytomedicine9 :3 −8,2002 .[Medline]
- Tian WX, Li LC, Wu XD, Chen CC: Weight reduction by Chinese medicinal herbs may be related to inhibition of fatty acid synthase. Life Sci74 :2389 −2399,2004 .[Medline]
- Dulloo AG, Seydoux J, Girardier L, Chantre P, Vandermander J: Green tea and thermogenesis: interactions between catechin-polyphenols, caffeine and sympathetic activity. Int J Obes Relat Metab Disord24 :252 −258,2000 .[Medline]
- Kovacs EM, Lejeune MP, Nijs I, Westerterp-Plantenga MS: Effects of green tea on weight maintenance after body-weight loss. Br J Nutr91 :431 −437,2004 .[Medline]
- Wu CH, Lu FH, Chang CS, Chang TC, Wang RH, Chang CJ: Relationship among habitual tea consumption, percent body fat, and body fat distribution. Obes Res11 :1088 −1095,2003a .[Medline]
- Anderson RA, Polansky MM: Tea enhances insulin activity. J Agric Food Chem50 :7182 −7186,2002 .[Medline]
- Wu LY, Juan CC, Hsu YP, Hwang LS: Effect of tea green supplementation on insulin sensitivity in Sprague-Dawley rats. J Agric Food Chem52 :643 −648,2004 .[Medline]
- Yee YK, Koo MWL, Szeto ML: Chinese tea consumption and lower risk of Helicobacter infection. J Gastroenterol Hepatol17 :552 −555,2002 .[Medline]
- Toda M, Okubo S, Ohnishi R, Shimamura T: Antibacterial and bactericidal activities of Japanese green tea. J Nippon Med Sch44 :669 −672,1989 .
- Weber JM, Ruzindana-Umunyana A, Sicar S, Cowan J: Adenovirus infection is inhibited in vitro by green tea catechins. J Clin Virol28 : S91 ,2003 .
- Muraki S, Yamamoto S, Ishibashi H, Horiuchi T, Hosoi T, Suzuki T, Orimo H, Nakamura K: Green tea drinking is associated with increased bone mineral density. J Bone Miner Res18 : S241 − S241,2003 .
- Park H, Ko S, Kim J, Kim S: Effects of green tea extracts and polyphenols on the proliferation and activity of bone cells. J Bone Miner Res18 : S342 ,2003 .
- Kakuda T: Neuroprotective effects of the tea components theanine and catechins. Biol Pharm Bull25 :1513 −1518,2002 .[Medline]
- Dajas F, Rivera F, Blasina F, Arredondo F, Echeverri C, Lafon L, Morkio A, Heizen H: Cell cultura protection and in vivo neuroprotective capacity of flavonoids. Neurotox Res5 :425 −432,2003 .[Medline]

- Weinreb O, Mandel S, Amit T, Youdim MB: Neurological mechanisms of green tea polyphenols in Alzheimer's and Parkinson's diseases. J Nutr Biochem15 :506 –516,2004 .[Medline]
- Dvorakova K, Dorr RT, Valcies S, Timmermann B, Apounderts DS: Pharmacokinetics of the green tea derivative, EGCG, by the topical route of administration in mouse and human skin. Cancer Chemother Pharmacol43 :331 –335,1999 .[Medline]
- Ishizuk H, Eguchi H, Oda T, Ogawa S, Nakagawa K, Honjo S, Kono S: Relation of coffee, green tea, and caffeine intake to gallstone disease in middle-age Japanese men. Eur J Epidemiol18 :401 –405,2003 .[Medline]
- Thiagarajan G, Chandani S, Sundari CS, Rao SH, Kulkarni AV, Balasubramanian D: Antioxidant properties of green and black tea, and their potential ability to retard the progression of eye lens cataract. Exp Eye Res73 :393 –401,2001 .[Medline]
- Gupta SK, Halder N, Srivastava S, Trivedi D, Joshi S, Varma SD: Green tea (Camellia sinensis) protects against selenite-induced oxidative stress in experimental cataractogenesis. Ophthalmic Res34 :258 –263,2002 .[Medline]

9 A sampling of supporting research:
- Dulloo AG, Duret C, Rohrer D, Girardier L, Mensi N, Fathi M, Chantre P, Vandermander J. Efficacy of a green tea extract rich in catechin polyphenols and caffeine in increasing 24-h energy expenditure and fat oxidation in humans. Am J Clin Nutr. 1999 Dec;70(6):1040-5. PubMed PMID: 10584049.
- Kao YH, Chang HH, Lee MJ, Chen CL. Tea, obesity, and diabetes. Mol Nutr Food Res. 2006 Feb;50(2):188-210. Review. PubMed PMID: 16416476
- Dulloo AG, Seydoux J, Girardier L, Chantre P, Vandermander J. Green tea and thermogenesis: interactions between catechin-polyphenols, caffeine and sympathetic activity. Int J Obes Relat Metab Disord. 2000 Feb;24(2):252-8. PubMed PMID: 10702779.

10 "Caffeine — You may like caffeine's effects, but how much is too much?—MayoClinic.com." Mayo Clinic. N.p., n.d. Web. 24 Dec. 2010. <http://www.mayoclinic.com/health/caffeine/NU00600>.

11 "Caffeine content for coffee, tea, soda and more—MayoClinic.com." Mayo Clinic. N.p., n.d. Web. & wwww.exergyfiend.com

12 Friedman M, Levin CE, Lee SU, Kozukue N. Stability of green tea catechins in commercial tea leaves during storage for 6 months. J Food Sci. 2009 Mar;74(2):H47-51. PubMed PMID: 19323750.

13 A sampling of supporting research:
- Green RJ, Murphy AS, Schulz B, Watkins BA, Ferruzzi MG. Common tea formulations modulate in vitro digestive recovery of green tea catechins. Mol Nutr Food Res. 2007 Sep;51(9):1152-62. PubMed PMID: 17688297.
- Manning J, Roberts JC. Analysis of catechin content of commercial green tea products. J Herb Pharmacother. 2003;3(3):19-32. PubMed PMID: 15277054.
- Seeram NP, Henning SM, Niu Y, Lee R, Scheuller HS, Heber D. Catechin and caffeine content of green tea dietary supplements and correlation with antioxidant capacity. J Agric Food Chem. 2006 Mar 8;54(5):1599-603. PubMed PMID: 16506807.

14 DiMeglio DP, Mattes RD. Liquid versus solid carbohydrate: effects on food intake and body weight. Int J Obes Relat Metab Disord. 2000 Jun;24(6):794-800. PubMed PMID: 10878689. & Malik VS, Schulze MB, Hu FB. Intake of sugar-sweetened beverages and weight gain: a systematic review. Am J Clin Nutr. 2006 Aug;84(2):274-88. Review. PubMed PMID: 16895873.

15 Nationwide Food Consumption Surveys (1965, 1977-78) and NHANES (1988-94, 1999-02); Duffey & Popkin, Obesity (Silver Spring) 2007

16 Paarlberg, Robert. Food Politics : What Everyone Needs to Know. London: Oxford University Press, 2010. Print.

17 A sampling of supporting research:
- Jenkins DJ, Wolever TM, Vuksan V, Brighenti F, Cunnane SC, Rao AV, Jenkins AL, Buckley G, Patten R, Singer W, et al. Nibbling versus gorging: metabolic advantages of increased meal frequency. N

Engl J Med. 1989 Oct 5;321(14):929-34. PubMed PMID: 2674713.

- Wilson J, Wilson GJ. Contemporary issues in protein requirements and consumption for resistance trained athletes. J Int Soc Sports Nutr. 2006 Jun 5;3:7-27. PubMed PMID: 18500966; PubMed Central PMCID: PMC2129150.
- Wolever TM. Metabolic effects of continuous feeding. Metabolism. 1990 Sep;39(9):947-51. PubMed PMID: 2202886.
- Layman DK. Dietary Guidelines should reflect new understandings about adult protein needs. Nutr Metab (Lond). 2009 Mar 13;6:12. PubMed PMID: 19284668; PubMed Central PMCID: PMC2666737.
- Obesity and leanness. Basic aspects. Stock, M., Rothwell, N., Author Affiliation: Dep. Physiology, St. George's Hospital Medical School, London Univ., London, UK.

18 http://www.nal.usda.gov/fnic/foodcomp/search/ & Chu YF, Sun J, Wu X, Liu RH. Antioxidant and antiproliferative activities of common vegetables. J Agric Food Chem. 2002 Nov 6;50(23):6910-6. PubMed PMID: 12405796.

19 "Protein: Moving Closer to Center Stage—What Should You Eat?—the Nutrition Source—Harvard School of Public Health ." Harvard School of Public Health—HSPH. N.p., n.d. Web. 31 May 2010. <http://www.hsph.harvard.edu/nutritionsource/what-should-you-eat/protein-full-story/index.html>.

20 http://www.nal.usda.gov/fnic/foodcomp/search/

21 http://www.nal.usda.gov/fnic/foodcomp/search/

22 "ESS Website ESS : Agricultural production." FAO: FAO Home. N.p., n.d. Web. <http://www.fao.org/economic/ess/ess-publications/ess-yearbook/ess-yearbook2010/yearbook2010-production/en/>. & World Bank, World Development Indicators, U.S. Census Bureau—Population Division, World Bank, World Development Indicators, "ESS Website ESS : Agricultural production." FAO: FAO Home. N.p., n.d. Web. <http://www.fao.org/economic/ess/ess-publications/ess-yearbook/ess-yearbook2010/yearbook2010-production/en/>.

23 "World Economic Outlook Database April 2011." IMF -- International Monetary Fund Home Page. N.p., n.d. Web. 11 May 2011. <http://imf.org/external/pubs/ft/weo/2011/01/weodata/index.aspx>.

24 A sampling of supporting research:
- http://apps.who.int/bmi/index.jsp
- "Obesity Explosion May Weigh on China's Future." Daily Nature and Science News and Headlines | National Geographic News. N.p., n.d. Web. 10 May 2011. <http://news.nationalgeographic.com/news/2006/08/060808-china-fat.html>.
- World Bank, World Development Indicators

Chapter 27

1 "How just six minutes of exercise can be as healthy as six hours | Scotsman (Edinburgh, Scotland), the Newspaper | Find Articles at BNET." Find Articles at BNET | News Articles, Magazine Back Issues & Reference Articles on All Topics. N.p., n.d. Web. 17 Aug. 2010. <http://findarticles.com/p/news-articles/scotsman-edinburgh-scotland-the/mi_7951/is_2005_June_6/just-minutes-exercise-healthy-hours/ai_n34034903/>.

2 A sampling of supporting research:
- Progression and Resistance Training http://www.fitness.gov/Digest-September2005.pdf
- Gibala M. Molecular responses to high-intensity interval exercise. Appl Physiol Nutr Metab. 2009 Jun;34(3):428-32. Review. PubMed PMID: 19448710.
- Eaton SB, Cordain L, Sparling PB. Evolution, body composition, insulin receptor competition, and insulin resistance. Prev Med. 2009 Oct;49(4):283-5. Epub 2009 Aug 15. PubMed PMID: 19686772.
- Craig BW, Everhart J, Brown R. The influence of high-resistance training on glucose tolerance in young and elderly subjects. Mech Ageing Dev. 1989 Aug;49(2):147-57. Review. PubMed PMID: 2677535.

- Miller WJ, Sherman WM, Ivy JL. Effect of strength training on glucose tolerance and post-glucose insulin response. Med Sci Sports Exerc. 1984 Dec;16(6):539-43. PubMed PMID: 6392812.
- "Metabolic syndrome—MayoClinic.com." Mayo Clinic medical information and tools for healthy living—MayoClinic.com. N.p., n.d. Web. 30 Nov. 2010. <http://www.mayoclinic.com/health/ metabolic+syndrome/DS00522>.
- Harrison BC, Leinwand LA. Fighting fat with muscle: bulking up to slim down. Cell Metab. 2008 Feb;7(2):97-8. Review. PubMed PMID: 18249167.

3 Lee SJ. Regulation of muscle mass by myostatin. Annu Rev Cell Dev Biol. 2004;20:61-86. Review. PubMed PMID: 15473835.

4 Kolata, Gina Bari. Ultimate Fitness: The Quest for Truth about Exercise and Health. New York: Farrar, Straus and Giroux, 2003. Print.

5 Kolata, Gina Bari. Ultimate Fitness: The Quest for Truth about Exercise and Health. New York: Farrar, Straus and Giroux, 2003. Print

6 A sampling of supporting research:

- Ades PA, Savage PD, Brochu M, Tischler MD, Lee NM, Poehlman ET. Resistance training increases total daily energy expenditure in disabled older women with coronary heart disease. J Appl Physiol. 2005 Apr;98(4):1280-5. PubMed PMID:15772059.
- Björntorp P. The regulation of adipose tissue distribution in humans. Int J Obes Relat Metab Disord. 1996 Apr;20(4):291-302. Review. PubMed PMID: 8680455.
- Blackburn GL, Wilson GT, Kanders BS, Stein LJ, Lavin PT, Adler J, Brownell KD. Weight cycling: The experience of human dieters. Am J Clin Nutr. 1989 May;49(5 Suppl):1105-9. PubMed PMID: 2718940.
- Candow DG, Chilibeck PD, Abeysekara S, Zello GA. Short-term Heavy Resistance Training Eliminates Age-Related Deficits in Muscle Mass and Strength in Healthy
- Calles-Escandón J, Arciero PJ, Gardner AW, Bauman C, Poehlman ET. Basal fat oxidation decreases with aging in women. J Appl Physiol. 1995 Jan;78(1):266-71. PubMed PMID: 7713822
- Gilliat-Wimberly M, Manore MM, Woolf K, Swan PD, Carroll SS. Effects of habitual physical activity on the resting metabolic rates and body compositions of women aged 35 to 50 years. J Am Diet Assoc. 2001 Oct;101(10):1181-8. PubMed PMID: 11678489.
- Gotshalk, L.A., et.al. (1996). Pituitary-gonadal hormonal responses of multi-set vs. single -set resistance training. Journal of Strength and Conditioning Research. 10(4):286.
- Harman SM, Metter EJ, Tobin JD, Pearson J, Blackman MR; Baltimore Longitudinal Study of Aging. Longitudinal effects of aging on serum total and free testosterone levels in healthy men. Baltimore Longitudinal Study of Aging. J Clin Endocrinol Metab. 2001 Feb;86(2):724-31. PubMed PMID: 11158037.
- http://www.cnn.com/2009/HEALTH/expert.q.a/06/05/building.muscle.nutrition.jampolis/index. html Dr. Steve Fleck, chair of the Sport Science Department at Colorado College and a member of the International Society of Sports Nutrition
- Hunter GR, Wetzstein CJ, Fields DA, Brown A, Bamman MM. Resistance training increases total energy expenditure and free-living physical activity in older adults. J Appl Physiol. 2000 Sep;89(3):977-84. PubMed PMID: 10956341.
- Ivy JL, Zderic TW, Fogt DL. Prevention and treatment of non-insulin-dependent diabetes mellitus. Exerc Sport Sci Rev. 1999;27:1-35. Review. PubMed PMID: 10791012.
- Kraemer WJ, Ratamess NA. Hormonal responses and adaptations to resistance training and training. Sports Med. 2005;35(4):339-61. Review. PubMed PMID:15831061.
- Kraemer WJ. Endocrine responses to resistance training. Med Sci Sports Exerc. 1988 Oct;20(5 Suppl):S152-7. Review. PubMed PMID: 3057315.
- Leibel RL, Rosenbaum M, Hirsch J. Changes in energy expenditure resulting from altered body weight. N Engl J Med. 1995 Mar 9;332(10):621-8. Erratum in: N Engl J Med 1995 Aug 10;333(6):399.

PubMed PMID: 7632212.

- Obesity and leanness. Basic aspects. Stock, M., Rothwell, N., Author Affiliation: Dep. Physiology, St. George's Hospital Medical School, London Univ., London, UK.
- Piers LS, Soares MJ, McCormack LM, O'Dea K. Is there evidence for an age-related reduction in metabolic rate? J Appl Physiol. 1998 Dec;85(6):2196-204. PubMed PMID: 9843543.
- Poehlman ET, Mepoundy C. Resistance training and energy balance. Int J Sport Nutr. 1998 Jun;8(2):143-59. Review. PubMed PMID: 9637193.
- Rasmussen BB, Wolfe RR. Regulation of fatty acid oxidation in skeletal muscle. Annu Rev Nutr. 1999;19:463-84. Review. PubMed PMID: 10448533.
- Schutz Y, Jequier E. Resting Energy Expenditure, thermic Effect of Food, and Total Energy Expenditure In: Bray GA, Couchard d, James WP, eds. Handbook of Obesity. New York: Marcel Dekker, 1997: 443-456.
- Simoneau JA. Kelly D. Skeletal Muscle and Obesity In: Bray GA, Couchard d, James WP, eds. Handbook of Obesity. New York: Marcel Dekker, 1997: 539-553.
- Snyder PJ. Decreasing testosterone with increasing age: more factors, more questions. J Clin Endocrinol Metab. 2008 Jul;93(7):2477-8. PubMed PMID: 18617703.
- Staley, Charles. Muscle Logic : Escalating Density Training. Emmaus, Pa.: Rodale Books, 2005. Print. Poehlman ET, Mepoundy C. Resistance training and energy balance. Int J Sport Nutr. 1998 Jun;8(2):143-59. Review. PubMed PMID: 9637193.
- Stárka L, Pospísilová H, Hill M. Free testosterone and free dihydrotestosterone throughout the life span of men. J Steroid Biochem Mol Biol. 2009 Aug;116(1-2):118-20. Epub 2009 May 22. PubMed PMID: 19465126.
- van Pelt RE, Dinneno FA, Seals DR, Jones PP. Age-related decline in RMR in physically active men: relation to exercise volume and energy intake. Am J Physiol Endocrinol Metab. 2001 Sep;281(3):E633-9. PubMed PMID: 11500320.
- Van Pelt RE, Jones PP, Davy KP, Desouza CA, Tanaka H, Davy BM, Seals DR. Regular exercise and the age-related decline in resting metabolic rate in women. J Clin Endocrinol Metab. 1997 Oct;82(10):3208-12. PubMed PMID: 9329340.
- Weigle DS, Sande KJ, Iverius PH, Monsen ER, Brunzell JD. Weight loss leads to a marked decrease in nonresting energy expenditure in ambulatory human subjects. Metabolism. 1988 Oct;37(10):930-6. PubMed PMID: 3173112.
- Ferrando AA, Sheffield-Moore M, Yeckel CW, Gilkison C, Jiang J, Achacosa A, Lieberman SA, Tipton K, Wolfe RR, Urban RJ. Testosterone administration to older men improves muscle function: molecular and physiological mechanisms. Am J Physiol Endocrinol Metab. 2002 Mar;282(3):E601-7. PubMed PMID: 11832363.
- Meirelles, Cláudia de Mello and GOMES, Paulo Sergio Chagas. Acute effects of resistance training on energy expenditure: revisiting the impact of the training variables. Rev Bras Med Esporte [online]. 2004, vol.10, n.2 [cited 2010-08-10], pp. 122-130 .

7 Izumiya Y, Hopkins T, Morris C, Sato K, Zeng L, Viereck J, Hamilton JA, Ouchi N, LeBrasseur NK, Walsh K. Fast/Glycolytic muscle fiber growth reduces fat mass and improves metabolic parameters in obese mice. Cell Metab. 2008 Feb;7(2):159-72. PubMed PMID: 18249175.

Chapter 28

1 Izumiya Y, Hopkins T, Morris C, Sato K, Zeng L, Viereck J, Hamilton JA, Ouchi N, LeBrasseur NK, Walsh K. Fast/Glycolytic muscle fiber growth reduces fat mass and improves metabolic parameters in obese mice. Cell Metab. 2008 Feb;7(2):159-72. PubMed PMID: 18249175.
2 Little, John, and Doug Mcguff. Body by Science: A Research Based Program to Get the Results You Want in 12 Minutes a Week. 1 ed. New York: McGraw-Hill, 2008.

3   Carpinelli RN, Otto RM. Strength training. Single versus multiple sets. Sports Med. 1998 Aug;26(2):73-84. Review. PubMed PMID: 9777681.

4   A sampling the research supporting the Deep exercise principle:
  - Saladin, Kenneth. Anatomy and Physiology: The Unity of Form and Function. 5 ed. New York: Mc-Graw-Hill Science/Engineering/Math, 2009. Print.
  - Henneman E, Olson Cb. Relations Between Structure And Function In the Design of Skeletal Muscles. J Neurophysiol. 1965 May;28:581-98. Pubmed Pmid: 14328455.
  - Harrison BC, Leinwand LA. Fighting fat with muscle: bulking up to slim down. Cell Metab. 2008 Feb;7(2):97-8. Review. PubMed PMID: 18249167.
  - Henneman E, Somjen G, Carpenter DO. Excitability and inhibitability of motoneurons of different sizes. J Neurophysiol. 1965 May;28(3):599-620. PubMed PMID: 5835487.
  - Progression and Resistance Training http://www.fitness.gov/Digest-September2005.pdf
  - Goto K, Ishii N, Kizuka T, Takamatsu K. The impact of metabolic stress on hormonal responses and muscular adaptations. Med Sci Sports Exerc. 2005 Jun;37(6):955-63. PubMed PMID: 15947720.
  - Costanzo, Linda S.. Physiology (Saunders Text and Review Series). 2nd ed. Philadelphia: W.B. Saunders Company, 2002. Print.
  - Wilcox G. Insulin and insulin resistance. Clin Biochem Rev. 2005 May;26(2):19-39. PubMed PMID: 16278749; PubMed Central PMCID: PMC1204764.
  - Milner-Brown HS, Stein RB, Yemm R. The orderly recruitment of human motor units during voluntary isometric contractions. J Physiol. 1973 Apr;230(2):359-70. PubMed PMID: 4350770; PubMed Central PMCID: PMC1350367.
  - Mendell LM. The size principle: a rule describing the recruitment of motoneurons. J Neurophysiol. 2005 Jun;93(6):3024-6. PubMed PMID: 15914463.
  - Cope TC, Sokoloff AJ. Orderly recruitment among motoneurons supplying different muscles. J Physiol Paris. 1999 Jan-Apr;93(1-2):81-5. Review. PubMed PMID: 10084711.
  - Pruves, Dale. Neuroscience, Fourth Edition. Fourth Edition ed. Sunderland: Sinauer Associates, Inc., 2007. Print.
  - Henneman E, Somjen G, Carpenter Do. Functional Significance of Cell Size In Spinal Motoneurons. J Neurophysiol. 1965 May;28:560-80. Pubmed Pmid: 14328454.

Chapter 29

1   A sampling of supporting research:
  - Kersten S. Mechanisms of nutritional and hormonal regulation of lipogenesis. EMBO Rep. 2001 Apr;2(4):282-6. Review. PubMed PMID: 11306547; PubMed Central PMCID: PMC1083868.
  - Obesity and leanness. Basic aspects. Stock, M., Rothwell, N., Author Affiliation: Dep. Physiology, St. George's Hospital Medical School, London Univ., London, UK.
  - Bengtsson BA, Edén S, Lönn L, Kvist H, Stokland A, Lindstedt G, Bosaeus I, Tölli J, Sjöström L, Isaksson OG. Treatment of adults with growth hormone (GH) deficiency with recombinant human GH. J Clin Endocrinol Metab. 1993 Feb;76(2):309-17. PubMed PMID: 8432773.

2   A sampling of supporting research:
  - Harrison BC, Leinwand LA. Fighting fat with muscle: bulking up to slim down. Cell Metab. 2008 Feb;7(2):97-8. Review. PubMed PMID: 18249167.
  - Izumiya Y, Hopkins T, Morris C, Sato K, Zeng L, Viereck J, Hamilton JA, Ouchi N, LeBrasseur NK, Walsh K. Fast/Glycolytic muscle fiber growth reduces fat mass and improves metabolic parameters in obese mice. Cell Metab. 2008 Feb;7(2):159-72. PubMed PMID: 18249175; PubMed Central PMCID: PMC2828690.
  - Ballor, D.L., Becque, M.D., & Katch, V.L. (1987). Metabolic responses during hydraulic resistance training. Medicine & Science in Sports & Exercise 19, 363-367.

- Kraemer,W.J. & Ratamess, N.A. (2005). Hormonal responses and adaptations to resistance training and training. Sports Medicine 35, 339-361.
- Kraemer WJ, Ratamess NA. Fundamentals of resistance training: progression and exercise prescription. Med Sci Sports Exerc. 2004 Apr;36(4):674-88. Review. PubMed PMID: 15064596.
- Pritzlaff CJ, Wideman L, Blumer J, Jensen M, Abbott RD, Gaesser GA, Veldhuis JD, Weltman A. Catecholamine release, growth hormone secretion, and energy expenditure during exercise vs. recovery in men. J Appl Physiol. 2000 Sep;89(3):937-46. PubMed PMID: 10956336.
- Pritzlaff CJ, Wideman L, Weltman JY, Abbott RD, Gutgesell ME, Hartman ML, Veldhuis JD, Weltman A. Impact of acute exercise intensity on pulsatile growth hormone release in men. J Appl Physiol. 1999 Aug;87(2):498-504. PubMed PMID: 10444604

3   A sampling of supporting research:
- Yeaman SJ. Hormone-sensitive lipase--new roles for an old enzyme. Biochem J. 2004 Apr 1;379(Pt 1):11-22. Review. PubMed PMID: 14725507; PubMed Central PMCID: PMC1224062.
- [|de Meijer J] (1998-05-01). Hormone sensitive lipase: structure, function and regulation. demeijer. com. http://demeijer.com/biology/scriptie.pdf. Retrieved 02-09-2010. A thesis written at the Biochemical Physiology Research Group, Department of Experimental Zoology, University of Utrecht, under supervision of dr. W. J. A. van Marrewijk
- Ades PA, Savage PD, Brochu M, Tischler MD, Lee NM, Poehlman ET. Resistance training increases total daily energy expenditure in disabled older women with coronary heart disease. J Appl Physiol. 2005 Apr;98(4):1280-5. PubMed PMID:15772059.
- Björntorp P. The regulation of adipose tissue distribution in humans. Int J Obes Relat Metab Disord. 1996 Apr;20(4):291-302. Review. PubMed PMID: 8680455.
- Blackburn GL, Wilson GT, Kanders BS, Stein LJ, Lavin PT, Adler J, Brownell KD. Weight cycling: The experience of human dieters. Am J Clin Nutr. 1989 May;49(5 Suppl):1105-9. PubMed PMID: 2718940.
- Candow DG, Chilibeck PD, Abeysekara S, Zello GA. Short-term Heavy Resistance Training Eliminates Age-Related Deficits in Muscle Mass and Strength in Healthy
- Calles-Escandón J, Arciero PJ, Gardner AW, Bauman C, Poehlman ET. Basal fat oxidation decreases with aging in women. J Appl Physiol. 1995 Jan;78(1):266-71. PubMed PMID: 7713822
- Gilliat-Wimberly M, Manore MM, Woolf K, Swan PD, Carroll SS. Effects of habitual physical activity on the resting metabolic rates and body compositions of women aged 35 to 50 years. J Am Diet Assoc. 2001 Oct;101(10):1181-8. PubMed PMID: 11678489.
- Gotshalk, L.A., et.al. (1996). Pituitary-gonadal hormonal responses of multi-set vs. single -set resistance training. Journal of Strength and Conditioning Research. 10(4):286.
- Harman SM, Metter EJ, Tobin JD, Pearson J, Blackman MR; Baltimore Longitudinal Study of Aging. Longitudinal effects of aging on serum total and free testosterone levels in healthy men. Baltimore Longitudinal Study of Aging. J Clin Endocrinol Metab. 2001 Feb;86(2):724-31. PubMed PMID: 11158037.
- http://www.cnn.com/2009/HEALTH/expert.q.a/06/05/building.muscle.nutrition.jampolis/index. html Dr. Steve Fleck, chair of the Sport Science Department at Colorado College and a member of the International Society of Sports Nutrition
- Hunter GR, Wetzstein CJ, Fields DA, Brown A, Bamman MM. Resistance training increases total energy expenditure and free-living physical activity in older adults. J Appl Physiol. 2000 Sep;89(3):977-84. PubMed PMID: 10956341.
- Ivy JL, Zderic TW, Fogt DL. Prevention and treatment of non-insulin-dependent diabetes mellitus. Exerc Sport Sci Rev. 1999;27:1-35. Review. PubMed PMID: 10791012.
- Kraemer WJ, Ratamess NA. Hormonal responses and adaptations to resistance training and training. Sports Med. 2005;35(4):339-61. Review. PubMed PMID:15831061.
- Kraemer WJ. Endocrine responses to resistance training. Med Sci Sports Exerc. 1988 Oct;20(5

Suppl):S152-7. Review. PubMed PMID: 3057315.

- Leibel RL, Rosenbaum M, Hirsch J. Changes in energy expenditure resulting from altered body weight. N Engl J Med. 1995 Mar 9;332(10):621-8. Erratum in: N Engl J Med 1995 Aug 10;333(6):399. PubMed PMID: 7632212.
- Obesity and leanness. Basic aspects. Stock, M., Rothwell, N., Author Affiliation: Dep. Physiology, St. George's Hospital Medical School, London Univ., London, UK.
- Piers LS, Soares MJ, McCormack LM, O'Dea K. Is there evidence for an age-related reduction in metabolic rate? J Appl Physiol. 1998 Dec;85(6):2196-204. PubMed PMID: 9843543.
- Poehlman ET, Mepoundy C. Resistance training and energy balance. Int J Sport Nutr. 1998 Jun;8(2):143-59. Review. PubMed PMID: 9637193.
- Rasmussen BB, Wolfe RR. Regulation of fatty acid oxidation in skeletal muscle. Annu Rev Nutr. 1999;19:463-84. Review. PubMed PMID: 10448533.
- Schutz Y, Jequier E. Resting Energy Expenditure, thermic Effect of Food, and Total Energy Expenditure In: Bray GA, Couchard d, James WP, eds. Handbook of Obesity. New York: Marcel Dekker, 1997: 443-456.
- Simoneau JA. Kelly D. Skeletal Muscle and Obesity In: Bray GA, Couchard d, James WP, eds. Handbook of Obesity. New York: Marcel Dekker, 1997: 539-553.
- Snyder PJ. Decreasing testosterone with increasing age: more factors, more questions. J Clin Endocrinol Metab. 2008 Jul;93(7):2477-8. PubMed PMID: 18617703.
- Staley, Charles. Muscle Logic : Escalating Density Training. Emmaus, Pa.: Rodale Books, 2005. Print. Poehlman ET, Mepoundy C. Resistance training and energy balance. Int J Sport Nutr. 1998 Jun;8(2):143-59. Review. PubMed PMID: 9637193.
- Stárka L, Pospísilová H, Hill M. Free testosterone and free dihydrotestosterone throughout the life span of men. J Steroid Biochem Mol Biol. 2009 Aug;116(1-2):118-20. Epub 2009 May 22. PubMed PMID: 19465126.
- van Pelt RE, Dinneno FA, Seals DR, Jones PP. Age-related decline in RMR in physically active men: relation to exercise volume and energy intake. Am J Physiol Endocrinol Metab. 2001 Sep;281(3):E633-9. PubMed PMID: 11500320.
- Van Pelt RE, Jones PP, Davy KP, Desouza CA, Tanaka H, Davy BM, Seals DR. Regular exercise and the age-related decline in resting metabolic rate in women. J Clin Endocrinol Metab. 1997 Oct;82(10):3208-12. PubMed PMID: 9329340.
- Weigle DS, Sande KJ, Iverius PH, Monsen ER, Brunzell JD. Weight loss leads to a marked decrease in nonresting energy expenditure in ambulatory human subjects. Metabolism. 1988 Oct;37(10):930-6. PubMed PMID: 3173112.

Chapter 30

1   Babraj JA, Vollaard NB, Keast C, Guppy FM, Cottrell G, Timmons JA. Extremely short duration high intensity interval training substantially improves insulin action in young healthy males. BMC Endocr Disord. 2009 Jan 28;9:3. PubMed PMID: 19175906; PubMed Central PMCID: PMC2640399.

2   A sampling of supporting research:
- Wernbom M, Augustsson J, Thomeé R. The influence of frequency, intensity, volume and mode of strength training on whole muscle cross-sectional area in humans. Sports Med. 2007;37(3):225-64. Review. PubMed PMID: 17326698.
- Kraemer,W.J. & Ratamess, N.A. (2004). Fundamentals of resistance training: progression and exercise prescription. Medicine & Science in Sports & Exercise 36, 674-688.
- Fry AC. The Role of Training Intensity in Resistance training Overtraining and Overreaching. In: Kreider RB. Fry AC, O'Toole ML, editors. Overtraining in sport. Champaign (IL): Human Kinetics, 1998: 107-27.

3   A sampling of supporting research:
- Golden CL, Graves JE, Buchanan P, Dudly G. Eccentric and Concentric Strength After Repeated Bouts of Intense Exercise. Med Sci Sports Exerc 1991; 23 (Suppl): 655A.
- Golden CL, Dudley GA. Strength after bouts of eccentric or concentric actions. Med Sci Sports Exerc. 1992 Aug;24(8):926-33. PubMed PMID: 1406179.
- Fridén J; Sjöström M; Ekblom B. Myofibrillar damage following intense eccentric exercise in man. Int J Sports Med. 1983; 4(3):170-6 (ISSN: 0172-4622)
- Cleak MJ, Eston RG. Muscle soreness, swelling, stiffness and strength loss after intense eccentric exercise. Br J Sports Med. 1992 Dec;26(4):267-72. PubMed PMID: 1490222; PubMed Central PMCID: PMC1479005.
- Newham DJ, McPhail G, Mills KR, Edwards RH. Ultrastructural changes after concentric and eccentric contractions of human muscle. J Neurol Sci. 1983 Sep;61(1):109-22. PubMed PMID: 6631446.
- O'Reilly KP, Warhol MJ, Fielding RA, Frontera WR, Meredith CN, Evans WJ. Eccentric exercise-induced muscle damage impairs muscle glycogen repletion. J Appl Physiol. 1987 Jul;63(1):252-6. PubMed PMID: 3624128.

Chapter 31

1   Wernbom M, Augustsson J, Thomeé R. The influence of frequency, intensity, volume and mode of strength training on whole muscle cross-sectional area in humans. Sports Med. 2007;37(3):225-64. Review. PubMed PMID: 17326698.
2   A sampling of supporting research:
- Parr JJ, Yarrow JF, Garbo CM, Borsa PA. Symptomatic and functional responses to concentric-eccentric isokinetic versus eccentric-only isotonic exercise. J Athl Train. 2009 Sep-Oct;44(5):462-8. PubMed PMID: 19771283; PubMed Central PMCID: PMC2742454.
- Keogh, J. W. L., G. J. Wilson, And R. P. Weatherby. A Crosssectional Comparison of Different Resistance Training Techniques In the Bench Press. J. Strength Cond. Res. 13:247–258, 1999.
- Tomberlin JP, Basford JR, Schwen EE, Orte PA, Scott SC, Laughman RK, Ilstrup DM. Comparative study of isokinetic eccentric and concentric quadriceps training. J Orthop Sports Phys ther. 1991;14(1):31-6. PubMed PMID: 18796832.
- Clarkson PM, Nosaka K, Braun B. Muscle function after exercise-induced muscle damage and rapid adaptation. Med Sci Sports Exerc. 1992 May;24(5):512-20. Review. PubMed PMID: 1569847.
- Colliander EB, Tesch PA. Effects of eccentric and concentric muscle actions in resistance training. Acta Physiol Scand. 1990 Sep;140(1):31-9. PubMed PMID:2275403.
- Hather BM, Tesch PA, Buchanan P, Dudley GA. Influence of eccentric actions on skeletal muscle adaptations to resistance training. Acta Physiol Scand. 1991 Oct;143(2):177-85. PubMed PMID: 1835816.
- Vikne H, Refsnes PE, Ekmark M, Medbø JI, Gundersen V, Gundersen K. Muscular performance after concentric and eccentric exercise in trained men. Med Sci Sports Exerc. 2006 Oct;38(10):1770-81. PubMed PMID: 17019299.
- Komi PV, Buskirk ER. Effect of eccentric and concentric muscle conditioning on tension and electrical activity of human muscle. Ergonomics. 1972 Jul;15(4):417-34. PubMed PMID: 4634421.
- Hortobágyi T, Dempsey L, Fraser D, Zheng D, Hamilton G, Lambert J, Dohm L. Changes in muscle strength, muscle fibre size and myofibrillar gene expression after immobilization and retraining in humans. J Physiol. 2000 Apr 1;524 Pt 1:293-304. PubMed PMID: 10747199; PubMed Central PMCID: PMC2269843.
- Seger, JY, Arvidson B, and Thorstensson A. Specific effects of eccentric and concentric training on muscle strength and morphology in humans. Eur J Appl Physiol 79: 49-57, 1998.
- Duncan PW, Chandler JM, Cavanaugh DK, Johnson KR, Buehler AG. Mode and speed specificity

of eccentric and concentric exercise training. J Orthop Sports Phys ther. 1989;11(2):70-5. PubMed PMID: 18796927.

- Farthing JP, Chilibeck PD. The effects of eccentric and concentric training at different velocities on muscle hypertrophy. Eur J Appl Physiol. 2003 Aug;89(6):578-86. Epub 2003 May 17. PubMed PMID: 12756571.

3   A sampling of supporting research:

- Dudley GA, Tesch PA, Miller BJ, Buchanan P. Importance of eccentric actions in performance adaptations to resistance training. Aviat Space Environ Med. 1991 Jun;62(6):543-50. PubMed PMID: 1859341.

- Watkins, P.H (2010) Augmented Eccentric Loading: Theoretical and Practical Applications for the Strength and Conditioning Professional. Professional Strength and Conditioning, UKSCA Issue 17, pp4-12

- Higbie EJ, Cureton KJ, Warren GL 3rd, Prior BM. Effects of concentric and eccentric training on muscle strength, cross-sectional area, and neural activation. J Appl Physiol. 1996 Nov;81(5):2173-81. PubMed PMID: 8941543.

- Nardone A, Romanò C, Schieppati M. Selective recruitment of high-threshold human motor units during voluntary isotonic lengthening of active muscles. J Physiol. 1989 Feb;409:451-71. PubMed PMID: 2585297; PubMed Central PMCID: PMC1190454.

- Henneman E, Somjen G, Carpenter Do. Functional Significance of Cell Size In Spinal Motoneurons. J Neurophysiol. 1965 May;28:560-80. Pubmed Pmid: 14328454.

- Wernbom M, Augustsson J, Thomeé R. The influence of frequency, intensity, volume and mode of strength training on whole muscle cross-sectional area in humans. Sports Med. 2007;37(3):225-64. Review. PubMed PMID: 17326698.

- Hortobágyi T, Barrier J, Beard D, Braspennincx J, Koens P, Devita P, Dempsey L, Lambert J. Greater initial adaptations to submaximal muscle lengthening than maximal shortening. J Appl Physiol. 1996 Oct;81(4):1677-82. PubMed PMID: 8904586.

- Enoka RM. Eccentric contractions require unique activation strategies by the nervous system. J Appl Physiol. 1996 Dec;81(6):2339-46. Review. PubMed PMID: 9018476

- Roig M, O'Brien K, Kirk G, Murray R, McKinnon P, Shadgan B, Reid WD. The effects of eccentric versus concentric resistance training on muscle strength and mass in healthy adults: a systematic review with meta-analysis. Br J Sports Med. 2009

4   A sampling of supporting research:

- Katz B. The relation between force and speed in muscular contraction. J Physiol. 1939 Jun 14;96(1):45-64. PubMed PMID: 16995114; PubMed Central PMCID:PMC1393840.

- Wernbom M, Augustsson J, Thomeé R. The influence of frequency, intensity, volume and mode of strength training on whole muscle cross-sectional area in humans. Sports Med. 2007;37(3):225-64. Review. PubMed PMID: 17326698.

- Reeves ND, Maganaris CN, Longo S, Narici MV. Differential adaptations to eccentric versus conventional resistance training in older humans. Exp Physiol. 2009 Jul;94(7):825-33. Epub 2009 Apr 24. PubMed PMID: 19395657.

Chapter 32

1   Tremblay A, Simoneau JA, Bouchard C. Impact of exercise intensity on body fatness and skeletal muscle metabolism. Metabolism. 1994 Jul;43(7):814-8. PubMed PMID: 8028502

2   Earnest CP. Exercise interval training: an improved stimulus for improving the physiology of pre-diabetes. Med Hypotheses. 2008 Nov;71(5):752-61. Epub 2008 Aug 15. PubMed PMID: 18707813.

3   Christmass MA, Dawson B, Arthur PG. Effect of work and recovery duration on skeletal muscle oxygenation and fuel use during sustained intermittent exercise. Eur J Appl Physiol Occup Physiol. 1999

Oct;80(5):436-47. PubMed PMID: 10502077.

4   Irving BA, Davis CK, Brock DW, Weltman JY, Swift D, Barrett EJ, Gaesser GA, Weltman A. Effect of exercise training intensity on abdominal visceral fat and body composition. Med Sci Sports Exerc. 2008 Nov;40(11):1863-72. PubMed PMID:18845966; PubMed Central PMCID: PMC2730190.

5   A sampling of supporting research:

• Gibala MJ, McGee SL. Metabolic adaptations to short-term high-intensity interval training: a little pain for a lot of gain? Exerc Sport Sci Rev. 2008 Apr;36(2):58-63. Review. PubMed PMID: 18362686.

• Gibala MJ, Little JP, van Essen M, Wilkin GP, Burgomaster KA, Safdar A, Raha S, Tarnopolsky MA. Short-term sprint interval versus traditional endurance training: similar initial adaptations in human skeletal muscle and exercise performance. J Physiol. 2006 Sep 15;575(Pt 3):901-11. Epub 2006 Jul 6. PubMed PMID: 16825308; PubMed Central PMCID: PMC1995688.

• "How just six minutes of exercise can be as healthy as six hours | Scotsman (Edinburgh, Scotland), the Newspaper | Find Articles at BNET." Find Articles at BNET | News Articles, Magazine Back Issues & Reference Articles on All Topics. N.p., n.d. Web. 17 Aug. 2010. <http://findarticles.com/p/news-articles/scotsman-edinburgh-scotland-the/mi_7951/is_2005_June_6/just-minutes-exercise-healthy-hours/ai_n34034903/>.

6   A sampling of supporting research

• Haram PM, Kemi OJ, Lee SJ, Bendheim MØ, Al-Share QY, Waldum HL, Gilligan LJ, Koch LG, Britton SL, Najjar SM, Wisløff U. Aerobic interval training vs. continuous moderate exercise in the metabolic syndrome of rats artificially selected for low aerobic capacity. Cardiovasc Res. 2009 Mar 1;81(4):723-32. Epub 2008 Dec 1. PubMed PMID: 19047339; PubMed Central PMCID: PMC2642601.

• Wisløff U, Støylen A, Loennechen JP, Bruvold M, Rognmo Ø, Haram PM, Tjønna AE, Helgerud J, Slørdahl SA, Lee SJ, Videm V, Bye A, Smith GL, Najjar SM, Ellingsen Ø, Skjaerpe T. Superior cardiovascular effect of aerobic interval training versus moderate continuous training in heart failure patients: a randomized study. Circulation. 2007 Jun 19;115(24):3086-94. Epub 2007 Jun 4. PubMed PMID: 17548726.

• King, J., Panton, L., Broeder, C., Browder, K., Quindry, J., & Rhea, L. (2001). A comparison of high intensity vs. low intensity exercise on body composition in overweight women. Medicine and Science in Sports & Exercise, 33, A2421

• Wisløff U, Ellingsen Ø, Kemi OJ. High-intensity interval training to maximize cardiac benefits of exercise training? Exerc Sport Sci Rev. 2009 Jul;37(3):139-46. Review. PubMed PMID: 19550205.

• Wisløff U, Nilsen TI, Drøyvold WB, Mørkved S, Slørdahl SA, Vatten LJ. A single weekly bout of exercise may reduce cardiovascular mortality: how little pain for cardiac gain? 'The HUNT study, Norway'. Eur J Cardiovasc Prev Rehabil. 2006 Oct;13(5):798-804. PubMed PMID: 17001221.

• Babraj JA, Vollaard NB, Keast C, Guppy FM, Cottrell G, Timmons JA. Extremely short duration high intensity interval training substantially improves insulin action in young healthy males. BMC Endocr Disord. 2009 Jan 28;9:3. PubMed PMID: 19175906; PubMed Central PMCID: PMC2640399.

• Talanian JL, Galloway SD, Heigenhauser GJ, Bonen A, Spriet LL. Two weeks of high-intensity aerobic interval training increases the capacity for fat oxidation during exercise in women. J Appl Physiol. 2007 Apr;102(4):1439-47. Epub 2006 Dec 14. PubMed PMID: 17170203.

• Burgomaster KA, Howarth KR, Phillips SM, Rakobowchuk M, Macdonald MJ, McGee SL, Gibala MJ. Similar metabolic adaptations during exercise after low volume sprint interval and traditional endurance training in humans. J Physiol. 2008 Jan 1;586(1):151-60. Epub 2007 Nov 8. PubMed PMID: 17991697; PubMed Central PMCID: PMC2375551.

• Rakobowchuk M, Tanguay S, Burgomaster KA, Howarth KR, Gibala MJ, MacDonald MJ. Sprint interval and traditional endurance training induce similar improvements in peripheral arterial stiffness and flow-mediated dilation in healthy humans. Am J Physiol Regul Integr Comp Physiol. 2008 Jul;295(1):R236-42. Epub 2008 Apr 23.PubMed PMID: 18434437; PubMed Central PMCID: PMC2494806.

- Perry CG, Heigenhauser GJ, Bonen A, Spriet LL. High-intensity aerobic interval training increases fat and carbohydrate metabolic capacities in human skeletal muscle. Appl Physiol Nutr Metab. 2008 Dec; 33(6):1112-23. PubMed PMID: 19088769.
7 Sesso HD, Paffenbarger RS Jr, Lee IM. Physical activity and coronary heart disease in men: The Harvard Alumni Health Study. Circulation. 2000 Aug 29;102(9):975-80. PubMed PMID: 10961960.
8 Paffenbarger RS Jr, Lee IM. Intensity of physical activity related to incidence of hypertension and all-cause mortality: an epidemiological view. Blood Press Monit. 1997 Jun;2(3):115-123. PubMed PMID: 10234104.
9 Lee IM, Sesso HD, Oguma Y, Paffenbarger RS Jr. Relative intensity of physical activity and risk of coronary heart disease. Circulation. 2003 Mar 4;107(8):1110-6. PubMed PMID: 12615787.
10 Haskell WL, Lee IM, Pate RR, Powell KE, Blair SN, Franklin BA, Macera CA, Heath GW, Thompson PD, Bauman A; American College of Sports Medicine; American Heart Association. Physical activity and public health: updated recommendation for adults from the American College of Sports Medicine and the American Heart Association. Circulation. 2007 Aug 28;116(9):1081-93. Epub 2007 Aug 1. PubMed PMID: 17671237.
11 Haram PM, Kemi OJ, Lee SJ, Bendheim MØ, Al-Share QY, Waldum HL, Gilligan LJ, Koch LG, Britton SL, Najjar SM, Wisløff U. Aerobic interval training vs. continuous moderate exercise in the metabolic syndrome of rats artificially selected for low aerobic capacity. Cardiovasc Res. 2009 Mar 1;81(4):723-32. Epub 2008 Dec 1. PubMed PMID: 19047339; PubMed Central PMCID: PMC2642601.
12 A sampling of supporting research:
- Swain DP, Franklin BA. Comparison of cardioprotective benefits of vigorous versus moderate intensity aerobic exercise. Am J Cardiol. 2006 Jan 1;97(1):141-7. Epub 2005 Nov 16. Review. PubMed PMID: 16377300.
- Coyle EF. Very intense exercise-training is extremely potent and time efficient: a reminder. J Appl Physiol. 2005 Jun;98(6):1983-4. PubMed PMID:15894535.
- Kemi OJ, Haram PM, Loennechen JP, Osnes JB, Skomedal T, Wisløff U, Ellingsen Ø. Moderate vs. high exercise intensity: differential effects on aerobic fitness, cardiomyocyte contractility, and endothelial function. Cardiovasc Res. 2005 Jul 1;67(1):161-72. Epub 2005 Apr 20. PubMed PMID: 15949480.
13 A sampling of supporting research:
- Helgerud J, Høydal K, Wang E, Karlsen T, Berg P, Bjerkaas M, Simonsen T, Helgesen C, Hjorth N, Bach R, Hoff J. Aerobic high-intensity intervals improve VO2max more than moderate training. Med Sci Sports Exerc. 2007 Apr;39(4):665-71. PubMed PMID: 17414804.
- Tanasescu M, Leitzmann MF, Rimm EB, Willett WC, Stampfer MJ, Hu FB. Exercise type and intensity in relation to coronary heart disease in men. JAMA. 2002 Oct 23-30;288(16):1994-2000. PubMed PMID: 12387651.
- Tyldum GA, Schjerve IE, Tjønna AE, Kirkeby-Garstad I, Stølen TO, Richardson RS, Wisløff U. Endothelial dysfunction induced by post-prandial lipemia: complete protection afforded by high-intensity aerobic interval exercise. J Am Coll Cardiol. 2009 Jan 13;53(2):200-6. PubMed PMID: 19130989; PubMed Central PMCID:PMC2650775.
- Tremblay A, Després JP, Leblanc C, Craig CL, Ferris B, Stephens T, Bouchard C. Effect of intensity of physical activity on body fatness and fat distribution. Am J Clin Nutr. 1990 Feb;51(2):153-7. PubMed PMID: 2305702.
- Myers J, Gullestad L, Vagelos R, Do D, Bellin D, Ross H, Fowler MB. Clinical, hemodynamic, and cardiopulmonary exercise test determinants of survival in patients referred for evaluation of heart failure. Ann Intern Med. 1998 Aug 15;129(4):286-93. PubMed PMID: 9729181.
- Treuth MS, Hunter GR, Williams M. Effects of exercise intensity on 24-h energy expenditure and substrate oxidation. Med Sci Sports Exerc. 1996 Sep;28(9):1138-43. PubMed PMID: 8883001.
- King, J., Panton, L., Broeder, C., Browder, K., Quindry, J., & Rhea, L. (2001). A comparison of high

intensity vs. low intensity exercise on body composition in overweight women. Medicine and Science in Sports & Exercise, 33, A2421

14 Oliver, J. Eric. Fat Politics: The Real Story behind America's Obesity Epidemic. New Ed ed. New York: Oxford University Press, USA, 2006. Print.

15 A sampling of supporting research:
- Wang Z, Heshka S, Zhang K, Boozer CN, Heymsfield SB. Resting energy expenditure: systematic organization and critique of prediction methods. Obes Res. 2001 May;9(5):331-6. Review. PubMed PMID: 11346676.
- 1998: Poehlman E T; Mepoundy C Resistance training and energy balance. International journal of sport nutrition 1998;8(2):143-59.
- Whitehead, Saffron A.; Nussey, Stephen (2001). Endocrinology: an integrated approach. Oxford: BIOS. pp. 122. ISBN 1-85996-252-1.
- FAO/OMS/UNU. Necessidades de energia e proteína: Série de relatos técnicos 724. Genebra: Organização Mundial da Saúde, 1998.

16 Michael Jenson MD in: Spiker, Ted, and David Zinczenko. The Abs Diet: The Six-Week Plan to Flatten Your Stomach and Keep You Lean for Life. Emmaus, Pa.: Rodale Books, 2005. Print.

17 A sampling of supporting research:
- Prentice AM, Black AE, Coward WA, Cole TJ. Energy expenditure in overweight and obese adults in affluent societies: an analysis of 319 doubly-labelled water measurements. Eur J Clin Nutr. 1996 Feb;50(2):93-7. PubMed PMID: 8641251.
- Stofan JR, DiPietro L, Davis D, Kohl HW III, Blair SN. Physical activity patterns associated with cardiorespiratory fitness and reduced mortality: The Aerobics Center Longitudinal Study. Am J Public Health 1998;88:1807-1813.
- Johnson JL, Slentz CA, Houmard JA, Samsa GP, Duscha BD, Aiken LB, McCartney JS, Tanner CJ, Kraus WE. Exercise training amount and intensity effects on metabolic syndrome (from Studies of a Targeted Risk Reduction Intervention through Defined Exercise). Am J Cardiol. 2007 Dec 15;100(12):1759-66. Epub 2007 Oct 29. PubMed PMID: 18082522; PubMed Central PMCID: PMC2190779.
- Manson JE, Hu FB, Rich-Edwards JW, Colditz GA, Stampfer MJ, Willett WC, Speizer FE, Hennekens CH. A prospective study of walking as compared with vigorous exercise in the prevention of coronary heart disease in women. N Engl J Med 1999;341:650-658.
- Oguma Y, Sesso HD, Paffenbarger RS Jr, Lee IM. Physical activity and all cause mortality in women: a review of the evidence. Br J Sports Med. 2002 Jun;36(3):162-72. Review. PubMed PMID: 12055109; PubMed Central PMCID: PMC1724493.
- Löllgen H, Böckenhoff A, Knapp G. Physical activity and all-cause mortality: an updated meta-analysis with different intensity categories. Int J Sports Med. 2009 Mar;30(3):213-24. Epub 2009 Feb 6. PubMed PMID: 19199202.
- Blair SN, Kohl HW 3rd, Paffenbarger RS Jr, Clark DG, Cooper KH, Gibbons LW. Physical fitness and all-cause mortality. A prospective study of healthy men and women. JAMA. 1989 Nov 3;262(17):2395-401. PubMed PMID: 2795824.
- Kesaniemi YK, Danforth E Jr, Jensen MD, Kopelman PG, Lefèbvre P, Reeder BA. Dose-response issues concerning physical activity and health: an evidence-based symposium. Med Sci Sports Exerc. 2001 Jun;33(6 Suppl):S351-8. PubMed PMID:11427759.
- Morris JN, Heady JA, Raffle PA, Roberts CG, Parks JW. Coronary heart-disease and physical activity of work. Lancet 1953;265:1111-1120.
- Paffenbarger RS, Hale WE. Work activity and coronary heart mortality. N Engl J Med 1975;292:545-550.
- Manson JE, Greenland P, LaCroix AZ, Stefanick ML, Mouton CP, Oberman A, Perri MG, Sheps DS, Pettinger MB, Siscovick DS. Walking compared with vigorous exercise for the prevention of cardio-

vascular events in women. N Engl J Med 2002;347:716-725.

- Hu FB, Sigal RJ, Rich-Edwards JW, Colditz GA, Solomon CG, Willett WC, Speizer FE, Manson JE. Walking compared with vigorous physical activity and risk of type 2 diabetes in women: a prospective study. JAMA 1999;282:1433-1439.

- Wei M, Gibbons LW, Mitchell TL, Kampert JB, Lee CD, Blair SN. The association between cardiorespiratory fitness and impaired fasting glucose and type 2 diabetes mellitus in men. Ann Intern Med 1999;130:89-96.

- Wei M, Kampert JB, Barlow CE, Nichaman MZ, Gibbons LW, Paffenbarger RS Jr, Blair SN. Relationship between low cardiorespiratory fitness and mortality in normal-weight, overweight, and obese men. JAMA 1999;282:1547-1553.

- Hu FB, Willett WC, Li T, Stampfer MJ, Colditz GA, Manson JE. Adiposity as compared with physical activity in predicting mortality among women. N Engl J Med 2004;351:2694-2703.

- Kannel WB, Wilson P, Blair SN. Epidemiological assessment of the role of physical activity and fitness in development of cardiovascular disease. Am Heart J 1985;109:876-885.

- Feinstein AR. The treatment of obesity: an analysis of methods, results, and factors which influence success. J Chronic Dis. 1960 Apr;11:349-93. PubMed PMID: 13821960.

Chapter 33

1 Haskell WL, Lee IM, Pate RR, Powell KE, Blair SN, Franklin BA, Macera CA, Heath GW, Thompson PD, Bauman A; American College of Sports Medicine; American Heart Association. Physical activity and public health: updated recommendation for adults from the American College of Sports Medicine and the American Heart Association. Circulation. 2007 Aug 28;116(9):1081-93. Epub 2007 Aug 1. PubMed PMID: 17671237.

2 Email correspondence with researcher John Little at on September 01, 2010. & Kolata, Gina Bari. Ultimate Fitness: The Quest for Truth about Exercise and Health. New York: Farrar, Straus and Giroux, 2003. Print.

3 Carpinelli RN. Berger in retrospect: effect of varied strength training programmes on strength. Br J Sports Med. 2002 Oct;36(5):319-24. Review. PubMed PMID: 12351327; PubMed Central PMCID: PMC1724552

4 A sampling of supporting research:

- Taaffe DR, Duret C, Wheeler S, Marcus R. Once-weekly resistance training improves muscle strength and neuromuscular performance in older adults. J Am Geriatr Soc. 1999 Oct;47(10):1208-14. PubMed PMID: 10522954.

- Burt J, Wilson R, Willardson JM. A comparison of once versus twice per week training on leg press strength in women. J Sports Med Phys Fitness. 2007 Mar;47(1):13-7. PubMed PMID: 17369792.

- Candow, Darren G., and Darren G. Burke. "Effect of short-term equal-volume resistance training with different workout frequency on muscle mass and strength in untrained men and women." Journal of Strength and Conditioning Research 21.1 (2007): 204+. Expanded Academic ASAP. Web. 9 Dec. 2009. <http://find.galegroup.com/gtx/start.do?prodId=EAIM&userGroupName=kcls_web>.

- Wernbom M, Augustsson J, Thomeé R. The influence of frequency, intensity, volume and mode of strength training on whole muscle cross-sectional area in humans. Sports Med. 2007;37(3):225-64. Review. PubMed PMID: 17326698.

- Carpinelli RN. Berger in retrospect: effect of varied strength training programmes on strength. Br J Sports Med. 2002 Oct;36(5):319-24. Review. PubMed PMID: 12351327; PubMed Central PMCID: PMC1724552.

- Hass CJ, Garzarella L, de Hoyos D, Pollock ML. Single versus multiple sets in long-term recreational weightlifters. Med Sci Sports Exerc. 2000 Jan;32(1):235-42. PubMed PMID: 10647555.

- Ostrowski, K. J., G. J. Wilson, R. Weatherby, P. W. Murphy, And A. D. Lyttle. The Effect of Strength training Volume On Hormonal Output And Muscular Size And Function. J. Strength Cond. Res. 11:148–154, 1997.

- D. Starkey, M. Welsch, and M. Pollock, "Equivalent Improvement in Strength Following High Intensity, Low and High Volume Training," (Paper presented at the annual meeting of the American College of Sports Medicine, Indianapolis, IN, Jone 2, 1994).)
- W. Wescott, K. Greenberger, and D. Milius, "Strength Training Research: Sets and Repetitions," Scholastic Coach 58 (1989): 73-84.
- Effect of resistance training volume and complexity on EMG, strength, and regional body composition Journal European Journal of Applied Physiology Publisher Springer Berlin / Heidepounderg ISSN 1439-6319 (Print) 1439-6327 (Online) Issue Volume 90, Numbers 5-6 / November, 2003 Category Original Article DOI 10.1007/s00421-003-0930-3 Pages 626-632 Subject Collection Biomedical and Life Sciences SpringerLink Date Thursday, February 19, 2004
- Berger RA. Effect of varied strength training programs on strength. Res Q 1962;33:168–81.
- Dudley, G.A. & Djamil, R. (1985). Incompatibility of endurance- and strength-training modes of exercise. Journal of Applied Physiology 59, 1446-1455.
- Berger, R.A. (1962). Optimum repetitions for the development of strength. Research Quarterly 33, 334-338.
- Campos, G.E.R., Luecke, T.J.,Wendeln, H.K., et al. (2002). Muscular adaptations in response to three different resistance-training regimens: specificity of repetition maximum training zones. European Journal of Applied Physiology 88, 50-60.
- Dudley, G.A., Tesch, P.A., Miller, B.J., & Buchanan, M.D. (1991). Importance of eccentric actions in performance adaptations to resistance training. Aviation, Space & Environmental Medicine 62, 543-550.
- Sale, D.G., Jacobs, I., MacDougall, J.D., & Garner, S. (1990). Comparisons of two regimens of concurrent strength and endurance training. Medicine & Science inSports & Exercise 22, 348-356.
- Starkey DB, Pollock ML, Ishida Y, Welsch MA, Brechue WF, Graves JE, Feigenbaum MS. Effect of resistance training volume on strength and muscle thickness. Med Sci Sports Exerc. 1996 Oct;28(10):1311-20. PubMed PMID: 8897390.

5   A sampling of supporting research:
- Wernbom M, Augustsson J, Thomeé R. The influence of frequency, intensity, volume and mode of strength training on whole muscle cross-sectional area in humans. Sports Med. 2007;37(3):225-64. Review. PubMed PMID: 17326698.
- Kraemer WJ, Ratamess NA. Fundamentals of resistance training: progression and exercise prescription. Med Sci Sports Exerc. 2004 Apr;36(4):674-88. Review. PubMed PMID: 15064596.
- Robinson, J.M., Stone, M.H., Johnson, R.L., et al. (1995). Effects of different strength training exercise/rest intervals on strength, power, and high intensity exercise endurance. Journal of Strength & Conditioning Research 9, 216-221.
- Pincivero, D.M., Lephart, S.M., & Karunakara, R.G. (1997). Effects of rest interval on isokinetic strength and functional performance after short term high intensity training. British Journal of Sports Medicine 31, 229-234.

6   Hansen S, Kvorning T, Kjaer M, Sjøgaard G. The effect of short-term strength training on human skeletal muscle: The importance of physiologically elevated hormone levels. Scand J Med Sci Sports. 2001 Dec;11(6):347-54. PubMed PMID: 11782267.

Chapter 34

1   Izumiya Y, Hopkins T, Morris C, Sato K, Zeng L, Viereck J, Hamilton JA, Ouchi N, LeBrasseur NK, Walsh K. Fast/Glycolytic muscle fiber growth reduces fat mass and improves metabolic parameters in obese mice. Cell Metab. 2008 Feb;7(2):159-72. PubMed PMID: 18249175.

2 Kraemer WJ, Ratamess NA. Fundamentals of resistance training: progression and exercise prescription. Med Sci Sports Exerc. 2004 Apr;36(4):674-88. Review. PubMed PMID: 15064596.

Chapter 36

1 Babraj JA, Vollaard NB, Keast C, Guppy FM, Cottrell G, Timmons JA. Extremely short duration high intensity interval training substantially improves insulin action in young healthy males. BMC Endocr Disord. 2009 Jan 28;9:3. PubMed PMID: 19175906; PubMed Central PMCID: PMC2640399.

Conclusion

1 Ravnskov, Uffe, and Joel M. Kauffman. Fat and Cholesterol Are Good for You. [S.l.]: GP, 2009. Print.
2 A sampling of supporting research:
  • http://en.wikipedia.org/wiki/List_of_countries_by_Muslim_population
  • http://en.wikipedia.org/wiki/Jewish_population
  • http://en.wikipedia.org/wiki/Hinduism
  • http://www.raw-food-health.net/NumberOfVegetarians.html
  • http://www.who.int/diabetes/facts/world_figures/en/
  • Longley, Robert. "Americans Now Spend Over 100 Hours a Year Commuting." U.S. Government Info—Resources. N.p., n.d. Web. 1 Dec. 2010. <http://usgovinfo.about.com/od/censusandstatistics/a/commutetimes.htm>.
  • "One Day in America—TIME." Breaking News, Analysis, Politics, Blogs, News Photos, Video, Tech Reviews—TIME.com. N.p., n.d. Web. 1 Dec. 2010. <http://www.time.com/time/2007/america_numbers/commuting.html>.

Appendices

1 Rattay, Wolfgang. "Protein pulls ahead on the post-workout menu—USATODAY.com." News, Travel, Weather, Entertainment, Sports, Technology, U.S. & World—USATODAY.com. N.p., n.d. Web. 26 Aug. 2010. <http://www.usatoday.com/news/health/2009-02-11-protein-recovery_N.htm>.
2 A sampling of supporting research:
  • Tipton KD, Rasmussen BB, Miller SL, Wolf SE, Owens-Stovall SK, Petrini BE, Wolfe RR. Timing of amino acid-carbohydrate ingestion alters anabolic response of muscle to resistance training. Am J Physiol Endocrinol Metab. 2001 Aug;281(2):E197-206. PubMed PMID: 11440894.
  • Tang JE, Moore DR, Kujbida GW, Tarnopolsky MA, Phillips SM. Ingestion of whey hydrolysate, casein, or soy protein isolate: effects on mixed muscle protein synthesis at rest and following resistance training in young men. J Appl Physiol. 2009 Sep;107(3):987-92. Epub 2009 Jul 9. PubMed PMID: 19589961.
  • Levenhagen DK, Gresham JD, Carlson MG, Maron DJ, Borel MJ, Flakoll PJ. Postexercise nutrient intake timing in humans is critical to recovery of leg glucose and protein homeostasis. Am J Physiol Endocrinol Metab. 2001;280:E982-93.
  • Biolo G, Tipton KD, Klein S, Wolfe RR. An abundant supply of amino acids enhances the metabolic effect of exercise on muscle protein. Am J Physiol. 1997 Jul;273(1 Pt 1):E122-9. PubMed PMID: 9252488.
  • Wilson J, Wilson GJ. Contemporary issues in protein requirements and consumption for resistance trained athletes. J Int Soc Sports Nutr. 2006 Jun 5;3:7-27. PubMed PMID: 18500966; PubMed Central PMCID: PMC2129150.
  • Manninen, A.H. (2002) Protein metabolism in exercising humans with special reference to protein supplementation. Master thesis. Department of Physiology, Faculty of Medicine, University of Kuo-

pio, Finland.

- Vukovich, Matthew D. FACSM; Tausz, Shawn M.; Ballard, Tasha L.; Stevermer, Cheryl L.; Gerlach, Amanda M.; VanderWeerd, Marie K.; Binkley, Teresa L.; Specker, Bonny L. Effect of Protein Supplementation During a 6-month Strength and Conditioning Program on Muscular Strength. Medicine & Science in Sports & Exercise: May 2004—Volume 36—Issue 5—p S193
- Wilson J, Wilson GJ. Contemporary issues in protein requirements and consumption for resistance trained athletes. J Int Soc Sports Nutr. 2006 Jun 5;3:7-27. PubMed PMID: 18500966; PubMed Central PMCID: PMC2129150.

3   A sampling of supporting research:

- Pascoe DD, Costill DL, Fink WJ, Robergs RA, Zachwieja JJ. Glycogen resynthesis in skeletal muscle following resistive exercise. Med Sci Sports Exerc. 1993 Mar;25(3):349-54. PubMed PMID: 8455450.
- Roy BD, Fowles JR, Hill R, Tarnopolsky MA. Macronutrient intake and whole body protein metabolism following resistance exercise. Med Sci Sports Exerc. 2000 Aug;32(8):1412-8. PubMed PMID: 10949007.
- Burke LM. Nutrition for post-exercise recovery. Aust J Sci Med Sport. 1997 Mar;29(1):3-10. Review. PubMed PMID: 9127682.
- Zawadzki KM, Yaspelkis BB 3rd, Ivy JL. Carbohydrate-protein complex increases the rate of muscle glycogen storage after exercise. J Appl Physiol. 1992 May;72(5):1854-9. PubMed PMID: 1601794.
- Pascoe DD, Gladden LB. Muscle glycogen resynthesis after short term, high intensity exercise and resistance exercise. Sports Med. 1996 Feb;21(2):98-118. Review. PubMed PMID: 8775516.
- Roy BD, Tarnopolsky MA. Influence of differing macronutrient intakes on muscle glycogen resynthesis after resistance exercise. J Appl Physiol. 1998 Mar;84(3):890-6. PubMed PMID: 9480948.
- Rasmussen BB, Tipton KD, Miller SL, Wolf SE, Wolfe RR. An oral essential amino acid-carbohydrate supplement enhances muscle protein anabolism after resistance exercise. J Appl Physiol. 2000 Feb;88(2):386-92. PubMed PMID: 10658002.
- Ivy JL, Katz AL, Cutler CL, Sherman WM, Coyle EF. Muscle glycogen synthesis after exercise: effect of time of carbohydrate ingestion. J Appl Physiol. 1988 Apr;64(4):1480-5. PubMed PMID: 3132449.
- Jentjens R, Jeukendrup A. Determinants of post-exercise glycogen synthesis during short-term recovery. Sports Med. 2003;33(2):117-44. Review. PubMed PMID: 12617691.

4   Arciero PJ, Gentile CL, Martin-Pressman R, Ormsbee MJ, Everett M, Zwicky L, Steele CA. Increased dietary protein and combined high intensity aerobic and resistance training improves body fat distribution and cardiovascular risk factors. Int J Sport Nutr Exerc Metab. 2006 Aug;16(4):373-92. PubMed PMID: 17136940.

5   McCullough ML, Feskanich D, Stampfer MJ, Giovannucci EL, Rimm EB, Hu FB, Spiegelman D, Hunter DJ, Colditz GA, Willett WC. Diet quality and major chronic disease risk in men and women: moving toward improved dietary guidance. Am J Clin Nutr. 2002 Dec;76(6):1261-71. PubMed PMID: 12450892.

6   A sampling of supporting research:

- Howarth NC, Saltzman E, Roberts SB. Dietary fiber and weight regulation. Nutr Rev. 2001 May;59(5):129-39. Review. PubMed PMID: 11396693.
- Ludwig DS, Pereira MA, Kroenke CH, Hilner JE, Van Horn L, Slattery ML, Jacobs DR Jr. Dietary fiber, weight gain, and cardiovascular disease risk factors in young adults. JAMA. 1999 Oct 27;282(16):1539-46. PubMed PMID: 10546693.
- Bazzano LA, He J, Ogden LG, Loria CM, Whelton PK; National Health and Nutrition Examination Survey I Epidemiologic Follow-up Study. Dietary fiber intake and reduced risk of coronary heart disease in U.S. men and women: The National Health and Nutrition Examination Survey I Epidemiologic Follow-up Study. Arch Intern Med. 2003 Sep 8;163(16):1897-904. PubMed PMID: 12963562.

7   Lasker DA, Evans EM, Layman DK. Moderate carbohydrate, moderate protein weight loss diet reduces cardiovascular disease risk compared to high carbohydrate, low protein diet in obese adults: A randomized clinical trial. Nutr Metab (Lond). 2008 Nov 7;5:30. PubMed PMID: 18990242; PubMed Central

PMCID: PMC2585565.

8   Frassetto LA, Schloetter M, Mietus-Synder M, Morris RC Jr, Sebastian A. Metabolic and physiologic improvements from consuming a paleolithic, hunter-gatherer type diet. Eur J Clin Nutr. 2009 Aug;63(8):947-55. Epub 2009 Feb 11. PubMed PMID: 19209185.

9   A sampling of supporting research:

  • Layman DK. Dietary Guidelines should reflect new understandings about adult protein needs. Nutr Metab (Lond). 2009 Mar 13;6:12. PubMed PMID: 19284668; PubMed Central PMCID: PMC2666737.

  • Farnsworth E, Luscombe ND, Noakes M, Wittert G, Argyiou E, Clifton PM. Effect of a high-protein, energy-restricted diet on body composition, glycemic control, and lipid concentrations in overweight and obese hyperinsulinemic men and women.Am J Clin Nutr. 2003 Jul;78(1):31-9.

  • McAuley KA, Hopkins CM, Smith KJ, McLay RT, Williams SM, Taylor RW, Mann JI. Comparison of high-fat and high-protein diets with a high-carbohydrate diet in insulin-resistant obese women. Diabetologia. 2005 Jan;48(1):8-16.

  • Nuttall FQ, Gannon MC. The metabolic response to a high-protein, low-carbohydrate diet in men with type 2 diabetes mellitus. Metabolism. 2006 Feb;55(2):243-51.

  • Nuttall FQ, Gannon MC. Metabolic response of people with type 2 diabetes to a high protein diet. Nutr Metab (Lond). 2004 Sep 13;1(1):652.

  • McAuley KA, Smith KJ, Taylor RW, McLay RT, Williams SM, Mann JI. Long-term effects of popular dietary approaches on weight loss and features of insulin resistance. Int J Obes (Lond). 2006 Feb;30(2):342-9.

  • Brand-Miller J. Diets with a low glycemic index: From theory to practice. Nutrition Today. 1999;34:64–72.

  • Gannon MC, Nuttall FQ, Saeed A, Jordan K, Hoover H. An increase in dietary protein improves the blood glucose response in persons with type 2 diabetes. Am J Clin Nutr. 2003 Oct;78(4):734-41. PubMed PMID: 14522731.

  • Børsheim E, Bui Q-UT, Tissier S, Kobayashi H, Ferrando AA, Wolfe RR. Effect of amino acid supplementation in insulin sensitivity in elderly. Fed Proc (in press).

  • Frost G, Keogh B, Smith D, Akinsanya K, Leeds A. (1996). The effect of low-glycemic carbohydrate on insulin and glucose response in vivo and in vitro in patients with coronary heart disease. Metabolism, 45: 669-672.

  • Arora SK, McFarlane SI. The case for low carbohydrate diets in diabetes management. Nutr Metab (Lond). 2005 Jul 14;2:16. PubMed PMID: 16018812; PubMed Central PMCID: PMC1188071.

  • Augustin LS, Franceschi S, Jenkins DJ, Kendall CW, La Vecchia C. Glycemic index in chronic disease: a review. Eur J Clin Nutr. 2002 Nov;56(11):1049-71.Review. PubMed PMID: 12428171.

  • Layman DK, Boileau RA, Erickson DJ, Painter JE, Shiue H, Sather C, Christou DD. A reduced ratio of dietary carbohydrate to protein improves body composition and blood lipid profiles during weight loss in adult women. J Nutr. 2003 Feb;133(2):411-7. PubMed PMID: 12566476.

  • Skov, A. R., Toubro, S., Ronn, B., Holm, L. & Astrup, A. (1999) Randomized trial on protein vs carbohydrate in ad libitum fat reduced diet for the treatment of obesity. Int. J. Obes. 23:528-536.

  • Parker, B., Noakes, M., Luscombe, N. & Clifton, P. (2002) Effect of a high-protein, monounsaturated fat weight loss diet on glycemic control and lipid levels in type 2 diabetes. Diabetes Care 25:425-430.

  • Piatti PM, Monti F, Fermo I, Baruffaldi L, Nasser R, Santambrogio G, Librenti MC, Galli-Kienle M, Pontiroli AE, Pozza G. Hypocaloric high-protein diet improves glucose oxidation and spares lean body mass: comparison to hypocaloric high-carbohydrate diet. Metabolism. 1994 Dec;43(12):1481-7. PubMed PMID: 7990700.

10   Arciero PJ, Gentile CL, Martin-Pressman R, Ormsbee MJ, Everett M, Zwicky L, Steele CA. Increased dietary protein and combined high intensity aerobic and resistance training improves body fat distribution and cardiovascular risk factors. Int J Sport Nutr Exerc Metab. 2006 Aug;16(4):373-92. PubMed PMID: 17136940.

11 Westerterp-Plantenga MS. The significance of protein in food intake and body weight regulation. Curr Opin Clin Nutr Metab Care. 2003 Nov;6(6):635-8. Review. PubMed PMID: 14557793.

12 A sampling of supporting research:
- Noakes M, Keogh JB, Foster PR, Clifton PM. Effect of an energy-restricted, high-protein, low-fat diet relative to a conventional high-carbohydrate, low-fat diet on weight loss, body composition, nutritional status, and markers of cardiovascular health in obese women. Am J Clin Nutr. 2005 Jun;81(6):1298-306.
- Weigle DS, Breen PA, Matthys CC, Callahan HS, Meeuws KE, Burden VR, Purnell JQ. A high-protein diet induces sustained reductions in appetite, ad libitum caloric intake, and body weight despite compensatory changes in diurnal plasma leptin and ghrelin concentrations. Am J Clin Nutr. 2005 Jul;82(1):41-8
- Skov AR, Toubro S, Rønn B, Holm L, Astrup A. Randomized trial on protein vs carbohydrate in ad libitum fat reduced diet for the treatment of obesity. Int J Obes Relat Metab Disord. 1999 May;23(5):528-36. PubMed PMID: 10375057.
- Lasker DA, Evans EM, Layman DK. Moderate carbohydrate, moderate protein weight loss diet reduces cardiovascular disease risk compared to high carbohydrate, low protein diet in obese adults: A randomized clinical trial. Nutr Metab (Lond). 2008 Nov 7;5:30. PubMed PMID: 18990242; PubMed Central PMCID: PMC2585565.
- Wolfe RR. The underappreciated role of muscle in health and disease. Am J Clin Nutr. 2006 Sep;84(3):475-82. Review. PubMed PMID: 16960159.
- Westerterp-Plantenga MS, Lejeune MP, Nijs I, van Ooijen M, Kovacs EM. High protein intake sustains weight maintenance after body weight loss in humans. Int J Obes Relat Metab Disord. 2004 Jan;28(1):57-64.
- Lejeune MP, Kovacs EM, Westerterp-Plantenga MS. Additional protein intake limits weight regain after weight loss in humans. Br J Nutr. 2005 Feb;93(2):281-9. PubMed PMID: 15788122.
- Baba NH, Sawaya S, Torbay N, Habbal Z, Azar S, Hashim SA: High protein vs high carbohydrate hypoenergetic diet for the treatment of obese hyperinsulinemic subjects. Int J Obes23 :1202 –1206,1999.
- Brehm BJ, Seeley RJ, Daniels SR, D'Alessio DA: A randomized trial comparing a very low carbohydrate diet and a calorie restricted low fat diet on body weight and cardiovascular risk factors in healthy women. J Clin Endocrinol Metab88 :1617 –1623,2003
- Foster GD, Wyatt HR, Hill JO, McGuckin BG, Brill C, Mohammed S: A randomized trial of a low-carbohydrate diet. N Eng J Med348 :2082 –2090,2003
- Samaha FF, Iqbal N, Seshadri P, Chicano KL, Daily D, Mcgrory J: A low carbohydrate as compared with a low fat diet in severe obesity. N Eng J Med348 :2074 –2081,2003 .
- Worthington BS, Taylor LE: Balanced low calorie vs high protein, low carbohydrate reducing diets. J Am Diet Assoc64 :47 –51,1974 .
- Yancy Jr WS, Olsen MK, Guyton JR, Bakst RP, Westman EC: A low-carbohydrate, ketogenic diet versus a low-fat diet to treat obesity and hyperlipidemia. Ann Intern Med140 :769 –777,2004

13 Layman DK, Boileau RA, Erickson DJ, Painter JE, Shiue H, Sather C, Christou DD. A reduced ratio of dietary carbohydrate to protein improves body composition and blood lipid profiles during weight loss in adult women. J Nutr. 2003 Feb;133(2):411-7. PubMed PMID: 12566476.

14 A sampling of supporting research:
- Due A, Toubro S, Skov AR, Astrup A. Effect of normal-fat diets, either medium or high in protein, on body weight in overweight subjects: a randomised 1-year trial. Int J Obes Relat Metab Disord. 2004 Oct;28(10):1283-90. PubMed PMID:15303109.
- Despres JP, Moorjani S, Lupien PJ, Tremblay A, Nadeau A, Bouchard C. Regional distribution of body fat, plasmalipoproteins, and cardiovascular disease. rteriosclerosis 1990;10: 497–511.
- Despres JP. Dyslipidaemia and obesity. Baillieres Clin Endocrinol Metab 1994; 8: 629–660.

- Kissebah AH, Krakower GR. Regional adiposity and morbidity. Physiol Rev 1994; 74: 761–811.

15 Frisch S, Zittermann A, Berthold HK, Götting C, Kuhn J, Kleesiek K, Stehle P, Körtke H. A randomized controlled trial on the efficacy of carbohydrate-reduced or fat-reduced diets in patients attending a tele-medically guided weight loss program. Cardiovasc Diabetol. 2009 Jul 18;8:36. PubMed PMID: 19615091; PubMed Central PMCID: PMC2722581.

16 Meckling KA, Sherfey R. A randomized trial of a hypocaloric high-protein diet, with and without exercise, on weight loss, fitness, and markers of the Metabolic Syndrome in overweight and obese women. Appl Physiol Nutr Metab. 2007 Aug;32(4):743-52. PubMed PMID: 17622289.

17 Low-carbohydrate diet in type 2 diabetes. Stable improvement of bodyweight and glycemic control during 22 months follow-up Jørgen Vesti Nielsen and Eva Joensson Nutr Metab (Lond). 2006; 3: 22. Published online 2006 June 14. doi: 10.1186/1743-7075-3-22. PMCID: PMC1526736

18 P.J. Skerrett, and W.C. Willett. Eat, Drink, and Be Healthy: The Harvard Medical School Guide to Healthy Eating. Free Press Trade Pbk. Ed ed. New York City: Free Press, 2005. Print.

19 Albert CM, Hennekens CH, O'Donnell CJ, Ajani UA, Carey VJ, Willett WC, Ruskin JN, Manson JE. Seafood consumption and risk of sudden cardiac death. JAMA. 1998 Jan 7;279(1):23-8. PubMed PMID: 9424039.

20 A sampling of supporting research:
- Williams GM, Williams CL, Weisburger JH. Diet and cancer prevention: The fiber first diet. Toxicol Sci. 1999 Dec;52(2 Suppl):72-86. Review. PubMed PMID: 10630594.
- Trock B, Lanza E, Greenwald P. Dietary fiber, vegetables, and colon cancer: critical review and meta-analyses of the epidemiologic evidence. J Natl Cancer Inst. 1990 Apr 18;82(8):650-61. PubMed PMID: 2157027.
- Singh RB, Dubnov G, Niaz MA, et al. Effect of an Indo-Mediterraneandiet on progression of coronary artery disease in high risk patients (Indo-Mediterranean Diet Heart Study): a randomized single-blind trial. Lancet. 2002;360:1455-1461.
- de Lorgeril M, Salen P, Martin JL, Monjaud I, Delaye J, Mamelle N. Mediterranean diet, traditional risk factors, and the rate of cardiovascular complications after myocardial infarction: final report of the Lyon Diet Heart Study. Circulation. 1999;99:779-785.
- Hickey JT, Hickey L, Yancy WS, Hepburn J, Westman EC. Clinical use of a carbohydrate-restricted diet to treat the dyslipidemia of the metabolic syndrome.Metab Syndr Relat Disord. 2003 Sep;1(3):227-32. PubMed PMID: 18370666.
- Anderson JW, Tietyen-Clark J. Dietary fiber. Am J Gastroenterol. 1986;81:907-919.
- Rimm EB, Ascherio A, Giovannucci E, et al. Vegetable, fruit, and cereal fiber intake and risk of coronary heart disease among men. JAMA. 1996;275:447-451.
- Jenkins DJ, Wolever TM, Kalmusky J, et al. Low glycemic index carbohydrate foods in the management of hyperlipidemia. Am J Clin Nutr. 1985;42:604-617.
- Frost G, Leeds AA, Dore CJ, et al. Glycaemic index as a determinant of serum HDL-cholesterol concentration. Lancet. 1999;353:1045-1048.
- Anderson JW, Garrity TF, Wood CL, Whitis SE, Smith BM, Oeltgen PR. Prospective, randomized, controlled comparison of the effects of low-fat and low-fat plus high-fiber diets on serum lipid concentrations. Am J Clin Nutr. 1992 Nov;56(5):887-94. PubMed PMID: 1329482.
- Boden G, Sargrad K, Homko C, Mozzoli M, Stein TP. Effect of a low-carbohydrate diet on appetite, blood glucose levels, and insulin resistance in obese patients with type 2 diabetes. Ann Intern Med. 2005 Mar 15;142(6):403-11. PubMed PMID:15767618.
- Volek JS, Feinman RD. Carbohydrate restriction improves the features of Metabolic Syndrome. Metabolic Syndrome may be defined by the response to carbohydrate restriction. Nutr Metab (Lond). 2005 Nov 16;2:31. PubMed PMID:16288655; PubMed Central PMCID: PMC1323303. Citing: Rickman et al. 1974, LaRosa et al. 1980, Phinney et al. 1980, Phinney et al. 1983, Newbold, 1988, Volek et al. 2000, Sharman et al. 2002, Meckling et al. 2002, Westman et al. 2002, Dashti et al. 2003, Hays

et al. 2003, Dashti et al. 2004, Boden et al. 2005, Brehm et al. 2003, Sondike et al. 2003, Samaha et al. 2003, Foster et al. 2003, Volek et al. 2004, Sharman et al. 2004, Brehm et al. 2004, Meckling et al. 2004, Stern et al. 2004, Yancy et al. 2004, Aude et al. 2004, Seshadri et al. 2004, McAuley et al. 2004, Dansinger et al. 2004.

- Salmerón J, Ascherio A, Rimm EB, Colditz GA, Spiegelman D, Jenkins DJ, Stampfer MJ, Wing AL, Willett WC. Dietary fiber, glycemic load, and risk of NIDDM in men. Diabetes Care. 1997 Apr;20(4):545-50. PubMed PMID: 9096978.
- Salmerón J, Manson JE, Stampfer MJ, Colditz GA, Wing AL, Willett WC. Dietary fiber, glycemic load, and risk of non-insulin-dependent diabetes mellitus in women. JAMA. 1997 Feb 12;277(6):472-7. PubMed PMID: 9020271.
- Volek JS, Feinman RD. Carbohydrate restriction improves the features of Metabolic Syndrome. Metabolic Syndrome may be defined by the response to carbohydrate restriction. Nutr Metab (Lond). 2005 Nov 16;2:31. PubMed PMID:16288655; PubMed Central PMCID: PMC1323303.
- Fukagawa NK, Anderson JW, Hageman G, Young VR, Minaker KL. High-carbohydrate, high-fiber diets increase peripheral insulin sensitivity in healthy young and old adults. Am J Clin Nutr. 1990;52:524-528.
- Arora SK, McFarlane SI. The case for low carbohydrate diets in diabetes management. Nutr Metab (Lond). 2005 Jul 14;2:16. PubMed PMID: 16018812; PubMed Central PMCID: PMC1188071.
- Liu S, Willett WC, Stampfer MJ, Hu FB, Franz M, Sampson L, Hennekens CH, Manson JE. A prospective study of dietary glycemic load, carbohydrate intake, and risk of coronary heart disease in U.S. women. Am J Clin Nutr. 2000 Jun;71(6):1455-61. PubMed PMID: 10837285.
- Willett WC, McCullough ML. Dietary pattern analysis for the evaluation of dietary guidelines. Asia Pac J Clin Nutr. 2008;17 Suppl 1:75-8. Review. PubMed PMID: 18296306.
- Katan MB, Zock PL, Mensink RP. Effects of fats and fatty acids on blood lipids in humans: an overview. Am J Clin Nutr. 1994 Dec;60(6 Suppl):1017S-1022S. Review. PubMed PMID: 7977143.
- Sharman MJ, Kraemer WJ, Love DM, Avery NG, Gómez AL, Scheett TP, Volek JS. A ketogenic diet favorably affects serum biomarkers for cardiovascular disease in normal-weight men. J Nutr. 2002 Jul;132(7):1879-85. PubMed PMID: 12097663.
- Ascherio A. Epidemiologic studies on dietary fats and coronary heart disease. Am J Med. 2002;113(suppl 9B):9S-12S.
- Hu FB, Stampfer MJ, Manson JE, Rimm E, Colditz GA, Rosner BA, Hennekens CH, Willett WC. Dietary fat intake and the risk of coronary heart disease in women. N Engl J Med. 1997 Nov 20;337(21):1491-9. PubMed PMID: 9366580.
- Gramenzi A, Gentile A, Fasoli M, Negri E, Parazzini F, La Vecchia C. Association between certain foods and risk of acute myocardial infarction in women. BMJ. 1990 Mar 24;300(6727):771-3. PubMed PMID: 2322737; PubMed CentralPMCID: PMC1662535.
- World Cancer Research Fund and American Institute for Cancer Research. Food, nutrition and the prevention of cancer: a global perspective. Washington, DC: American Institute for Cancer Research, 1997.
- Appel LJ, Moore TJ, Obarzanek E, et al. A clinical trial of the effects of dietary patterns on blood pressure. N Engl J Med 1997;336: 1117–24.
- Key TJ, Thorogood M, Appleby PN, Burr ML. Dietary habits and mortality in 11,000 vegetarians and health conscious people: resultsof a 17-year follow-up. BMJ 1996;313:775–9.
- Hu F, Stampfer MJ, Manson JE, et al. Frequent nut consumption and risk of coronary heart disease in women: prospective cohort study. BMJ 1998;317:1341–5.
- Fraser GE, Sabate J, Beeson WL, Strahan TM. A possible protective effect of nut consumption on risk of coronary heart disease. The Adventist Health Study. Arch Intern Med 1992;152:1416–24.
- Ludwig DS, Pereira MA, Kroenke CH, Hilner JE, Van Horn L, Slattery ML, Jacobs DR Jr. Dietary fiber, weight gain, and cardiovascular disease risk factors in young adults. JAMA. 1999 Oct

27;282(16):1539-46. PubMed PMID: 10546693.
- Ascherio A, Rimm EB, Giovannucci EL, Spiegelman D, Stampfer M, Willett WC. Dietary fat and risk of coronary heart disease in men: cohort follow up study in the United States. BMJ. 1996 Jul 13;313(7049):84-90. PubMed PMID: 8688759; PubMed Central PMCID: PMC2351515.
- Levine AS, Billington CJ. Dietary fiber: does it affect food intake and body weight? In: Fernstrom JD, Miller GD, eds. Appetite and body weight regulation: sugar, fat, and macronutrient substitutes. Boca Raton, FL: CRC Press, 1994:191–200.
- Non-starchy vegetables
- World Cancer Research Fund and American Institute for Cancer Research. Food, nutrition and the prevention of cancer: a global perspective. Washington, DC: American Institute for Cancer Research, 1997.
- Appel LJ, Moore TJ, Obarzanek E, et al. A clinical trial of the effects of dietary patterns on blood pressure. N Engl J Med 1997;336: 1117–24.
- Gramenzi A, Gentile A, Fasoli M, Negri E, Parazzini F, La Vecchia C. Association between certain foods and risk of acute myocardial infarction in women. BMJ 1990;300:771–3.
- Fruit and nuts:
- Appel LJ, Moore TJ, Obarzanek E, et al. A clinical trial of the effects of dietary patterns on blood pressure. N Engl J Med 1997;336: 1117–24.
- Key TJ, Thorogood M, Appleby PN, Burr ML. Dietary habits and mortality in 11,000 vegetarians and health conscious people: results of a 17-year follow-up. BMJ 1996;313:775–9.
- Hu F, Stampfer MJ, Manson JE, et al. Frequent nut consumption and risk of coronary heart disease in women: prospective cohort study. BMJ 1998;317:1341–5.
- Fraser GE, Sabate J, Beeson WL, Strahan TM. A possible protective effect of nut consumption on risk of coronary heart disease. The Adventist Health Study. Arch Intern Med 1992;152:1416–24.
- Seafood and chicken:
- Kromhout D, Bosscheiter EB, de Lezenne Coulander C. The inverse relation between seafood consumption and 20-year mortality from coronary heart disease. N Engl J Med 1985;312:1205–9.
- Ascherio A, Rimm EB, Stampfer MJ, Giovannucci E, Willett WC. Dietary intake of marine n3 fatty acids, seafood intake and the risk of coronary disease among men. N Engl J Med 1995;332:977–82.
- Key TJ, Fraser GE, Thorogood M, Appleby PN, Beral V, Reeves G, Burr ML, Chang-Claude J, Frentzel-Beyme R, Kuzma JW, Mann J, McPherson K. Mortality in vegetarians and nonvegetarians: detailed findings from a collaborative analysis of 5 prospective studies. Am J Clin Nutr. 1999 Sep;70(3 Suppl):516S-524S. PubMed PMID: 10479225.
21 Halton TL, Hu FB. The effects of high protein diets on thermogenesis, satiety and weight loss: a critical review. J Am Coll Nutr. 2004 Oct;23(5):373-85. Review. PubMed PMID: 15466943.
22 A sampling of supporting research:
- Boden G, Sargrad K, Homko C, Mozzoli M, Stein TP. Effect of a low-carbohydrate diet on appetite, blood glucose levels, and insulin resistance in obese patients with type 2 diabetes. Ann Intern Med. 2005 Mar 15;142(6):403-11. PubMed PMID:15767618.
- Weigle DS, Breen PA, Matthys CC, Callahan HS, Meeuws KE, Burden VR, Purnell JQ. A high-protein diet induces sustained reductions in appetite, ad libitum caloric intake, and body weight despite compensatory changes in diurnal plasma leptin and ghrelin concentrations. Am J Clin Nutr. 2005 Jul;82(1):41-8. PubMed PMID: 16002798.
- Yancy WS, Vernon MC, Westman EC: A pilot trial of low carbohydrate ketogenic diet in patients with type 2 diabetes. Metabolic syndrome and related disorders 2003, 1:239-243.
- Freedman MR, King J, Kennedy E: Popular diets: a scientific review. Obes Res 2001, 9 Suppl 1:1S-40S.
- Brehm BJ, Seeley RJ, Daniels SR, D'Alessio DA: A randomized trial comparing a very low carbohydrate diet and a calorie-restricted low fat diet on body weight and cardiovascular risk factors in healthy women. J Clin Endocrinol Metab 2003, 88:1617-1623.

- Volek J, Sharman M, Gomez A, Judelson D, Rubin M, Watson G, Sokmen B, Silvestre R, French D, Kraemer W: Comparison of energy-restricted very low-carbohydrate and low-fat diets on weight loss and body composition in overweight men and women.
- Meckling KA, O'Sullivan C, Saari D: Comparison of a low-fat diet to a low-carbohydrate diet on weight loss, body composition, and risk factors for diabetes and cardiovascular disease in free-living, overweight men and women. J Clin Endocrinol Metab 2004, 89:2717-2723.
- Stevens J. Does dietary fiber affect food intake and body weight? J Am Diet Assoc. 1988;88:939-942, 945.
- Paddon-Jones D, Westman E, Mattes RD, Wolfe RR, Astrup A, Westerterp-Plantenga M. Protein, weight management, and satiety. Am J Clin Nutr. 2008 May;87(5):1558S-1561S. Review. PubMed PMID: 18469287. And
- Astrup A. The satiating power of protein—a key to obesity prevention? Am J Clin Nutr 2005;82:1–2.
- Mori TA, Bao DQ, Burke V, Puddey IB, Watts GF, Beilin LJ. Dietary seafood as a major component of a weight-loss diet: effect on serum lipids, glucose, and insulin metabolism in overweight hypertensive subjects. Am J Clin Nutr. 1999 Nov;70(5):817-25. PubMed PMID: 10539741.

23 Layman DK. Dietary Guidelines should reflect new understandings about adult protein needs. Nutr Metab (Lond). 2009 Mar 13;6:12. PubMed PMID: 19284668; PubMed Central PMCID: PMC2666737.

24 A sampling of supporting research:
- Eaton SB, Eaton SB 3rd, Konner MJ. Paleolithic nutrition revisited: a twelve-year retrospective on its nature and implications. Eur J Clin Nutr. 1997 Apr;51(4):207-16. Review. PubMed PMID: 9104571.
- Paddon-Jones D, Sheffield-Moore M, Urban RJ, Sanford AP, Aarsland A, Wolfe RR, Ferrando AA. Essential amino acid and carbohydrate supplementation ameliorates muscle protein loss in humans during 28 days bedrest. J Clin Endocrinol Metab. 2004 Sep;89(9):4351-8. PubMed PMID: 15356032.
- Lasker DA, Evans EM, Layman DK. Moderate carbohydrate, moderate protein weight loss diet reduces cardiovascular disease risk compared to high carbohydrate, low protein diet in obese adults: A randomized clinical trial. Nutr Metab (Lond). 2008 Nov 7;5:30. PubMed PMID: 18990242; PubMed Central PMCID: PMC2585565.
- Paddon-Jones D, Westman E, Mattes RD, Wolfe RR, Astrup A, Westerterp-Plantenga M. Protein, weight management, and satiety. Am J Clin Nutr. 2008 May;87(5):1558S-1561S. Review. PubMed PMID: 18469287.
- Hoffer LJ, Bistrian BR, Young VR, Blackburn GL, Matthews DE. Metabolic effects of very low calorie weight reduction diets. J Clin Invest. 1984 Mar;73(3):750-8. PubMed PMID: 6707202; PubMed Central PMCID: PMC425077.
- Krieger JW, Sitren HS, Daniels MJ, Langkamp-Henken B. Effects of variation in protein and carbohydrate intake on body mass and composition during energy restriction: a meta-regression 1. Am J Clin Nutr. 2006 Feb;83(2):260-74. PubMed PMID: 16469983.
- Dauncey MJ, Bingham SA. Dependence of 24 h energy expenditure in man on the composition of the nutrient intake. Br J Nutr 1983;50:1–13.
- Hill JO, Peters JC, Reed GW, Schlundt DG, Sharp T, Greene HL. Nutrient balance in humans: effects of diet composition. Am J Clin Nutr 1991;54:10–7.
- Whitehead JM, McNeill G, Smith JS. The effect of protein intake on 24-h energy expenditure during energy restriction. Int J Obes Relat Metab Disord 1996;20:727–32.
- Layman DK, Boileau RA, Erickson DJ, Painter JE, Shiue H, Sather C, Christou DD. A reduced ratio of dietary carbohydrate to protein improves body composition and blood lipid profiles during weight loss in adult women. J Nutr. 2003 Feb;133(2):411-7. PubMed PMID: 12566476.
- Willi SM, Oexmann MJ, Wright NM, Collop NA, Key LL Jr. The effects of a high-protein, low-fat, ketogenic diet on adolescents with morbid obesity: body composition, blood chemistries, and sleep abnormalities. Pediatrics. 1998 Jan;101(1 Pt 1):61-7. PubMed PMID: 9417152.
- Layman DK, Evans EM, Erickson D, Seyler J, Weber J, Bagshaw D, Griel A, Psota T, Kris-Etherton P.

A moderate-protein diet produces sustained weight loss and long-term changes in body composition and blood lipids in obese adults. J Nutr. 2009 Mar;139(3):514-21. Epub 2009 Jan 21. PubMed PMID: 19158228.

- Piatti PM, Monti F, Fermo I, Baruffaldi L, Nasser R, Santambrogio G, Librenti MC, Galli-Kienle M, Pontiroli AE, Pozza G. Hypocaloric high-protein diet improves glucose oxidation and spares lean body mass: comparison to hypocaloric high-carbohydrate diet. Metabolism. 1994 Dec;43(12):1481-7. PubMed PMID: 7990700.
- Baba NH, Sawaya S, Torbay N, Habbal Z, Azar S, Hashim SA. High protein vs high carbohydrate hypoenergetic diet for the treatment of obese hyperinsulinemic subjects. Int J Obes Relat Metab Disord. 1999 Nov;23(11):1202-6. PubMed PMID:10578211

Glossary

1   Castelli WP. Concerning the possibility of a nut... Arch Intern Med. 1992 Jul;152(7):1371-2. PubMed PMID: 1303626.
2   A sampling of supporting research:
- Kersten S. Mechanisms of nutritional and hormonal regulation of lipogenesis. EMBO Rep. 2001 Apr;2(4):282-6. Review. PubMed PMID: 11306547; PubMed Central PMCID: PMC1083868.
- Jump DB, Clarke SD, Thelen A, Liimatta M. Coordinate regulation of glycolytic and lipogenic gene expression by polyunsaturated fatty acids. J Lipid Res. 1994 Jun;35(6):1076-84. PubMed PMID: 8077846.
- Lopez-Garcia E, Schulze MB, Manson JE, Meigs JB, Albert CM, Rifai N, Willett WC, Hu FB. Consumption of (n-3) fatty acids is related to plasma biomarkers of inflammation and endothelial activation in women. J Nutr. 2004 Jul;134(7):1806-11. PubMed PMID: 15226473.
- Sands SA, Reid KJ, Windsor SL, Harris WS. The impact of age, body mass index, and fish intake on the EPA and DHA content of human erythrocytes. Lipids 2005;40:343-347.
3   Friedman JM. A war on obesity, not the obese. Science. 2003 Feb7;299(5608):856-8. PubMed PMID: 12574619.

CPSIA information can be obtained at www.ICGtesting.com
Printed in the USA
LVOW111104180213

320578LV00004B/46/P

9 780983 520801